DCOMPLETE GUIDE TO DOCUMENTATION

Second Edition

COMPLETE GUIDE TO DOCUMENTATION

Second Edition

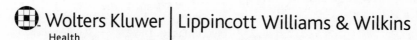

Wolters Kluwer | Lippincott Williams & Wilkins
Health

Philadelphia · Baltimore · New York · London
Buenos Aires · Hong Kong · Sydney · Tokyo

Staff

Executive Publisher
Judith A. Schilling McCann, RN, MSN

Editorial Director
H. Nancy Holmes

Clinical Director
Joan M. Robinson, RN, MSN

Art Director
Mary Ludwicki

Editorial Project Manager
Ann E. Houska

Clinical Manager
Collette Bishop Hendler, RN, BS, CCRN

Clinical Project Manager
Kathryn Henry, RN, BSN, CCRC

Editors
Linda Hager, Julie Munden

Clinical Editor
Cynthia Brophy, RN, BSN, CPAN

Copy Editor
Marna Poole

Digital Composition Services
Diane Paluba (manager), Joyce Rossi Biletz,
Donna S. Morris (project manager)

Manufacturing
Beth J. Welsh

Editorial Assistants
Megan L. Aldinger, Karen J. Kirk,
Linda K. Ruhf

Indexer
Ellen Brennan

CGD010507

FOCUS CHARTING is a registered trademark of Creative Healthcare Management, Inc.

**Library of Congress
Cataloging-in-Publication Data**

Complete guide to documentation. — 2nd ed.
    p. ; cm.
  Includes bibliographical references and index.
  1. Nursing records. 2. Nursing care plans. I. Lippincott Williams & Wilkins. II. Title: Documentation.
  [DNLM: 1. Nursing Records. 2. Documentation. 3. Forms and Records Control. WY 100.5 C737 2008]
  RT50.C65 2008
  651.5'04261—dc22
ISBN-13: 978-1-58255-556-0 (alk. paper)
ISBN-10: 1-58255-556-7 (alk. paper)   2007005720

Contents

CONTRIBUTORS AND CONSULTANTS

Diana Beck, RN, MSN, CNOR
Perioperative Education Specialist
St. Mary's Good Samaritan, Inc.
Centralia, Ill.

Susan Boggs, RN, BSN
Director of Professional Services
Complete Home Health Care
Clarksville, Tenn.

Janice Gasho Brennan, RN, MSOM, MSN,
   CPHQ
Outcomes Manager
CareScience, Inc., a Quovadx Company
Cooper University Hospital
Camden, N.J.

Alex Bux, RN, MS, APRN, BC
Clinical Inservice Instructor
Montefiore Medical Center
Bronx, N.Y.

Kim Cooper, RN, MSN
Nursing Department Program Chair
Ivy Tech Community College
Terre Haute, Ind.

Christine Greenidge, RN, BSN, MSN, BC
Director of Nursing Professional Practice
Montefiore Medical Center
Bronx, N.Y.

Joy L. Herzog, RN
Director Nursing Services
Beverly Healthcare of Phoenixville
Phoenixville, Pa.

Mary Ellen Howell, MN, RNC
Clinical Assistant Professor
University of South Carolina
Columbia

Lisa Kosits, RN, BC, MSN, CCRN, CEN
Clinical Inservice Instructor
Montefiore Medical Center
Bronx, N.Y.

Pamela Moody, PhD, APRN-BC, NHA
Nurse Administrator
Alabama Department of Public Health
Tuscaloosa

Carol Okupniak, RN, MSN
Nursing Instructor
Episcopal Hospital School of Nursing
Philadelphia

Dana Reeves, RN, MSN
Assistant Professor
University of Arkansas
Fort Smith

Maria Rodriguez, *RN, BS, CMSRN*
Director of Education
Kindred Hospital
San Diego

Donna Scemons, *RN, MSN, FNP-C, CNS,*
  CWOCN
President
Healthcare Systems Inc.
Castaic, Calif.

Elliot Stetson, *RN, BC, MSN, CCRN*
Assistant Professor
Raritan Valley Community College
Somerville, N.J.

Rita M. Wick, *RN, BSN*
Education Specialist
Berkshire Medical Center
Pittsfield, Mass.

FOREWORD

An ethically, legally, and procedurally laden task, documentation is the timely recording and validation of events that have occurred during the course of providing health care. As a nurse, your appropriate and accurate documentation is required by health care, government, insurance, and legal systems. But as a *busy* nurse, how can you find the time to appropriately and accurately document your actions?

The second edition of the *Complete Guide to Documentation* holds the answers to this question. Written expressly for those who are pressed for time, this is the only tool you'll need to document the delivery of health care. You won't waste valuable time reading or searching through long, complicated guidelines to understand the health record or to learn how to document clearly and effectively. Explanations of basic documentation methods, such as recording routine nursing care and procedures, move smoothly and easily into explanations of more complicated kinds of documentation, such as the recording of specific events, incidents, or conditions by using templates, forms, and system-tailored grids.

Historically, nursing documentation has followed a medical format, focusing on the patient's initial symptoms and a comprehensive assessment of body systems. Many facilities still organize their nursing assessment forms using this format, but some have adopted documentation formats that reflect the nursing process. These formats are based on human response patterns or functional health care patterns. Other documentation formats are modeled on specific conceptual framework or evidence-based

documentation. The *Complete Guide to Documentation*, Second Edition, compares the different kinds of documentation formats, making it easy to understand the circumstances in which each is used. Additionally, the Joint Commission's National Patient Safety Goals are included wherever appropriate throughout the text.

The book offers straightforward and practical information, saving you valuable time because of its user-friendly organization and clear writing style. Throughout the book are examples of completed forms that instantly help to clarify the use of these forms. What better way to learn to use a complex form such as the Minimum Data Set (MDS) than to study the completed form and use the helpful hints provided for completing it?

In Part I, Fundamentals, five chapters guide you through the basics of documentation. This section also provides an overview of the legal and ethical implications of documentation, performance improvement and reimbursement, documentation systems, and documentation of the nursing process.

Part II, Documentation in Practice Settings, contains four chapters, each focusing on one specific practice area: acute care, long-term care, home health care, and ambulatory care.

Part III, Documentation in Action, has three chapters covering procedures—with clarifying examples—of documentation of everyday events; documentation in selected clinical specialties (critical care, emergency, maternal-neonatal, pediatric, psychiatric, surgical); and legally perilous charting practices.

Thoroughly expanded and updated in this edition, Part IV, Electronic documentation, has a chapter on electronic medical records and another on electronic nursing documentation.

What's more, you'll turn often to the back of the book to augment your knowledge in your own nursing practice. Here you'll find NANDA-I nursing diagnoses, the Joint Commission nursing care and documentation standards, outcomes and interventions for common nursing diagnoses, and a detailed index. This text is a "must have" for nurses in any kind of health care unit or continuing education or orientation program.

Rose E. Constantino, *PhD, JD, RN, FAAN, FACFE, SANE*
Associate Professor
University of Pittsburgh (Pa.) School of Nursing

FUNDAMENTALS

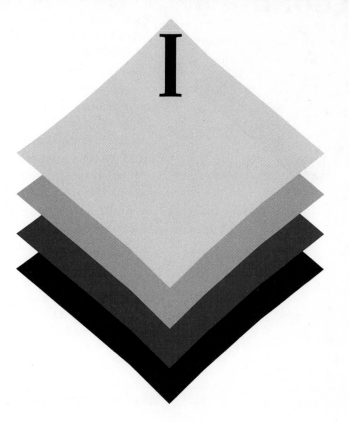

I

Nursing Documentation and the Medical Record

1

Broadly speaking, documentation refers to the preparation and maintenance of records that describe a patient's care. If you document with attention to detail, you'll clearly show the quality of care your patient received, the outcome of that care, and the treatment he still needs.

The detailed information you assemble will be scrutinized by many reviewers, including many other health care team members; accrediting, certifying, and licensing organizations; performance improvement monitors; peer reviewers; and Medicare and insurance company reviewers. Your documentation may also be examined by attorneys and judges. Researchers and educators may use it to improve patient care and to provide continuing education.

This chapter spells out what you need to document for these reviewers and to enhance the quality of patient care. After summarizing the history of documentation, it describes the development of the medical record and covers documentation systems and formats. Next, the chapter reviews the principles of sound documentation, including using computers to promote efficiency. It then discusses current nursing documentation requirements, policies, and trends.

Overview of documentation

Traditionally, nurses recorded their observations of patients, creating documents only under the direction of physicians. The chief purposes of these documents were to demonstrate that physicians' orders had been followed, that the facility's policies had been observed, and that all requisite care had been provided. Charting began as a checklist of cursory observations, such as whether the patient "ate well" or "slept well."

Beyond such simple notations, nurses were reluctant to record their own ideas.

Florence Nightingale, the 19th-century British nurse, is customarily regarded as the founder of nursing documentation. In *Notes on Nursing,* she stressed the importance of gathering patient information in a clear, concise, organized manner. As her theories gained acceptance, nurses began to be trained in her concept of lucid, formal nursing documentation. Gradually, nurses' perceptions and observations about patient care gained credence and respect.

Much later, in the 1970s, nurses began to create their own vocabulary for documentation based on *nursing diagnoses.* This was the first attempt to answer the increasingly urgent call for standards based on nursing data and nursing interventions. Nursing diagnosis terminology is now developed by the North American Nursing Diagnosis Association-International (NANDA-I). The new and revised terminology describes the important judgments nurses make in providing patient care and is recognized as well-established diagnosis terminology. Recognized by the American Nurses Association (ANA) and available in several languages, the diagnoses continue to be refined and are the basis for nursing interventions and outcomes. However, insurance companies and Medicare still don't reimburse for nursing services rendered under a nursing diagnosis.

Currently, NANDA-I's Taxonomy II provides a classification of nursing diagnoses and, in conjunction with the Nursing Intervention Classification (NIC) and Nursing Outcomes Classification (NOC), facilitates structure for nursing practice. The goal to develop a common structure for nursing continues, and each step strengthens the relationship among nursing diagnoses, nursing interventions, and nursing outcomes.

The current reimbursement trend is to compensate advanced practice nurses for skilled care that meets eligibility requirements. This care includes assessing a patient's condition, creating a care plan, and following a strict treatment regimen. Reimbursement to the health care facility for patient services depends on accurate documentation to support the necessity of services and verify the provision of services.

In today's health care environment, regulatory agencies—such as The Joint Commission and the Centers for Medicare and Medicaid Services (CMS), previously known as the Health Care Financing Administration (HCFA)—require meticulous documentation to support patient care that meets the standards set for compliance with their regulations. This helps to ensure patient safety, quality care, and reimbursement from insurance companies, Medicare, and Medicaid, and avoidance of litigation. More than ever before, nursing documentation plays a vital role in verifying—and justifying—safe, timely patient care to meet these standards and the nursing standards set by the ANA and your state board.

Understanding the medical record

Management of patient information is a complex integrated system that facilitates the flow of information throughout a health care system and the patient's episodes of care. Medical records are an important resource for health care providers and today may be paper-based, electronic, or a combination of both. The patient's main medical record should contain an organized collection of all data and information relating to the services provided to a patient. Although the main medical record is available for reference,

What makes up the medical record?

Each health care facility has its own medical record-keeping system. The patient-specific data in the record provides information appropriate to the care, treatment, and services provided to the patient. Some of the documents typically found in an acute care medical record include:

FACE SHEET
The first page of the medical record, this form includes demographic information identifying the patient's name, birth date, sex, social security number, address, and marital status. It also lists his closest relative or guardian, food or drug allergies, admitting diagnosis, assigned diagnosis-related group, the attending practitioner, insurance information and address, and language and communication needs.

ADVANCE DIRECTIVES
Each patient must be asked about advance directives when he is admitted to the health care facility. Advance directive forms include information about a health care proxy or durable power of attorney for health care or a living will. These documents, when available, should become part of the patient's medical record. If the patient chooses not to complete an advance directive, documentation in the medical record must reflect that information was provided and explained to the patient, but he declined.

NURSING DATABASE
This document contains nursing data, including the patient's health history, physical and psychosocial assessments, baseline functional status, demographics, and pertinent social environment information. The assessment should also address the patient's risk for falling and for developing pressure ulcers.

MEDICAL HISTORY AND PHYSICAL EXAMINATION
Completed by a qualified practitioner, this form contains the patient's medical history, description of the patient's chief complaint and initial medical examination and evaluation data. The form should also contain a list of the medications and dosages that the patient is currently taking.

PRACTITIONER'S ORDER SHEET
This is the record of the practitioner's medical orders.

PROGRESS NOTES
This record details patient care information and notes on the patient's progress in a sequential, time-oriented fashion. The notes are documented by practitioners, nurses, and other health care providers responsible for the patient's care, treatment, and services.

GRAPHIC FLOW SHEET
Known by various titles assigned by the health care facility, this form is a type of flow sheet that tracks the patient's temperature, pulse rate, respiratory rate, blood pressure and, if needed, daily weight. Additional graphic sheets may be designed for recording such information as skin care, blood glucose levels, test results, neurologic assessment data, patient intake and output, as well as frequent vitals signs and hemodynamic parameters when necessary. These forms allow the

a separate record of care is started upon each patient admission to the acute care setting and is incorporated into the main medical record after discharge.

Typically, a patient's inpatient medical record contains many forms, including the initial assessment and demographic forms, daily assessment flow sheets, problem or nursing diagnosis lists, care plan or clinical pathways, and other nurse to show that a certain task or assessment was completed by simply dating, initialing, or checking off the appropriate column.

MEDICATION ADMINISTRATION RECORD
This document contains a record of each medication a patient receives, including the date and time it was ordered, the name of the practitioner who prescribed it, and the dosage, administration route, site, date, and time.

DIAGNOSTIC REPORTS
These forms contain diagnostic and laboratory data—for example, radiology, hematology, and pathology test results.

CONSULTATION SHEETS
These forms contain evaluations made by practitioners, clinical specialists, and others consulted for diagnostic and treatment recommendations.

OPERATIVE REPORTS
Operative reports include preadmission, operating room (OR), postanesthesia care, and ambulatory surgery care forms that are collectively filed in the medical record. These forms are used to document patient care through the surgical process.

DISCHARGE PLAN AND SUMMARY
This document presents a brief summary of the patient's time in the health care facility and plans for care after discharge. Pertinent data may include dietary and medication instructions, follow-up care, or referrals. A transfer form will be completed if the patient is being transferred to another facility for extended care.

flow sheets. Forms vary according to the individual facility's policies and procedures and in response to a wealth of organizational, regulatory, and patient-related requirements. (See *What makes up the medical record?*)

Because of the medical record's complexity, many nurses organize the data by category, placing undue focus on format over content. However, a medical record is more than a dry summary of a patient's illness and recovery. It's an incremental record of a patient's daily care and a road map of actual and potential patient care problems and appropriate interventions. In addition to being well organized, the record also should be easy to read and accessible to all members of the health care team and, ultimately, the reviewers.

Many nurses approach the medical record with trepidation—needlessly. Think of the medical record as an ally, not an enemy. It serves as a focus for organizing your thoughts about patient care and recording your actions. Used properly, it can help you identify problem areas, plan better patient care, and evaluate the care given.

Nursing documentation makes up one critical part of the complete medical record, which contains contributions from all health care team members. Your contribution has many purposes. It communicates your assessments and the care you gave, and it allows you, the nurse, to take credit for what you have observed and done. It also assists all caregivers in coordinating treatment, ensures reimbursement, and provides legal protection for you and your employer. (See *Guarding against liability,* page 6.)

Purpose of the medical record
The medical record provides a comprehensive and accurate record of patient-specific data and information for both inpatient and outpatient care. It provides evidence to support all aspects of the patient's care, and it's used by various groups to evaluate and enhance the quality of that care. Besides communicating information and facilitating services, care, and treatment for the patient, the medical record is used for reim-

Legal eagle

Guarding against liability

Good documentation should offer legal protection to you, the patient's other caregivers, and the health care facility.

Admissible in court as a legal document, the medical record provides proof of the care received by the patient and the standards by which the care was provided. Medical records typically serve as evidence in disability, personal injury, and mental competence cases. They're also used in malpractice cases, and how and what you document—or don't document—can mean the difference between winning and losing a case, not only for you but also for your employer.

For the best legal protection, make sure that your documentation shows that you not only adhere to professional standards of nursing care but also follow your employer's policies and procedures—especially in high-risk situations.

bursement, for research, to support decision analysis, to guide performance improvement, and as a legal record.

EVIDENCE OF THE QUALITY OF CARE

To verify the quality of your care, you must describe what you've done for your patient and provide evidence that it was necessary. You also should describe your patient's response to the care and any changes made in his care plan. You must be sure to document this information in accordance with professional practice standards—those published by the American Nurses Association and The Joint Commission, for instance.

Another organization, the National Committee for Quality Assurance (NCQA), performs several functions, including accreditation of managed care plans and certification of quality assurance specialists, either through the national office or through state affiliates. Although the NCQA doesn't mandate a specific method of quality evaluation, it does reinforce the importance of using The Joint Commission, Medicare, and other standards to evaluate and improve patient care in all health care settings.

ACCREDITATION, CERTIFICATION, AND LICENSURE

Organizations, most notably The Joint Commission, accredit health care facilities that meet their standards. (Some states require all health care facilities to become licensed.) Health care facilities need The Joint Commission accreditation not only to demonstrate that they provide quality care but also to ensure their eligibility for government funds. The federal government also contracts with state organizations that certify health care facilities as being eligible to receive Medicare reimbursement.

In deciding whether a facility should receive accreditation, an accrediting organization looks at the structure and function of the facility and reviews medical records to ensure that the facility meets the required standards. Then, at regular intervals, the organization checks the facility for compliance. The accrediting organization conducts surveys to assess the standard and quality of care and audits the facility to ensure that it's complying with those standards.

Most accrediting organizations have some common standards for documentation. For example, most require that each patient's medical record contains an assessment, a care plan, medical orders, progress notes, and a discharge summary. Several organizations even spell out what these components must contain. Then the nurse-manager must establish and implement documentation guidelines that meet the accrediting organization's requirements. These guidelines should specify the format that must be used as well as the topics that must be covered in the documentation.

PERFORMANCE IMPROVEMENT

Mandated by state, The Joint Commission regulations, and other regulating agencies, such as the CMS, performance improvement activities are designed, conducted, and analyzed by designated employees of the health care facility. The performance improvement committee traditionally included physicians, nurses, and administrative personnel but has since expanded to include pharmacists, physical therapists and, often, consumers (such as a patient, family member, or community representative).

This committee seeks, develops, monitors, and evaluates new ways to improve the quality of patient care. Committee members must choose well-defined, objective, readily measurable indicators and collect data systematically over time to measure how often a performance standard is being followed and how well it's working. They may need to develop new indicators or even new standards, or they may need to redesign old ones. They then use statistical techniques to translate the data into useful information for assessment. Improvement actions are based on results of the measurement and evaluation process, and successful performance improvement depends on effective teamwork.

Performance improvement has been steadily changing since the mid-1980s because of a perception that improvement efforts were ineffective and not far-reaching enough, targeting only individuals and regulators. The trend has now shifted toward emphasizing clinical outcomes as a way to create meaningful improvement both clinically and financially. Regulatory agencies now mandate that facilities submit certain performance improvement indicators to them on a regular basis for review and to establish a continuous accreditation process. The need to manage costs has become everybody's responsibility. Through proper documentation, each member of the health care team is held accountable for the care given to the patient.

Peer review

Peer review organizations are mandated by federal law to evaluate the quality of care provided in health care facilities. These organizations cosist of employees who are paid by the federal government. They evaluate a sample of a health care facility's medical records and compare their findings with established generic standards or *screens*—a list of basic conditions that a group of similar health care facilities should meet. The reviewers use these screens to determine whether the health care facility or particular caregivers provided appropriate care. (See *How PROs evaluate performance,* page 8.)

REIMBURSEMENT REQUIREMENTS

Documentation helps determine the amount of reimbursement a health care facility receives. The federal government, for instance, uses a prospective payment system based on diagnosis-related groups (DRGs) to determine its Medicare reimbursements, paying a fixed amount for a particular diagnosis.

For your facility to receive payment, the patient's medical record at discharge must contain the correct DRG codes and show that the patient received the proper care for his DRGs. Your documentation should support your nursing diagnoses and indicate that appropriate patient teaching and discharge planning were provided.

How PROs evaluate performance

Your nursing documentation is vitally important to peer review organizations (PROs), which can fine or sanction a health care facility that fails to provide quality care. Using established screens, PROs scrutinize medical records to determine whether a health care facility or particular caregivers have provided appropriate patient care. The screens identify the following problem areas:

NECESSARY ADMISSION

Reviewers look at the medical record to determine whether a health care facility justifiably admitted a particular patient and whether the patient received appropriate treatment.

NOSOCOMIAL INFECTION

If the reviewers find that a health care facility has an excessive rate of nosocomial infection, the reviewers must examine the medical records to determine the causes.

MEDICAL STABILITY

If the record shows that a patient has a pattern of elevated temperature after insertion of an indwelling catheter, reviewers may question whether health care personnel have contributed to the patient's medical instability.

UNSCHEDULED RETURNS TO SURGERY

Reviewers are alert for unscheduled surgery such as repeat surgery for infection.

DISCHARGE PLANNING

Reviewers check whether the health care facility provides a formal discharge planning process, as evidenced by the forms that the facility uses.

AVOIDABLE TRAUMA AND DEATH

When a patient dies unexpectedly during or after surgery or after a return to the critical care unit within 24 hours of being transferred out of the unit, PROs must determine whether the health care facility could have prevented the death. If they find that the facility or specific caregivers were negligent, they can discipline those at fault and suggest steps to minimize the recurrence of such incidents.

MEDICARE COMPLAINTS

PROs review complaints made by Medicare patients about care received at health care facilities. If they find problems with the quality of care a patient received, they can impose fines or sanctions or deny reimbursement for care provided.

Faulty documentation can have a direct impact on the amount of reimbursement a facility receives. For example, a home health care agency can be denied payment retroactively for home care visits deemed unreasonable and unnecessary—a determination strongly influenced by documentation.

Numerous patients have been discharged from home health care plans because the payer would no longer agree to pay for improperly documented care. This has the added negative effect of denying patients the care they need. (For more information, see chapter 3, Performance Improvement and Reimbursement.)

Organization of the medical record

The medical record can be organized in many different ways. Each health care facility selects the method—or a variation of it—that best suits

its needs and the current legal and regulatory requirements.

NARRATIVE RECORD

The narrative method requires members of each discipline to record assessment, care interventions, and patient progress in chronological order in the patient's medical record. The narrative note is commonly entered in the progress notes, using a specific format. In the past, members of each discipline recorded information in a separate section of the chart, making information seem disjointed.

Because narrative charting takes considerable time but rarely provides a quantifiable measure of a patient's condition, most health care facilities have implemented more efficient narrative documentation systems: subjective-objective-assessment-planning (SOAP) charting, problem-intervention-evaluation (PIE) charting, assessment-intervention-response (AIR) charting, FOCUS CHARTING, and others. Each facility chooses a format that best fits its documentation needs. Activities of daily living (ADLs) flow sheets are commonly used along with the above charting methods.

SOAP charting, a vital component of the problem-oriented medical record, organizes record keeping by subjective, objective, assessment, and planning data. A variation, SOAPIE charting, adds two more categories: intervention and evaluation. FOCUS CHARTING provides a specific structure for progress notes and is best suited for reporting a patient's rapidly changing condition. (For more information on these formats, see chapter 4, Documentation Systems.)

There will always be a place for narrative documentation, especially in source-oriented, subjective evaluation charting. However, narrative entries should be concise and relevant to the topic; they shouldn't duplicate material already written on a flow sheet or care plan.

CHARTING BY EXCEPTION

Charting by exception (CBE), which is most appropriate for summarizing patient care, is currently being used successfully at many facilities. This type of charting consists of baseline data, a problem-oriented care plan, flow sheets, and progress notes. Baseline data include significant demographics, health history, and functional status. Initial and ongoing health and psychosocial assessments are documented only as exceptions to preprinted guidelines prepared for each body system.

If a patient is assessed as being "within normal limits" according to the standard, "WNL" is entered in the chart. Otherwise, whatever is charted reflects what's deemed as *not* normal—the exception.

The care plan depends heavily on clearly written standards of routine nursing care throughout the facility and within a particular unit. Only deviations from these standards need to be documented in a narrative fashion. Evaluations of patient status and response to care can be easily documented on a well-designed flow sheet with a few concise narrative notes to clarify any deviations from the expected outcome.

The only drawback to CBE is that sometimes the standards are inaccessible to staff who are responsible for the charting and to those who review the information.

PROBLEM-ORIENTED MEDICAL RECORD

The problem-oriented medical record (POMR) consists of baseline data, a problem list, a care plan for each problem, and progress notes. Baseline data, which are obtained from all departments involved in patient care, focus on the patient's present complaints and illness. They include the patient's social and emotional status, medical status, health history, initial assessment findings, and diagnostic test results.

A problem list is then distilled from this baseline data to construct a care plan. The care plan addresses each of the patient's problems; the status of these problems is routinely updated both in the care plan and in the part of the medical record known as progress notes.

OTHER SYSTEMS AND FORMATS

Many health care facilities have adapted the traditional narrative method or the problem-oriented method to better meet their documentation needs. In the home health care setting, for example, nurses have created many documentation forms—including the initial assessment form, problem list, day-visit sheet, and discharge summary—to better reflect the services and essential quality of care they provide. These forms were designed to meet the nurse's documentation needs while at the same time complying with state and federal laws and other regulations.

Several effective documentation systems currently in use were developed to respond to the expanded purposes and functions of the medical record—a result of the changes within the health care delivery system and the technological advances in health care.

Clinical pathways can successfully combine the recording of data, the Kardex, and the traditional care plan. Careful development of the pathway and the forms reflecting its implementation is crucial to the success of this format.

Each of these documentation systems has advantages, disadvantages, and distinguishing features that may make it more or less suitable for a given situation.

ELECTRONIC CHARTING

Today, computers play an increasing role in completing the medical record from admission through discharge. Nursing care plans, progress notes, medication records, vital signs records, intake and output sheets, and patient acuity may be recorded on computers. Some hospitals have installed bedside workstations to allow quick entry of information and access to it. Other facilities even have individualized forms for each area of nursing practice and provide a computer form that allows the nurse to select the assessment finding for a given patient and add information as needed. (For more detailed information on charting by computer, see Part IV, "Electronic Documentation.")

▶

Elements of sound documentation

Sound documentation demonstrates a logical approach to problem solving. Nursing documentation typically begins with initial assessment data, which provide a baseline definition of the patient's current health care needs or problems. Next, nursing documentation provides evidence that patient care has been planned, and it continues by reflecting nursing interventions and the patient's response and progress.

Essentially, effective documentation is a systematic, accurate, well-written account of nursing practice. To produce sound documentation, you'll need to set aside time for completing charts and other forms. Try to schedule a regular time for charting so that your records are current and updated. You'll need to use proper forms to ensure accuracy and consistency.

Legible, accurate, and clearly written charts that demonstrate professionalism and diligence will withstand litigation, ensure reimbursement, and satisfy reviewer requirements of the medical record.

Besides learning and applying documentation fundamentals, mastering documentation skills may involve improving existing documentation habits, using more efficient methods, adopting new systems, and applying new technology to documentation.

Of course, your documentation requirements will differ depending on where you work—in a hospital, nursing home, home health care agency, or other community facility. For instance, perioperative, critical, and emergency care areas have specialized criteria and forms for documenting nursing care. Requirements may change depending on the patient population— for example, requirements in obstetric settings differ from those in geriatric settings.

Three Cs

Documentation is both demanding and complex, a professional challenge for novice and expert alike. When documenting, remember the three Cs of good charting—clarity, conciseness, and consistency. Make sure that you use correct spelling and approved abbreviations and symbols. Don't alter notations; if you make an error when recording data, follow your facility's policy for correcting the error, and write legibly and neatly. Include your signature along with the date and time of posting.

Documentation should demonstrate the nursing process—from assessment, nursing diagnosis, outcome identification, and planning care to nursing interventions and evaluation. It should also demonstrate attention to precharting plans (such as the care plan, Kardex, or activity sheets). What's more, it must comply with standards established by accrediting and licensing organizations, state and federal agencies, insurance companies, and your health care facility.

Efficient methods

To ensure thoroughness and accuracy, you must adopt efficient documentation methods according to your facility's policy. Such methods may include tape-recorded dictation and transcription services, electronic documentation, and special charting forms, such as standardized flow sheets, checklists, admission forms, initial care plans, and progress notes.

These methods provide data about the intensity of nursing care given and the patient's condition. They help you make precise entries and supply information that can be retrieved easily.

Requirements of nursing documentation

State and professional organizations mandate certain documentation requirements. Some requirements are incorporated into laws, such as nurse practice acts, which vary from state to state. Other requirements—for example, evidence of accountability or a health care facility's documentation policies—aren't mandated by law but are accepted under the general scope of nursing as practiced today.

Adherence to nurse practice acts

Nurse practice acts are state laws designating the specific activities that nurses can perform in that state. Cumulative changes in the regulations that govern nursing have led to substantial redefinitions or revisions of the acts in many states. Today, state regulations consider nurses to be managers of care as well as being practitioners.

These and other revisions in state laws and regulations require that complete descriptions of nursing judgment and provision of care be documented in nurses' records as evidence that nurses have complied with standards.

Accountability

Proper nursing documentation provides evidence that the nurse has acted as required or ordered. She must demonstrate her accountability by complying with the documentation requirements established by the health care facility, regulatory agencies, professional organizations, and state law.

Policies affecting documentation

Health care facilities usually establish documentation policies that meet the requirements of insurance agencies and accrediting bodies. A facility's board of trustees typically appoints a committee to investigate various documentation systems and to make recommendations on adopting a particular format and style of documentation.

The health care facility may then decide to adopt a new system or modify an existing system to support its goals and preserve its accreditation and licenses.

Meeting requirements in special settings

In acute or critical care, long-term care, intermediate care, or home care environments, documentation requirements may be considerably more demanding. In such environments, be especially careful to review your facility's documentation policies and follow them accurately.

ACUTE OR CRITICAL CARE

Documentation policies in acute or critical care settings generally require you to record assessment findings, nursing interventions, patient responses, and patient outcomes. Much of critical care unit documentation is entered on flow sheets accompanied by commentary and critical data such as an electrocardiogram strip.

LONG-TERM AND INTERMEDIATE CARE

These settings offer more time to document, but documentation is highly regulated. State laws and Medicare's conditions of participation determine to a large extent what must be recorded. Some institutions choose the CBE documentation system for these settings.

HOME CARE

Again, Medicare's conditions of participation strongly influence the documentation required. To increase efficiency and avoid licensing, accreditation, and reimbursement difficulties, most home health care agencies have abandoned narrative notes in favor of individualized visit sheets and physical discomfort forms.

Understanding length of stay and patient awareness

As the average patient's length of hospitalization continues to decline, documentation must include all exceptional problems and interventions. This becomes particularly important when reimbursing agents and insurance companies insist on evidence to justify a patient's extended stay in the health care facility.

Patient awareness also influences documentation. Patients today are increasingly aware of the nurse's role in documentation and of their own right to view the medical record. More and more patients may ask you for a copy of the medical record. Though the patient is entitled to this information, you should always consult your legal department for advice. The practitioner also should be notified and should be present when the patient reviews the chart to answer any questions and explain terms. Keep in mind that the request to see the medical record may be preliminary to a lawsuit.

Understanding utilization review

Reimbursing agents maintain control over health care providers through utilization review programs that focus on length of stay, treatment regimen, validation of diagnostic tests and procedures, and verification that medical supplies and equipment were used. To determine whether utilization is proper, they commonly rely on nursing documentation.

Among specific data you may need to document (to comply with utilization review policy) are the types and quantity of I.V. access devices, infusion pumps, drains, tubes, and other equipment that you've used. Unfortunately, practitioners don't usually record their use of supplies. Utilization review policies can also affect where treatment occurs—in the hospital, practitioner's office, or patient's home, for example.

Current trends in documentation

The Joint Commission no longer requires a formal care plan, concluding that it doesn't necessarily affect patient outcomes. As a result, new documentation tools have arisen, including standardized care plans, clinical pathways, and patient-outcome time lines.

Standardized care plans

Today, standardized care plans that correspond with a medical diagnosis, DRG, or nursing diagnosis are growing in use. The emphasis is on concise care plans that reflect the patient's needs. Here, home health care nurses are on the cutting edge because Medicare's conditions of participation require that care plans be tailored to specific patient needs.

Clinical pathways

The clinical pathway (also known as *critical pathway, care map,* or *care track*) is a blend of evidence-based medical and nursing care plans. It's a sequence of processes and events that moves a patient toward an expected outcome. As a road map to care, it outlines such key elements as expected patient outcomes, essential medical and nursing interventions, and other patient variables for specific health-related conditions (usually based on a DRG).

Physicians and nurses are responsible for establishing a clinical pathway for each condition or DRG. The clinical pathway defines a patient's daily care requirements and desired outcomes that are consistent with the average length of stay for the specified condition or DRG.

Clinical pathways are the patient care plan of the future. They ensure that patient care is consistent and carried out in an appropriate sequence. They also demonstrate quality and consistency of care to third-party payers and enable the health care industry to prepare for the effects of prospective payment and managed care on reimbursement for services. They are especially useful when moving toward an automated system because they provide a structured approach in manageable categories.

Patient-outcome time lines

Another valuable documentation tool, the patient-outcome time line allows all practitioners to note essential diagnostic tests, interventions, patient outcomes, and other parameters to attain the average length of stay for each DRG.

For example, the patient-outcome time line for a patient who has had abdominal surgery might recommend that he be out of bed and into a chair the day after surgery and walking in the hallway 4 days after surgery. This plan will also list key interventions needed to achieve the expected outcomes and will be used to monitor the patient's progress during each shift.

Conclusion

Documentation will continue to change rapidly, which makes it all the more essential for you to understand and explore new approaches as documentation systems become more efficient and improve communication among health care personnel. New technology—and new ways of organizing your observations—should help you save time, eliminate confusion and, most importantly, improve patient care.

Selected references

Allen, R., Ventura, N. "Advance Directives Use in Acute Care Hospitals," *JONA's Healthcare Law, Ethics & Regulation* 7(3):86-91, July/September 2005.

Austin, S. "Ladies & Gentlemen of the Jury, I Present … the Nursing Documentation," *Nursing* 36(1):56-63, January 2006.

Charting Made Incredibly Easy, 3rd ed. Philadelphia: Lippincott Williams & Wilkins, 2005.

Chart Smart: The A-to-Z Guide to Better Nursing Documentation, 2nd ed. Philadelphia: Lippincott Williams & Wilkins, 2007.

Iyer, P., et al. *Medical Legal Aspects of Medical Records.* Tucson, AZ: Lawyers & Judges Publishing Company, Inc., 2006.

Lippincott Manual of Nursing Practice Series: Documentation. Philadelphia: Lippincott Williams & Wilkins, 2007.

The Joint Commission: *Comprehensive Accreditation Manual for Hospitals: The Official Handbook,* 2005.

LEGAL AND ETHICAL IMPLICATIONS OF DOCUMENTATION

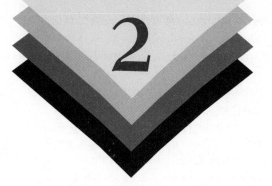

2

Nurses are ethically and legally accountable to all of their patients. The scope of your professional responsibility is set out by your state's Nurse Practice Act and by other state and federal regulations. Documenting the nursing care provided in the patient's medical record is one way of accepting that responsibility and of being accountable to the patient and your profession. Your documentation demonstrates that the patient care you provide meets the needs of the patient at a specific point in time and meets the accepted standards of nursing practice mandated by law, your profession, and the health care facility in which you practice. It also assures the patient that every effort has been made to guarantee his well-being.

The purpose of the medical record is to communicate important clinical information to your patient's other caregivers. Documentation is a form of communication that's more important today than ever before because of the increasing number and variety of providers who see the patient. If you deliver the appropriate standard of nursing care and chart that information in an acceptable and timely manner, you'll protect your patient's interests as well as your own. Failure to document appropriately has been a pivotal issue in many malpractice cases. The adage "If it isn't documented, it wasn't done" holds true in court.

Although the actual medical record, X-rays, laboratory reports, and other records belong to the institution, the *information* contained in them belongs to the patient, who has a right to obtain a copy of the materials. If a health care facility refuses to release a patient's records, the perceived reluctance may not bode well for the facility if the case comes to trial. In *Deford and Thompson v. Westwood Hills Health Care Center, Inc., Doctors Regional Medical Center and Barnes Hospital,* St. Louis City, Missouri Circuit Court, Case No. 922-9564 (1992), a patient died after

15

a nurse attempted to insert a feeding tube. Seven months later, when the family requested the patient's records, Westwood Hills staff mistakenly believed they weren't authorized to release them and so refused. Copies of the records were finally released more than 1 year later. The case resulted in an $80,000 verdict against Westwood Hills on a wrongful death claim.

Knowing your legal and ethical obligations and scrupulously documenting to show that the care you provide meets these standards are keys to conveying information, meeting your patient's health care needs, and protecting yourself legally.

This chapter discusses the important legal and ethical issues involved when documenting your patient's condition and your nursing care. These include the legal relevance of the medical record, malpractice litigation, how policies and procedures affect legal decisions, risk management programs, quality assurance programs, and ethical considerations in patient care.

Legal relevance of medical records

Accurately and completely documenting your nursing care helps other members of the health care team confirm their impressions of the patient's condition and progress—or may signal the need for adjustments in the therapeutic regimen. Your clinical account of a patient's condition, treatment, and responses may also be used as evidence in the courtroom—for example, in malpractice suits, workers' compensation litigation, personal injury cases and, possibly, criminal cases.

If you think of the medical record first and foremost as a tool for clinical communication, and you document carefully, you need not panic

if the court subpoenas it. However, if you think only of legal implications or document to protect yourself, your part of the medical record will sound self-serving and defensive. Such documentation tends to have a negative impact on a judge and jury.

Standards of documentation

The type of nursing information that appears in a medical record isn't dictated by standards set by the courts. It's governed by standards developed over the years by the nursing profession, state laws, and regulatory agencies.

Documentation that meets these standards communicates the patient's status, medical treatment, and nursing care. Professional organizations such as the American Nurses Association (ANA) and accrediting organizations, such as The Joint Commission and the Centers for Medicare and Medicaid Services (CMS), have established that documentation must include ongoing assessment, variations from the assessment, patient teaching, responses to therapy, and relevant statements made by the patient.

Although documentation goals have changed little since their inception, documentation methods have changed dramatically. For example, nurses no longer need to spend valuable time writing long narrative notes. Instead, many facilities today use such methods as flow sheets, graphic records, checklists, and charting by exception (in which only exceptions from articulated standards of care are charted). While flow sheets save valuable nursing time, they've been criticized as being too abbreviated and lacking important narrative information about the patient's condition. If used prudently, however, flow sheets can trigger or remind a nurse what actions are indicated. Point-of-care technology has also enabled nurses to document quickly in the patient's electronic medical record, giving other members of the health care team immediate access to patient information.

Timely communication

One purpose of charting is communication, with an emphasis on timeliness. When the patient's condition deteriorates or changes in therapy are clearly indicated, you must not only chart this information but also contact the responsible practitioner as soon as possible and chart the fact that you contacted the practitioner, the time the contact was made, and the practitioner's response and any orders received. If the practitioner isn't responding appropriately, in your opinion, you must contact the next individual in the chain of command. Failure to do so is a breach of duty to the patient and leaves you vulnerable to a malpractice lawsuit.

There are numerous legal cases involving failure of the nurse to notify the physician of changes in the patient's condition. When such notification isn't documented, it's nearly impossible to prove that the physician was called in a timely manner and that all critical information was communicated. These cases are often extremely serious, resulting in death or permanent disability.

In a California case, *Malovec v. Santa Monica Hospital,* Los Angeles County, California Superior Court, Case No. SC 019-167 (1994), a woman in labor repeatedly asked the charge nurse to call the chief of obstetrics because her obstetrician refused to perform a cesarean delivery despite guarded fetal heart tracings. The charge nurse refused, and the baby was born with cerebral palsy and spastic quadriplegia. A confidential settlement was reached.

Errors or omissions

Errors or omissions can severely undermine your credibility in court. A jury could reasonably conclude that you didn't perform a function if it wasn't charted. If you failed to chart something and need to enter a late entry, date it the day you entered it.

In the case of *Anonymous v. Anonymous,* Suffolk Superior Court, Boston (1993), failure to chart led to a $1 million settlement. A 2-year-old was admitted to Children's Hospital for correction of a congenital urinary tract defect. Postoperative orders required blood pressure, pulse, and temperature readings to be taken every 4 hours, and respiratory rate and reaction to analgesia every hour. However, the child's care wasn't charted for 5 hours. The child was found in cardiorespiratory arrest and died from an overdose of an opioid infusion. The responsible nurse admitted failing to assess the child strictly according to the orders; she also claimed that she had assessed the child adequately but had been "too busy" to chart her observations.

Failure to comply with a facility's policy can also constitute an omission. In *Wallace v. Sacred Heart Hospital,* Escambia County, Florida (1997), a nurse failed to apply Posey restraints to a patient who had a history of stroke and seizure disorder and was at high risk for falls. Early one morning, the patient was discovered trying to walk to the bathroom. The nurse who found her helped her back to bed but neglected to apply restraints. One hour later, the patient was found on the floor with a fractured left hip. The nurses involved failed to follow the facility's policy for patients at high risk for falls and the physician's order for restraints. A confidential settlement was reached during mediation.

Corrections and alterations

Any necessary corrections to the medical record should be made *only* by drawing a line through the initial charting, signing it, and dating it. Then you can proceed to supply the proper entry. *Never erase, obliterate, or otherwise alter a record.* Completely defensible malpractice cases have been lost because of chart alterations. The jury simply concluded the nurse was covering up something. Also, *never try to make the record "better" after you learn a malpractice case has been filed.* Attorneys have methods for analyzing papers and inks and can easily detect discrepancies.

Malpractice and documentation

Although you document first to serve your patient and to convey information, you must also be aware of documentation's legal import. Depending on how well you administer care and document your activities and observations, the records may or may not support a plaintiff's accusation of nursing malpractice. Legally, malpractice focuses on these four elements: duty, breach of duty, causation, and damages.

Duty and breach of duty

The term *duty* refers to your obligation to provide patient care and to follow appropriate standards. The courts have ruled that a nurse has a duty to provide care after a nurse-patient relationship is established. The relationship may be established in person—at admission, for example—or at a distance—say, during a telephone conversation. (Even telephone calls must be carefully documented, especially with outpatient care and telephone triage on the rise.)

Breach of duty, a failure to fulfill your nursing obligations, can be difficult to prove because nursing responsibilities typically overlap those of physicians and other health care providers. A key question asked when a possible breach of duty is being investigated is "How would a reasonable, prudent nurse with comparable training and experience have acted in the same or similar circumstances?" In judging a nurse to have breached her duty, the courts must prove that the nurse failed to provide the appropriate care—as they did in the following case.

In *Collins v. Westlake Community Hospital,* 312 N.E. 2d 614 (Ill. 1974), a 6-year-old boy was hospitalized for a fractured leg, which was put in a cast and placed in traction. Although the physician ordered the nurse on duty to monitor the condition of the boy's toes, the medical record lacked documentation that she did so. In fact, 7 hours elapsed between documented nursing entries in the medical record. The boy's leg was later amputated, and the parents sued on behalf of their son. Because a nurse is responsible for continually assessing patients and because documentation of these assessments didn't appear in the record, the nurse was found to have breached her duty to this child.

In another case, *Wickliffe v. Sunrise Hospital,* Clark County, Nevada District Court, Case No. 185939 (1988), a 13-year-old girl underwent Harrington rod surgery for scoliosis without complications. In the postanesthesia care unit, she was found without pulse or respiration. Although she was resuscitated, she remained comatose and eventually died. The family accused the nurses of failing to check the girl's vital signs every 15 minutes as required by facility policy. The authenticity of two pages of nursing notes was in dispute, with one page having entries of 11:20, 11:30, and 12:40 and another page covering from 11:50 to 12:40. The notes had different tab forms, were irregular in context, and were unlike other pages in the medical record. The jury concluded that the second page of notes was a later addition to the record and that a breach of duty had occurred when vital signs weren't recorded between 11:30 and 12:40. The jury awarded the family $1.75 million.

Causation

After the plaintiff establishes a breach of duty, he must then prove that this breach caused the injury. Of the four malpractice elements, causation is the most difficult to prove. For the nurse to be liable, she must have *proximately caused* the injury by an act or an oversight. The principle of *proximity* is important because, in a typical health care facility, so many caregivers are involved in a patient's care. Even if a nurse did commit malpractice, it's conceivable that the patient's injury was caused by something other than the nursing intervention. For instance, even if a nurse gave a patient an overdose of a medication, and the patient later vomited blood, the cause of the vomiting might actually be a surgical error and have nothing to do with the medication.

It's important to distinguish between bad outcomes and malpractice. A bad outcome isn't malpractice per se. Health care has many inherent risks, such as an adverse reaction to a blood transfusion received during surgery. If the medical record indicates that the blood was the correct type, that all policies and procedures were properly followed, and that the facility policy set a reasonable standard, the patient has no cause for a claim—he simply had an unexpected reaction to the blood transfusion.

Some patients assume that a bad outcome is due to malpractice because they had unrealistic expectations or received an inadequate explanation of a condition or procedure. That's why careful communication before and during treat-

ment is crucial. Many patients sue because they believe the health care provider didn't communicate with them enough, and they're unhappy with the results of their care. Again, they won't be successful in suing for malpractice unless they can prove that the standard of care wasn't met. Nurses and other providers can help prevent some lawsuits simply by communicating well with their patients to establish realistic expectations of care.

Damages

To show malpractice, the patient's attorney must prove that injury occurred because of breach of duty and causation. It isn't sufficient that the patient be disgruntled or dissatisfied; usually the injury must be physical, not just emotional or mental. If the patient has sustained a true physical injury, the attorney can then sue for *damages*. These damages represent the amount of money the court orders the defendant to pay to the plaintiff when a case is decided in the plaintiff's favor.

Policies and documentation

Although most discussions about documentation center on writing in the patient's chart, other types of documentation also affect nurses. One example is the documentation of policies and procedures contained in health care facility employee and nursing manuals. Deviation from these rules suggests that an employee failed to meet the facility's standards of care. Another is documentation of mandatory nursing education and competency verification.

Whether such policies establish a standard of care has been debated in some malpractice cases. But in *every* nursing malpractice case, the actions of the nurse are compared with the appropriate nursing standard of care. The jury measures the nurse's actions or omissions against the performance of a reasonable, prudent nurse with comparable training and experience, using accepted, regularly updated national standards as guidelines. Keep in mind, however, that the defense can always challenge the presumption of the standard by introducing expert testimony or by other methods.

In a case related to a health care facility's policies, the court was pressed to distinguish between a facility's policies and its "goals." In *H.C.A. Health Services v. National Bank,* 1745 S.W. 2d 120 (Ark. 1988), three nurses were working in a nursery composed of three connecting rooms. One nurse cared for a baby in the first (admissions) room. The other two nurses went into the second room, which housed 11 babies (two of whom were premature and one of whom was jaundiced). There was no documentation for 1½ hours that any of the nurses went into the third room, which had six babies. Documentation did show that when the first nurse finally entered the third room, she found that one of the infants had stopped breathing and had no heartbeat.

Both the facility's executive director and the nurse who found the baby testified that, according to the facility's manual, no infant is ever to be left alone without a member of the nursery staff present. However, they also testified that this was a goal—not a policy. Another physician testified that the baby's problem would have been avoided if a nurse had been present. The court disagreed with the distinction between policies and goals and ruled against the facility and nurses and in favor of the plaintiff.

Risk management and documentation

Sometimes documentation reveals potential problems within a health care facility—for example, a particular procedure that repeatedly leads to patient injury or another type of accident. To reduce injuries and accidents, minimize financial loss, and meet the guidelines of The Joint Commission and other regulatory agencies, health care facilities have instituted risk management programs. Based on similar programs first used in industry, risk management programs initially focused on maintaining and improving facilities and equipment and ensuring the safety of employees, visitors, and patients. Today, however, risk management and performance improvement efforts focus on identifying, evaluating, and reducing the risk of patient injury throughout the health care system.

The primary objectives of a risk management program are:
▶ to ensure optimal patient care
▶ to reduce the frequency of preventable injuries and accidents leading to liability claims by maintaining or improving quality of care
▶ to decrease the chance of a claim being filed by promptly identifying and following up on adverse events (incidents)
▶ to help control costs related to claims by identifying trouble spots early and intervening with the patient and his family.

Coordinating risk management and performance improvement
Rather than support two separate programs, many health care facilities now coordinate their risk management and performance improvement programs to ensure that they fulfill their legal duty to provide reasonable care. In doing so, the

facility may also coordinate the programs' educational efforts—for example, in reaching out to a specific employee, such as a nurse, physician, or other practitioner, who has been identified as having a particular problem, or to a larger population, such as new residents and nurses.

The health care facility should place a high priority on teaching new residents and nurses about risk management and performance improvement. Teaching topics for new employees may include malpractice claims, staff members' reporting obligations, proper informational and reporting channels, and principles of risk management and performance improvement.

Keep in mind, however, that a coordinated system usually continues its dual focus on different aspects of health care delivery. Risk management focuses more on the patients' and families' perception of the care provided, whereas performance improvement focuses on the role and functions of the health care provider. (For more information on performance improvement programs, see chapter 3, Performance Improvement and Reimbursement.)

A reputation for safe, reliable, effective service is a health care facility's primary defense against liability claims. Systematic, well-coordinated risk management and performance improvement programs demonstrate to the public that the facility is managed in a legally responsible way. When complaints do arise, risk managers handle them promptly to contain the damage and minimize liability claims.

Identifying adverse events

A key part of a risk management program involves developing a system for identifying *adverse events*—events such as patient falls that would be considered an abnormal consequence of a patient's condition or treatment. These events may or may not be caused by a health care provider's

breach of duty or the standard of care. The purpose of event reporting is to identify problem areas and implement solutions. Many institutions have adopted a blame-free environment and focus on identifying and correcting system issues to eliminate future events.

The most common "early-warning systems" for detecting adverse events are incident reporting and occurrence screening. These systems are crucial because they permit early investigation and intervention, thus helping to minimize additional adverse consequences and legal action. They also provide valuable databases for building strategies to prevent repeated incidents.

INCIDENT REPORTING

In *incident reporting,* events are reported by physicians, nurses, or other health care staff, either when they're observed or shortly after. Events should be reported whether or not harm occurs. Incident reports have become a tool for identifying safety issues. Examples of such events include a patient or visitor fall, equipment failure, blood exposure, the unplanned return of a patient to the operating room, and a medication error requiring intervention. *All errors must be reported* because it's impossible to predict which ones will require intervention.

OCCURRENCE SCREENING

In contrast, *occurrence screening* flags adverse events through a review of all or some of the medical charts. These reviews use generic criteria (such as a hospital-acquired infection, a fall, or an unexpected death). More specific reviews may focus on specialty- or service-specific criteria such as an incorrect sponge count during surgery. Over the years, generic and focused criteria have been developed for reporting and screening systems, and a growing body of literature exists to compare the effectiveness of various approaches.

Although these early-warning systems pinpoint much useful information, they aren't effective without a strong organizational structure, the commitment of key staff (such as practitioners, nurses, administrators, and chiefs of high-risk services such as perinatal care) to analyze the information and develop an action plan. They also require cooperation between risk management and performance improvement departments.

OTHER SOURCES OF INFORMATION
In addition to incident reports and occurrence screening, nurses and patient representatives are a primary source of information for identifying adverse events as well as health care dangers or trends.

Nurses
Nurses are typically the first to recognize potential problems because they spend so much time with patients and their families. They can identify patients who are dissatisfied with their care, particularly those with complications that might result in injuries.

Patient representatives
Another information source is the patient representative's office, which keeps a file of patient concerns and complaints. By evaluating these concerns and complaints for trends, patient representatives can provide an early-warning signal of health care problems that need to be addressed, ranging from staffing to faulty equipment. They are also trained to recognize litigious patients, and they maintain communication with the patient and family after an incident has occurred.

Other departments
Other departments also can provide information about adverse events. For example, the billing department may become aware of a patient who threatens to sue after receiving his bill. Or the first clue of an impending lawsuit may come from the medical records office, when a patient or attorney requests a copy of the medical record.

Reports from the engineering department about the safety of the hospital environment and from purchasing, biomedical engineering, and the pharmacy on the safety and adequacy of products and equipment are also informative.

Trending reports of adverse events from various departments can identify areas that need attention more quickly than a focused departmental review. For instance, medication errors may correlate with new nurses or decreased staffing. Patient falls may correlate with staffing problems, problems with history taking in fall-prone patients, safety hazards, or a combination of these factors.

Of course, reports from all sources should be documented thoroughly. For nurses, this means charting on the patient's medical record and filling out incident reports and related nursing documents.

Managing adverse events
The health care facility may appoint one key department or an employee as responsible for risk management. When the risk manager learns of a potential or actual lawsuit, he or she notifies the medical records department and the facility's insurance carrier or attorney (or both). The medical records department makes copies of the patient's chart and files the original in a secure place to prevent tampering.

A claim notice should also trigger a performance improvement peer review of the medical record. This review may be conducted by the chairperson of the department involved, the risk management or performance improvement de-

Smarter charting

Tips for writing an incident report

When a malpractice lawsuit reached the courtroom in years past, the plaintiff's attorney wasn't allowed to see incident reports. Today, however, the plaintiff in many states is legally entitled to a record of the incident if he requests it through proper channels.

When writing an incident report, keep in mind the people who may read it, and follow these guidelines:

WRITE OBJECTIVELY
Record the details of the incident in objective terms, describing exactly what you saw and heard. For example, unless you actually saw a patient fall, write: "Found patient lying on the floor." Then describe only the actions you took to provide care at the scene, such as helping the patient get back into bed or assessing him for injuries.

INCLUDE ONLY ESSENTIAL INFORMATION
Document the time and place of the incident and the name of the practitioner who was notified.

AVOID OPINIONS
Don't commit your opinions to writing in the incident report. Rather, verbally share your suggestions or opinions on how an incident may be avoided with your supervisor and risk manager.

ASSIGN NO BLAME
Don't admit to liability, and don't blame or point your finger at colleagues or administrators. Steer clear of such statements as "Better staffing would have prevented this incident." State only what happened.

AVOID HEARSAY AND ASSUMPTIONS
Each staff member involved in the incident should write a separate incident report. If one of your patients is injured in another department, the staff members in that department are responsible for documenting the details of the incident.

FILE THE REPORT PROPERLY
Don't document in the medical record that an incident report was completed, and don't file the incident report with the medical record. Send the report to the person designated to review it according to your facility's policy.

---

partment, or an external reviewer to measure the health care provider's conduct against the professional standards of conduct for the particular situation. This review helps the risk manager determine the claim's merit and also helps to define the facility's responsibility for care in particular situations. It also identifies areas where changes are needed, such as policy, training, staffing, or equipment.

COMPLETING INCIDENT REPORTS
An incident report is a formal report, written by practitioners, nurses, or other staff members, that informs facility administrators about an adverse event suffered by a patient. Incident reports are continually being revised, and some may be electronic. (Electronic processing permits classifying and counting of incidents to indicate trends.) If you're filing an incident report and need more room than the form allows, check your facility's policy; additional blank pages may not be protected from disclosure to a patient's attorney. (See *Tips for writing an incident report.* See also *Completing an incident report,* page 24.)

State, federal, and military statutes protect performance improvement and peer review documents from disclosure to a patient's attorney

ChartWizard

Completing an incident report

When you witness or discover a reportable event, you must fill out an incident report. Forms vary, but most include the following information.

INCIDENT REPORT

Name of person involved *Greta Manning*
Address *7 Worth Way, Boston, MA*
Phone *(617) 555-1122*
Medical record number (if patient) _____

DATE OF INCIDENT	TIME OF INCIDENT
3-20-07	*1442*

EXACT LOCATION OF INCIDENT (Bldg, Floor, Room No, Area)
4-Main, Rm. 447

TYPE OF INCIDENT
(CHECK ONE ONLY)   ☐ PATIENT   ☐ EMPLOYEE   ☑ VISITOR   ☐ VOLUNTEER   ☐ OTHER (specify)

DESCRIPTION OF THE INCIDENT (WHO, WHAT, WHEN, WHERE, HOW, WHY)
(Use back of form if necessary)
Patient's wife found on floor next to bed. States, "I was trying to put the siderail of the bed down and I fell down."

Patient fall incidents	**FLOOR CONDITIONS** ☐ OTHER _____ ☑ CLEAN & SMOOTH ☐ SLIPPERY (WET)		**FRAME OF BED** ☑ LOW ☐ HIGH	**NIGHT LIGHT** ☐ YES ☑ NO
	WERE BED RAILS PRESENT? ☐ NO ☐ 1 UP ☐ 2 UP ☐ 3 UP ☑ 4 UP	**OTHER RESTRAINTS (TYPE AND EXTENT)** *N/A*		
	AMBULATION PRIVILEGE ☐ UNLIMITED ☐ LIMITED WITH ASSISTANCE ☐ COMPLETE BEDREST ☐ OTHER			
	WERE NARCOTICS, ANALGESICS, HYPNOTICS, SEDATIVES, DIURETICS, ANTIHYPERTENSIVES, OR ANTICONVULSANTS GIVEN DURING LAST 4 HOURS? ☐ YES ☑ NO DRUG _____ AMOUNT _____ TIME _____			

Patient incidents	**PHYSICIAN NOTIFIED** Name of Physician *J. Reynolds, MD*	DATE *3-20-07*	TIME *1445*	COMPLETE IF APPLICABLE
Employee incidents	**DEPARTMENT**	**JOB TITLE**		**SOCIAL SECURITY #**
	MARITAL STATUS			

All incidents	**NOTIFIED** *C. Jones, RN* DATE *3-20-07* TIME *1500*	**LOCATION WHERE TREATMENT WAS RENDERED**
	NAME, ADDRESS, AND TELEPHONE NUMBERS OF WITNESS(ES) OR PERSONS FAMILIAR WITH INCIDENT - WITNESS OR NOT *Janet Adams (617) 555-0912 1 Main St., Boston, MA*	

SIGNATURE OF PERSON PREPARING REPORT *Connie Smith, RN*	**TITLE** *RN*	**DATE OF REPORT** *3-20-07*

PHYSICIAN'S REPORT — To be completed for all cases involving injury or illness   (DO NOT USE ABBREVIATIONS) (Use back if necessary)

DIAGNOSIS AND TREATMENT
Received patient in Emergency Department after reported fall in husband's room. 12 cm x 12 cm ecchymotic area noted on right hip. X-rays negative for fracture. Good range of motion, no c/o pain. VAS 0/10. Ice pack applied. ———————   J. Reynolds, MD

DISPOSITION   *sent home, written instructions provided*

PERSON NOTIFIED OTHER THAN HOSPITAL PERSONNEL NAME AND ADDRESS *R. Manning (daughter), address same as pt*	**DATE** *3-20-07*	**TIME** *1500*
PHYSICIAN'S SIGNATURE *J. Reynolds, MD*	**DATE** *3-20-07*	

on the grounds that health care providers should be allowed to freely and thoroughly investigate claims of adverse events without having to worry about being sued for what they discover; however, incident reports may not be thus protected. Because the patient's attorney may be able to obtain a copy of an incident report, the document should be factual and succinct. Keep in mind that although names of individuals who know about the incident are important, placing those names on the report may result in their being called to testify or give a deposition regarding the incident. Still, the goal of completing the incident report is to be truthful, timely, and objective.

Historically, nurses have been reluctant to complete incident reports for such events as medication errors because they feared retribution. The problem with this is that failure to complete a report may create the appearance that you're intentionally hiding information.

DOCUMENTING AN INCIDENT IN THE MEDICAL RECORD

When documenting an incident in the patient's medical record, keep the following in mind:

▶ Write a factual account of the incident, including the treatment and follow-up care provided and the patient's response. Don't write in the progress notes that an incident report was filed. If you don't document the incident, the plaintiff's lawyer might think you're hiding something. This documentation shows that the patient was closely monitored after the incident. If the case goes to court, the jury may be asked to determine whether the patient received appropriate care after the incident.

▶ Include in the progress notes and in the incident report anything the patient or his family says about their role in the incident; for example, "Patient stated, 'The nurse told me to ask for help before I went to the bathroom, but I decided to go on my own.'" This kind of statement helps the defense attorney prove that the patient was guilty of contributory or comparative negligence. Contributory negligence is conduct that contributed to the patient's injuries. Comparative negligence involves determining the percentage of each party's fault. For example, the nurse might be found 25% negligent and the patient 75% negligent.

Overview of malpractice lawsuits

Over the past two decades, some claims data have revealed that the number of lawsuits naming the nurse as a specific defendant continues to increase. The expanding role of nurses, changes in managed care, shorter hospitalizations, and more acute home care have challenged the nurse-patient relationship. Nurses have less time to establish relationships with patients than they once did because patients now move out of the acute care system very quickly or are transferred to other units. All of this can lead to unfamiliarity, which may lead to errors. Try to establish rapport with your patients, but remember that nothing replaces good nursing care.

Although your chances of actually being sued are still small, the fear of a malpractice suit can produce stress. It's important to remember, however, that the majority of malpractice cases are settled out of court well before a trial date; of those that do go to trial, the vast majority are decided in favor of the health care provider.

Preliminary steps in a lawsuit

When a patient (the plaintiff) believes harm was caused by the action or negligence of a health care provider, he may file a lawsuit. Most of these claims are settled out of court. A plaintiff injured by the negligence of a health care provider deserves compensation without going through the stress and expense of litigation. Ideally, all parties named as defendants (usually a physician, facility, and nurse) as well as their insurance companies and attorneys try to work toward a fair settlement.

A patient's refusal to pay his bill is sometimes the facility's first sign that the patient was dissatisfied with his care. Depending on how the billing office is integrated with the performance improvement and risk management departments, steps may be taken at this time to investigate the patient's concerns. If they appear to be valid, a settlement offer may be made before litigation is even considered.

Sometimes a patient will try to obtain a copy of his medical record in an effort to learn about the care he received and then base a complaint on what he perceives as "mistakes." Although the patient has a right to a copy of the record, X-rays, and other reports, the facility can charge the patient for copying costs.

The first step for some patients may be to contact a malpractice attorney. The attorney will interview the patient. If the case appears to have merit, the attorney will probably order a copy of the medical record or a specific section dealing with the event in question.

The plaintiff's attorneys usually work on a contingency basis, meaning that they aren't paid for their work unless they win the case. This procedure is intended to prevent attorneys from taking meritless cases. However, the patient must pay for filing the case with the court, retaining expert witnesses, and other costs. Some cases with actual merit aren't filed because the expense of trying the case outweighs any dollar amount that could be awarded for damages.

Preparations for adjudication

If the parties can't agree on a settlement or if the plaintiff is dissatisfied with the settlement offer, the plaintiff may take his claim to court for *adjudication* (a judicial decision). If the case appears to have merit and records have been obtained, the plaintiff's attorney will send the records to an expert for a preliminary review. If the attorney fails to do this, he runs the risk that the case will be dismissed as a frivolous claim. Some attorneys have nurses working full time or on a contract basis to do preliminary reviews.

Activity on the defendant's side may begin when the medical records department receives an attorney's request for a copy of the medical record and notifies the risk management department. This department begins an immediate review of the situation, and the health care facility's insurance carrier is notified. The practitioner involved in the lawsuit also will be notified and given an opportunity to review the record.

Remember: No one should make changes in the medical record after a lawsuit has been initiated. If the record is incomplete or inaccurate, this should be clarified in a dated addendum. The jury will think that you were covering up something if you try to explain changes made to the medical record after it was requested by a lawyer.

Complaint

If the expert review indicates that the standard of practice was breached and injury occurred that can be proximately related to that breach, the attorney will file a *complaint*—a summary of what the injured party aims to prove. Most states allow patients to file a complaint up to 2 years from the time the alleged act of malpractice occurred or was discovered. In most jurisdictions, several years may elapse before the case goes to trial.

The complaint is filed in the courthouse, and copies are presented to each defendant or agent. This legal document notifies the defendant of the plaintiff's charges and gives the latest date on which an answer to the complaint can be filed.

In most jurisdictions, the complaint is assigned to a lower court judge. In jurisdictions with an arbitration system, an arbitration panel receives the complaint and initially hears the case. The case may then be appealed to the designated court. In cases involving the military or the Department of Veterans Affairs, the case will be filed in federal court.

Discovery

When the attorney files the complaint, the discovery period begins. Discovery has two purposes: to give each party time to gather evidence and learn all the facts and allegations involved in the case, and to encourage an out-of-court settlement when appropriate. In complex malpractice suits, the discovery period can last 1 to 2 years or even longer. When this period is over, both sides are ready to testify in court.

DEPOSITION

The most important type of discovery for a nurse-defendant is the deposition, or testimony under oath. During a deposition, attorneys question the defendants, plaintiffs, and witnesses one by one while a court stenographer records the questions and answers. The nurse will be asked questions by the plaintiff's lawyer and sometimes by other lawyers representing additional parties.

If the nurse has her own malpractice insurance, she'll be represented by the insurer's attorney to protect her interests. At a minimum, her employer's attorney will be present to protect the interests of the health care facility. Many nurses believe they're adequately protected by their employer's attorney. This isn't true; the interests of the employer and the nurse may diverge. For instance, if you fail to fulfill a policy or a procedure 100%, the facility could say you were outside the scope of employment; or you may no longer be employed by the facility when the suit is filed.

The deposition process may sound innocuous, but it isn't. Lawyers spend considerable time preparing defendants for it. The same goes for nurses who testify at depositions as fact witnesses (as opposed to named defendants). No one should ever go to a deposition without reviewing the medical record and without legal representation. If the case goes to trial, transcripts from the deposition may be introduced as evidence and compared with courtroom testimony for any discrepancies or contradictions.

INTERROGATORIES

During the deposition, some attorneys use interrogatories (lists of written questions) and formal requests for documents to determine what evidence is available. The plaintiff's attorney may ask the health care facility for all records, policies, procedures, and committee minutes pertaining to the plaintiff. These documents may be protected from discovery under peer review acts, but each jurisdiction has different statutes governing what may be made available to opposing counsel. Some state and federal statutes provide confidentiality for these documents under quality assurance provisions.

Not documented, not done

Even if you provide appropriate care, you risk a lawsuit if you fail to document. Consider the case of *Jarvis v. St. Charles Medical Center,* 713 P.2d 620 (Oregon 1986).

Concerned that his patient with a fractured leg was developing compartment syndrome, the patient's practitioner spread the cast and instructed the nurses on duty to perform hourly tests (assessments and observations) and to notify him if problems developed.

Two days later, at 2030 hours, the physician noticed that the patient's foot was white and pulseless. A nurse's entry on the progress notes at 1600 hours indicated no change in circulation, movement, or sensation.

Although emergency surgery was performed, the patient was left with restricted use of her leg.

COURT'S DECISION

In the malpractice suit that followed, the hospital argued that muscle death was gradual and that the physician didn't manage the patient appropriately. The physician claimed that a sudden change had occurred and that the nurses hadn't notified him.

The court ruled that the physician was negligent and added that because the progress notes indicated only sporadic testing, the nurses had contributed to the physician's negligence by failing to conduct regular examinations.

In this case, it didn't matter whether the nurses assessed the patient hourly and provided care as ordered. What mattered was that the records didn't demonstrate that the ordered care was provided. The result: a judgment of negligence.

Nurse's response

After being named in a malpractice suit, the nurse-defendant will need to devote considerable time to preparing her case. She'll work with her attorney to prepare for and respond to discovery requests from the plaintiff's attorney. In addition, the nurse's own attorney will rely on her to provide accurate information on the plaintiff's nursing care and other treatment issues.

The attorney may also ask for the nurse's help in selecting the right type of expert witnesses for the defense and in developing probing questions to ask the plaintiff's expert witnesses.

Courtroom hearings

When the case finally goes to trial, the jury hears from a variety of witnesses. Fact witnesses include people with knowledge of the actual incident. Expert witnesses offer opinions about the case based on their expertise in a specific subject that's relevant to the case. Family members may attest to the plaintiff's pain and suffering.

In cases heard in a court, rather than by an arbitration panel, a jury weighs the credibility of the people testifying, listens to all the evidence, and then decides whose testimony it believes.

In malpractice cases, the parties involved almost always make contradictory statements. For example, a nurse may chart ominous changes in a patient's signs and symptoms (such as tachycardia or projectile vomiting) and document that the practitioner was "notified." At trial, the practitioner may admit having been called on the phone but deny learning of any problem requiring an immediate trip to the hospital. To avoid this kind of problem, you can write, "Practitioner notified of these findings" (include the specific data reported), and chart the practitioner's response, such as "Will come to hospital" or "Practitioner gave these telephone orders." This type of charting can prevent a "he said, she said" controversy.

Discrepancies in testimony sometimes arise not from deliberate deception but simply from a poor memory of events that may have occurred months or years earlier. Incomplete documentation only adds to the problem. For example, a nurse can testify that she always performs dressing changes a certain way, always observes for abnormal signs, and always notes changes in vital signs, but if she didn't chart the intervention, she has no proof that it occurred.

ROLE OF DOCUMENTATION
Good documentation can save a nurse in a credibility dispute. In one case, a house physician didn't respond for more than 1 hour to a nurse's calls about a patient's deteriorating neurologic condition. After repeated calls, the nurse finally notified the neurosurgeon directly. The patient had an epidural hematoma and left-sided hemiparesis. The house physician claimed that he never received the calls, but the nurse had documented each one, noting the time and the physician's responses. The jury decided against the house physician.

Lack of documentation doesn't always imply negligence, but juries often believe it does. You've probably heard the expression, "If it wasn't charted, it wasn't done." Juries may think that this statement applies to all situations, when in reality, you can't possibly document every word and action. Fair or not, this misconception can lead to a negative outcome in a malpractice case when no negligence occurred. (See *Not documented, not done.*)

ROLE OF THE JUDGE
In a malpractice case, the judge's role is to monitor the testimony, to decide legal questions about how the evidence is presented, and to determine questions of law. After all testimony has been presented, the judge instructs the jury as to how the law should be applied.

ROLE OF THE JURY
The jury decides whether negligence has occurred and, if so, what compensation should be awarded. At any point before the jury's decision, the opposing parties can decide to settle the case out of court. Out-of-court settlements are usually kept confidential.

Bioethical dilemmas and documentation

As a nurse, you routinely take part in decisions involving ethical dilemmas. These may range from "innocent" discussions of confidential patient information in hospital elevators to removing life support. Ethical dilemmas appear to have grown proportionately with increased technology. Years ago, nurses didn't have to ponder such issues as a patient's right to die or refuse treatment, terminating use of life-prolonging equipment, human experimentation and research, organ donation, or surrogate motherhood.

At the same time, nurses today have access to many excellent resources for addressing bioethical dilemmas, including professional conferences, textbooks, articles, and consultants. This material underscores the significance of documentation when facing bioethical dilemmas.

The Joint Commission mandates that health care facilities address ethical issues in providing patient care. The facility must list patient rights and maintain a code of ethical behavior for the facility. A few states have incorporated patient rights into their state statutes, and most have codified statutes for nursing home patients. The ANA and other nursing organizations have their own ethical codes of conduct for nurses. (See *Ethical codes for nurses,* pages 30 and 31.)

Health care facilities should have an established framework to support ethical decision making. Many have bioethics committees with

Ethical codes for nurses

One of the most important ethical codes for registered nurses is the American Nurses Association (ANA) code. Licensed practical and vocational nurses (LPNs and LVNs) also have an ethical code, which is set forth in each state by the state's nurses association. The National Federation of Licensed Practical Nurses also has a code of ethics for its members. In addition, the International Council of Nurses, an organization based in Geneva, Switzerland that seeks to improve the standards and status of nursing worldwide, has published a code of ethics. Summaries of these codes appear below.

ANA CODE OF ETHICS

The ANA views both nurses and patients as individuals who possess basic rights and responsibilities and who should command respect for their values and circumstances at all times. The ANA code provides guidance for carrying out nursing responsibilities consistent with the ethical obligations of the profession. According to the ANA code, the nurse is responsible for the following actions:

► Provide services with respect for human dignity and the uniqueness of the patient unrestricted by considerations of social or economic status, personal attributes, or the nature of health problems.

► Safeguard the patient's right to privacy by judiciously protecting information of a confidential nature.

► Act to safeguard the patient and the public when health care and safety are affected by the incompetent, unethical, or illegal practice of any person.

► Assume responsibility and accountability for individual nursing judgments and actions.

► Maintain competence in nursing.

► Exercise informed judgment, and use individual competence and qualifications as criteria in seeking consultation, accepting responsibilities, and delegating nursing activities to others.

► Cooperate in activities that contribute to the ongoing development of the profession's body of knowledge.

► Participate in the profession's efforts to implement and improve standards of nursing.

► Take part in the profession's efforts to establish and maintain conditions of employment conducive to high-quality nursing care.

► Share in the profession's efforts to protect the public from misinformation and misrepresentation and to maintain the integrity of nursing.

► Collaborate with members of the health care professions and other citizens in promoting community and national efforts to meet the health needs of the public.

CODE FOR LPNs AND LVNs

The code for LPNs and LVNs seeks to provide a motivation for establishing, maintaining, and elevating professional standards. It includes the following imperatives:

► Know the scope of maximum utilization of the LPN and LVN, as specified by the nurse practice act, and function within this scope.

► Safeguard the confidential information acquired from any source about the patient.

► Provide health care to all patients regardless of race, creed, cultural background, disease, or lifestyle.

► Refuse to give endorsement to the sale and promotion of commercial products or services.

► Uphold the highest standards in personal appearance, language, dress, and demeanor.

► Stay informed about issues affecting the practice of nursing and delivery of health care and, where appropriate, participate in government and policy decisions.

► Accept the responsibility for safe nursing by keeping oneself mentally and physically fit and educationally prepared to practice.

► Accept responsibility for membership in the National Federation of Licensed Practical Nurses, and participate in its efforts to maintain the established standards of nursing practice and employment policies that lead to quality patient care.

Ethical codes for nurses (continued)

INTERNATIONAL COUNCIL OF NURSES CODE OF ETHICS

According to the International Council of Nurses, the fundamental responsibility of the nurse is four-fold: to promote health, to prevent illness, to restore health, and to alleviate suffering.

The International Council of Nurses further states that inherent in nursing is respect for life, dignity, and human rights and that nursing is unrestricted by considerations of nationality, race, creed, color, age, sex, politics, or social status. The key points of the code appear below.

NURSES AND PEOPLE
▶ The nurse's primary responsibility is to those who require nursing care.
▶ The nurse, in providing care, respects the beliefs, values, and customs of the individual.
▶ The nurse holds in confidence personal information and uses judgment in sharing this information.

NURSES AND PRACTICE
▶ The nurse carries personal responsibility for nursing practice and for maintaining competence by continual learning.
▶ The nurse maintains the highest standards of nursing care possible within the reality of a specific situation.

▶ The nurse uses judgment in relation to individual competence when accepting and delegating responsibilities.
▶ The nurse, when acting in a professional capacity, should at all times maintain standards of personal conduct that would reflect credit upon the profession.

NURSES AND SOCIETY
▶ The nurse shares with other citizens the responsibility for initiating and supporting action to meet the health and social needs of the public.

NURSES AND COWORKERS
▶ The nurse sustains a cooperative relationship with coworkers in nursing and other fields.
▶ The nurse takes appropriate action to safeguard the individual when his care is endangered by a coworker or any other person.

NURSES AND THE PROFESSION
▶ The nurse plays a major role in determining and implementing desirable standards of nursing practice and nursing education.
▶ The nurse is active in developing a core of professional knowledge.
▶ The nurse, acting through the professional organization, participates in establishing and maintaining equitable social and economic working conditions in nursing.

---

multidisciplinary representation. Nurses serve on these committees and can present ethical dilemmas to the committees.

Your facility should have adopted policies to implement The Joint Commission and state statutes regarding bioethical dilemmas. These policies can serve as guidelines that outline documentation needs. One significant document, a written statement of a patient's rights, should be delivered to every patient on admission.

Other bioethical issues involving documentation include:
▶ informed consent (including witnessing informed consent and informed refusal)
▶ advance directives (living wills and health care proxy)
▶ durable power of attorney
▶ do-not-resuscitate orders
▶ withdrawal of treatment
▶ confidentiality of the medical record.

Informed consent

Required before most treatments and procedures, *informed consent* means that the patient understands the proposed therapy and its risks and agrees to undergo it by signing a consent form. The practitioner who will perform the procedure is legally responsible for obtaining the patient's informed consent. Know the policy at your facility. In some situations, the practitioner may verbally explain the procedure, risks, and complications and delegate the duty to a nurse who may confirm information with the patient and, if there are no questions, obtain the actual signature of the patient on the consent form. However, the responsibility remains with the physician or practitioner. Depending on your facility's policy, you may be asked to witness the patient's signature.

LEGAL REQUIREMENTS

For informed consent to be legally binding, the patient must be mentally competent and the practitioner must:

▶ explain the patient's diagnosis as well as the nature, purpose, and likelihood of success of the treatment or procedure

▶ describe the risks and benefits associated with the treatment or procedure

▶ explain the possible consequences of not undergoing the treatment or procedure

▶ describe alternative treatments and procedures

▶ inform the patient that he has the right to refuse the treatment or procedure without having other care or support withdrawn; this includes withdrawing his consent after giving it

▶ identify who will perform the procedure

▶ identify who is responsible for the patient's care

▶ obtain consent without coercing the patient.

Informed consent has two elements: the information and the consent. To be *informed,* the patient must be provided with a description of the treatment or procedure, the name and qualifications of the person who will perform it, and an explanation of risks and alternatives—all in language the patient can understand. Based on this, the patient may *consent* to the treatment or procedure.

The Joint Commission mandates the elements of informed consent. In addition, most states have statutes that set out specific elements of informed consent. In a few states, the practitioner can explain the procedure and simply ask whether the patient has any questions. If the patient has none, the practitioner isn't obligated by state law to discuss alternatives and risks unless the patient requests the information. Although this policy is inconsistent with The Joint Commission guidelines, keep in mind that those guidelines aren't the law; they're a set of requirements for licensure and accreditation.

In life-threatening emergencies, informed consent may not be required. In such cases, the law assumes that every individual wants to live and allows the practitioner to intervene to save life without obtaining consent.

In many cases, a patient may attempt to clarify issues with a nurse after giving the practitioner his informed consent. If you're questioned in this way, be aware that you aren't obligated to answer the patient's questions; however, if you do, be careful to document your answers. You should also notify the practitioner and document that you have done so, including the date and time.

WITNESSING INFORMED CONSENT

When you witness the patient signing an informed consent document, you're *not* witnessing that he received or understood the information. You're simply witnessing that the person who signed the consent form is in fact the person he says he is. For this, verify the patient's identity using two patient identifiers. You don't need to be present when the practitioner gives the information because you're only witnessing that the patient is signing the document, not that the information was given. If the patient can't read the consent form, read it to him before he signs.

Before a procedure is performed, make sure the patient's record contains a signed informed consent form. (See *Informed consent,* page 34.) If the patient appears to be concerned about the procedure or the practitioner's explanation of it, notify your supervisor or the practitioner, and chart that you've done this. If the patient wants to change his mind, contact the practitioner as soon as possible, and chart the patient's comments, the date and time you contacted the practitioner, and the practitioner's response.

INFORMED REFUSAL
Just as the patient has a right to consent to medical treatment based on relevant information, he also has the right to refuse treatment based on knowledge of the outcomes and risks. The Joint Commission requires (and federal statutes mandate) that health care facilities (both acute and long-term care) inform patients soon after admission about their treatment options.

Discuss the patient's wishes with him, and document the discussion for use later, in case the patient becomes unable to participate in decision making. With a few exceptions, a *competent* patient has the right to refuse mechanical ventilation, tube feedings, antibiotics, fluids, and other treatments that will clearly result in his death if they're withheld.

Legal competence differs from the medical or psychiatric concept of competence. The law presumes all individuals to be competent unless deemed otherwise through a court proceeding. The patient must also have *capacity*—that is,

have mental skills, such as memory, logic, the ability to calculate, and make decisions for consent purposes under state law.

Some health care facilities have informed refusal forms. It's important to chart in the medical record progress notes the details about the information given (including the risks and consequences associated with his decision) and that the patient refused the treatment. (See *Witnessing refusal of treatment,* page 35.)

Exceptions to the right to informed refusal may include pregnant women (because the life of the unborn child is at risk) and parents' wishes to withhold treatment for their child.

Advance directives
The U.S. Constitution and case law have established that a patient has the right to determine what happens to his body. The Joint Commission mandates that patients have the right to participate in decisions regarding their care and that health care facilities have a policy or procedure in place addressing how they'll implement the requirement. The Joint Commission also requires that a facility address forgoing or withdrawing life-sustaining treatment and withholding resuscitative services and care at the end of life.

An *advance directive* is a document that allows the patient to decide—before he is incapacitated—the type of care he'll be given at the end of his life. The directive may be in the form of a living will or a durable power of attorney for healthcare. The directive becomes effective only when the patient becomes incapacitated. It may be written or oral, but to comply with most state statutes, it must be written. Some states have their own advance directive forms available for use.

Some patients and health care providers have hesitated to accept the concept of advance

ChartWizard

Informed consent

If the patient signs a consent form, this implies that he understands the risks of a procedure and agrees to undergo it. Here's a typical form.

CONSENT FOR OPERATION AND RENDERING OF OTHER MEDICAL SERVICES

1. I hereby authorize Dr. _____Wesley_____ to perform upon _____Joseph Smith_____ (Patient name), the following surgical and/or medical procedures: (State specific nature of the procedures to be performed)
   _____Exploratory laparotomy_____

2. I understand that the procedure(s) will be performed at Valley Medical Center by or under the supervision of Dr. _____Wesley_____, who is authorized to utilize the services of other physicians, or members of the house staff as he or she deems necessary or advisable.

3. It has been explained to me that during the course of the operation, unforeseen conditions may be revealed that necessitate an extension of the original procedure(s) or different procedure(s) than those set forth in Paragraph 1; I therefore authorize and request that the above named physician, and his or her associates or assistants, perform such medical surgical procedures as are necessary and desirable in the exercise of professional judgment.

4. I understand the nature and purpose of the procedure(s), possible alternative methods of diagnosis or treatment, the risks involved, the possibility of complications, and the consequences of the procedure(s). I acknowledge that no guarantee or assurance has been made as to the results that may be obtained.

5. I authorize the above named physician to administer local or regional anesthesia (for all other anesthesia management a separate consent must be signed by the patient or patient's authorized representative).

6. I understand that if it is necessary for me to receive a blood transfusion during this procedure or this hospitalization, the blood will be supplied by sources available to the hospital and tested in accordance with national and regional regulations. I understand that there are risks in transfusion, including but not limited to allergic, febrile, and hemolytic transfusion reactions, and the transmission of infectious diseases, such as hepatitis and AIDS (Acquired Immune Deficiency Syndrome). I hereby consent to blood transfusion(s) and blood derivative(s).

7. I hereby authorize representatives from Valley to photograph or videotape me for the purpose of research or medical education. It is understood and agreed that patient confidentiality shall be preserved.

8. I authorize the physician named above and his or her associates and assistants and Valley Medical Center to preserve for scientific purposes or to dispose of any tissue, organs, or other body parts removed during surgery or other diagnostic procedures in accordance with customary medical practice.

9. I certify that I have read and fully understand the above consent statement. In addition, I have been afforded an opportunity to ask whatever questions I might have regarding the procedure(s) to be performed, and they have been answered to my satisfaction.

_____Joseph Smith_____   _____02/21/01_____   _____C. Gurney, RN_____
Legal Patient or Authorized Representative   Date   Witness
(State Relationship to Patient)

If the patient is unable to consent on his or her own behalf, complete the following:

Patient _____ is unable to consent because _____

Legally Responsible Person _____   Physician Obtaining Consent _____M. Wesley, MD_____

ChartWizard

Witnessing refusal of treatment

If a patient refuses treatment, the physician must first explain the risks and consequences involved in making this choice. Then the physician asks the patient to sign a refusal-of-treatment release form, such as the one below, which you may be asked to sign as a witness. Your signature only validates the identity of the patient signing the form—not that the patient received sufficient information or understood that infor-

---

REFUSAL-OF-TREATMENT RELEASE FORM

I, _____*Brenda Lyndstrom*_____ refuse to allow anyone to
       (patient's name)

_____*administer parenteral nutrition*_____
      (insert treatment)

The risks attendant to my refusal have been fully explained to me, and I fully understand the benefits of this treatment. I also understand that my refusal of treatment seriously reduces my chances for regaining normal health and may endanger my life.

I hereby release _____*Mercy General,*_____
       (name of hospital)

its nurses and employees, together with all physicians in any way connected with me as a patient, from liability for respecting and following my express wishes and direction.

_____*Susan Reynolds, RN*_____   _____*Brenda Lyndstrom*_____
    (witness's signature)   (patient's or legal guardian's signature)

_____*04/12/07*_____   _____*76*_____
    (date)   (patient's age)

---

directives, fearing that the patient won't be allowed to change his mind later. It's important to remember that an advance directive *can* be revoked. If a competent patient enters the hospital in a terminally ill state and decides that he wants all possible life-prolonging measures to be applied despite an existing advance directive to the contrary, his oral declaration that the advance directive be ignored effectively revokes the document. The patient's current wishes must be documented in the medical record.

Some state statutes have guidelines for revoking a directive, but the patient's oral wishes will suffice until those requirements can be met. If the patient signs a new advance directive, the previous advance directive is revoked.

If an advance directive is in effect and the nurse or other health care provider fails to honor it, any subsequent care provided may be considered unconsented touching, assault and battery, negligence, or intentional infliction of emotional, physical, and financial distress and, as such,

ChartWizard

Advance directive checklist

The Joint Commission requires that information on advance directives be charted on the admission assessment form. However, many facilities also use a checklist like the one below.

ADVANCE DIRECTIVE CHECKLIST

I. DISTRIBUTION OF ADVANCE DIRECTIVE INFORMATION

A. Advance directive information was presented to the patient: . . . . ☑

   1. At the time of preadmission testing. . . . . ☑

   2. Upon inpatient admission . . . . ☐

   3. Interpretive services contacted . . . . ☐

   4. Information was read to the patient . . . . ☐

B. Advance directive information was presented to the next of kin as
the patient is incapacitated . . . . ☐

C. Advance directive information was not distributed as the patient is
incapacitated and no relative or next of kin was available . . . . ☐

Mary Barren, RN	_04/10/07_
RN	**DATE**

	Upon admission		Upon transfer to Intensive Care Unit	
II. ASSESSMENT OF ADVANCE DIRECTIVE UPON ADMISSION	**YES**	**NO**	**YES**	**NO**
A. Does the patient have an advance directive?	☐	☑	☐	☐
If yes, was the attending physician notified?	☐		☐	
B. If no advance directive, does the patient want to execute an advance directive?	☑	☐	☐	☐
If yes, was the attending physician notified?	☑		☐	
Was the patient referred to resources?	☑		☐	
	Mary Barren, RN			
	RN		**RN**	
	_04/10/01_			
	DATE		**DATE**	

III. RECEIPT OF AN ADVANCE DIRECTIVE AFTER ADMISSION

A. The patient has presented an advance directive after admission
and the attending physician has been notified.

RN	**DATE**

grounds for a malpractice suit. Also, the patient has the right to change advance directives at any time. Because the patient's request may differ from what the family or practitioner wants, document discrepancies carefully. Use social services or the legal department for advice on how to proceed. (See *Advance directive checklist.*)

PATIENT SELF-DETERMINATION ACT

The Patient Self-Determination Act of 1990 allows patients to use advance directives and to appoint a surrogate to make decisions if the patient loses the ability to do so. This act mandates that on admission, each patient be informed of his right to create an advance directive. The fact that the patient has been offered this information must be documented in the medical record. If the patient elects to create an advance directive, this document must be placed in the medical record and honored.

Power of attorney

An advance directive can designate a friend or family member to whom the patient has given *power of attorney.* Power of attorney is a legal document in which a competent person designates another to act or conduct legally binding transactions (such as writing checks or signing legal documents) on his behalf. This power may encompass all of a person's affairs, including health and financial matters, or it may be limited to one specific area. If the power of attorney covers health matters, it allows the designated person to express an opinion and make decisions about the kind of health care the patient would want.

A power of attorney ceases if the patient becomes incompetent or revokes the document, unless he has executed a durable power of attorney.

A *durable power of attorney* is a legal document in which a competent person designates another person to act on his behalf if he should become incapable of managing his own affairs. Some states have created a durable power of attorney specifically for health care. This document ensures that the patient's wishes regarding treatment will be carried out if he should ever become incompetent or unable to make decisions because of illness.

A copy of the written power of attorney should be placed in a conspicuous place in the patient record. As with advance directives, failure to honor the power of attorney can result in litigation.

Do-not-resuscitate orders

The physician writes a do-not-resuscitate (DNR) order when it's medically indicated—that is, when a patient is terminally ill and expected to die. In spite of the patient's autonomy and the requirement to honor the patient's wishes, the patient can't mandate that a facility provide futile treatment. Thus, a DNR order may be written regardless of the advance directive, but ideally, this decision should be thoroughly discussed with the patient or his legal surrogate. DNR orders should be reviewed as policy dictates or whenever a significant change occurs in the patient's clinical status.

Some facilities temporarily suspend DNR orders during surgery. Although the patient and physician aren't seeking heroic measures at the end of life, the physician won't allow the patient to bleed to death if he should hemorrhage during a palliative surgical procedure. Another exception is the concept of partial or "à la carte" resuscitation codes. These are legally precarious since the standard of care is to attempt full resuscitation through all means available, not partial resuscitation.

The patient's family members or friends don't have the legal authority to write an advance directive or to advise the physician regarding a DNR order unless they have a legal power of attorney or durable power of attorney. The patient is presumed to be competent and has the sole right to state what care he wishes, unless that care isn't indicated from a medical standpoint.

Withdrawal of treatment

Although health care facilities aren't required to provide medically futile treatment, they are reluctant to withdraw futile treatment unless the patient (or the patient's immediate family, if the patient isn't legally competent) agrees. Bioethics committees at academic medical centers are struggling to find an ethical and practical way to approach withdrawal of medically futile and costly treatment without inviting an even more costly lawsuit brought by a dissenting family member. Whether treatment is withdrawn because of medical futility or the patient's wishes, as expressed through an advance directive or a legal surrogate, it's important to document the patient's condition and prognosis.

Confidentiality

One of your documentation responsibilities includes protecting the confidentiality of the patient's medical record and related health care information. You can't reveal confidential information without the patient's permission. The Health Insurance Portability and Accountability Act (HIPAA) was signed into law in 1996. The law was passed not only to protect the privacy of patients but to also provide greater access to health care insurance and promote standardization and efficiency in health care. Most clinical entities had until April 14, 2003, to fully comply with privacy regulations. (See *Patient rights under HIPAA*.)

Besides your legal responsibilities, you also have professional and ethical responsibilities (as specified by the ANA, The Joint Commission, and other professional bodies in their codes and standards) to protect your patient's privacy.

THE NURSE'S ROLE

Nurses assume a primary role in maintaining confidentiality and in safeguarding the privacy of medical records. Breaches in confidentiality can result from unintentional release of information, unauthorized entry into a patient's record, or even a casual conversation that's overheard by others. In fact, breaches of patient confidentiality on the part of nursing staff are more likely to occur through inadvertent conversations in cafeterias and elevators than through a specific request for a patient's chart. The best way to prevent such breaches is to avoid discussing patient concerns in areas where you can be overheard.

Most requests for copies of the medical record will go through the medical records department rather than through nursing staff. However, if you're asked for a copy of the record or an opportunity to view it, don't release the record without the documented consent of a competent patient. Increasing use of computers for documentation creates a new avenue for unauthorized release of patient information. (See chapter 13, Electronic Patient Records.)

All patient information is confidential, even information that may seem innocent. The release of certain information—for example, mental health records as well as information about drug and alcohol abuse and infectious diseases—is further constrained by state statutes.

In the case of *Anonymous v. Chino Valley Medical Center,* San Bernardino County, California Superior Court (1997), a 35-year-old disabled inpatient underwent a blood test for human immunodeficiency virus (HIV). He specifically told the physician that he didn't want the results to be given to anyone but him. On

Patient rights under HIPAA

The goal of the Health Insurance Portability and Accountability Act (HIPAA) is to provide safeguards against the inappropriate use and release of personal medical information, including all medical records and identifiable health information in any form (electronic, on paper, or oral).

Patients are the beneficiaries of this privacy rule, which includes the following six rights:

▶ the right to give consent before information is released for treatment, payment, or health care operations
▶ the right to be educated to the provider's policy on privacy protection
▶ the right to access their medical records
▶ the right to request that their medical records be amended for accuracy
▶ the right to access the history of nonroutine disclosures (those disclosures that didn't occur in the course of treatment, payment, or health care operations, or those not specifically authorized by the patient)
▶ the right to request that the provider restrict the use and routine disclosure of information he has (providers aren't required to grant this request, especially if they think the information is important to the quality of care for the patient, such as disclosing HIV status to another medical provider who is providing treatment).

ENFORCEMENT OF HIPAA
Enforcement of HIPAA regulation resides with the United States Department of Health and Human Services (HHS) and is based primarily on significant financial fines. HHS can impose civil penalties up to $25,000 a year per plan for unintentional violations. With hundreds of requirements,

fines could quickly add up. Criminal penalties can also be imposed for intentional violations, including fines up to $250,000, 10 years of imprisonment, or both.

IMPACT ON NURSING PRACTICE
Keep in mind that HIPAA regulations aren't intended to prohibit health care providers from talking to one another or to patients. Instead, they exist to help protect the information communicated. The regulations require organizations to make "reasonable" accommodations to protect patient privacy and to employ "reasonable" safeguards to prevent inappropriate disclosure. Changes in nursing practice have been made to meet these reasonable accommodations and safeguards.

Employers must provide education to nurses regarding the policies and procedures to be followed at their individual institutions. Nurses should be aware of how infractions will be handled because they, as well as the institution, face penalties for violations. Some safeguards nurses can enact in their everyday practice include:

▶ ensuring that computer passwords are protected
▶ making sure computer screens aren't in public view
▶ keeping patient charts closed when not in use
▶ immediately filing loose patient records
▶ not leaving faxes and computer printouts unattended
▶ properly disposing of unneeded patient information in accordance with the facility's procedure
▶ ensuring that conversations among health care providers aren't overheard.

---

the day of discharge, his sister was present in the hospital room. A nurse asked the sister to come into the hall, so she could tell her about the patient's diet instructions upon discharge. When in the hallway, the nurse told the sister that the patient had a positive HIV test. A few moments later, the physician approached them

and also conveyed the test results. No action was filed against the physician. The nurse denied releasing the information. A trial court imposed a $5,000 statutory civil penalty against the medical center.

In the case of *Hobbs v. Lopes*, 645 N.E.2d 1261, Ohio App. 4 DST. (1994), a 21-year-old

Ohio woman was found to be pregnant after consulting a physician for another medical problem. Options, including abortion, were discussed. The physician instructed a nurse to call the woman to find out which option she had chosen. The nurse called the woman's parents' home and disclosed the fact that their daughter was pregnant and had sought advice about an abortion. The daughter sued for medical malpractice, invasion of privacy, breach of privilege, and infliction of emotional distress.

Both of these cases underscore the importance of documenting the patient's consent or nonconsent to release of information. The patient's consent to release information should be on an official facility form. This form is handled not by the nurse but by the medical records department or hospital attorney.

Keep in mind that the law requires you to disclose confidential information in certain situations—for example, in instances of alleged child abuse, matters of public health and safety, and criminal cases.

RIGHT TO INFORMATION

As stated earlier, the patient has the right to the information in his medical record. Although the facility owns the actual record, the patient has a legal right to a copy of his chart, X-rays, and other reports. Many state statutes grant patients an express right to access the medical record. In the absence of a statute, some states have recognized the facility's duty to allow the patient at least limited access to the medical record. Release of psychiatric records, records of minors, records with adoptive parent information, and records addressing drug and alcohol treatment or communicable diseases may be covered by special state statutes.

Patients treated in federal facilities also have the right of access to their medical records, as mandated by the Freedom of Information Act of 1966 and the Privacy Act of 1974. Some states have freedom of information acts called public records or open records laws. Third-party access to medical records is controlled by these and other statutes dealing with criminal law, domestic abuse, and third-party payer or Medicare claims.

Selected references

"2005 JONA's Healthcare, Law, Ethics, and Regulation," *LWW* 7(3):2-10, July/Sept. 2005.

Austin, S. "Ladies & Gentlemen of theJury, I Present...the Nursing Documentation," *Nursing* 36(1):57-62, January 2006.

Bofinger, R., and Rizk, K. "Point System Versus Legal System: An Innovative Approach to Clinical Evaluation," *Nurse Educator* 31(2):69-73, March 2006.

Cheevakasemsook, A., et al. "The Study of Nursing Documentation Complexities," *International Journal of Nursing Practice* 12(6):366-74, December 2006.

Ewancuk, M. and Brindley, P.G. "Perioperative do-not-resuscitate Orders—Doing 'nothing' When Something Can Be Done," *Critical Care* 10(4):219, 2006.

Karkkainen, O., and Eriksson, K. "A Theoretical Approach to Documentation of Care," *Nursing Science Quarterly* 17(3):268-72, July 2004.

Langowski, C. "The Times They Are A-Changing: Effects of Online Nursing Documentation Systems," *Quality Management Healthcare* 14(2):121-125, April-June 2005.

Murphy, E.K. "Charting by Exception," *AORN Journal* 78(5):821-3, November 2003.

Salyer, R. "Improving Medical/Surgical Practice With JCAHO's 2005 National Patient Safety Goals," *Nursing* Suppl:12-13, Fall 2005.

PERFORMANCE IMPROVEMENT AND REIMBURSEMENT

3

The impact of nursing documentation in reflecting the quality of patient care, meeting regulatory standards, and criteria for reimbursement for patient care extends throughout—and beyond—the patient's stay in a health care facility. What makes this documentation so important? Nursing documentation constitutes a major part of the medical record and serves as a means of communication for the health care team. It helps prove or disprove that a health care facility provides acceptable care, meets standards, and qualifies for reimbursement. This means that the various parties interested in quality health care, reimbursement standards, and legal practices will review a great deal of nursing documentation.

QUALITY WATCHDOGS

Who are these parties? Typically, they include representatives of The Joint Commission, Centers for Medicare and Medicaid Services (CMS), U.S. Department of Health and Human Services (HSS), peer review organizations (PROs), performance improvement committees, and others, such as those involved in assigning patients to appropriate diagnostic groups and meeting legal requirements. These parties are directly charged with improving quality and justifying government and insurance company disbursements for health care.

To accomplish their mission, they scrutinize medical records to evaluate care that they can't observe firsthand. Because what you document or don't document either supports or challenges the quality standards and appropriateness of care, your notes directly affect your health care facility's accreditation, financial reimbursement, and legal security.

Comparing Medicare and Medicaid

Medicare and Medicaid were established in 1966 under the Social Security Act. As the following table shows, the two organizations differ in their reimbursement policies, regulations, and documentation guidelines.

MEDICARE	MEDICAID
Federal health insurance benefits program for persons over age 65. Part A covers skilled nursing home and hospital care; Part B covers care by physicians, hospital equipment, and supplies.	Combined state and federal insurance and medical assistance plan for qualified needy individuals of any age; it encourages home care as an alternative to institutional care.
Benefits are uniform for eligible recipients nationwide.	Benefits differ from state to state.
The program pays for skilled medical and nursing care only.	The program pays for home nursing care (not necessarily skilled care).
Patients must be confined to their homes to receive reimbursement for part-time or intermittent skilled nursing care.	Patients aren't required to be confined to their homes.
Documentation is required to support the need for skilled medical and nursing care and its delivery.	Documentation is required to ensure payment, but the required content varies according to setting.
The program doesn't pay for custodial care.	The program pays for custodial care in specified care settings.
A physician order initiates service.	The patient's qualifying need initiates service.

Documentation and performance improvement

The Joint Commission, PROs, case managers, performance improvement committees, and the National Committee for Quality Assurance (NCQA) are just a few of the groups that will periodically evaluate your facility's quality of care and service and overall nursing competence. (For information on the NCQA, see chapter 8, Documentation in Home Health Care.)

The Joint Commission quality standards

The Joint Commission surveys U.S. health care facilities to make sure that they meet its standards as accredited health care providers. Health care facilities agree to these surveys to show that they provide high-quality, safe health care. They also seek The Joint Commission accreditation to qualify for government and insurance agency reimbursement and other funding. These agencies require health care facilities to hold The Joint Commission accreditation before they're eligible to receive Medicare, Medicaid, or private funds. (See *Comparing Medicare and Medicaid.*)

Besides requiring that documentation show a facility's measurable overall quality care and service, The Joint Commission insists that the documentation meet certain quality standards. In 2006, The Joint Commission began evaluating medical record documentation during the observation and interview process of the survey. If a deficiency is found, closed patient records are formally evaluated. Reviewers also examine personnel records, such as clinical nurse competence evaluations, nursing licenses and credentials, and nursing assignments.

Because The Joint Commission depends on nursing documentation to evaluate patient care, what and how you document is crucial to the accreditation process. To be accredited by The Joint Commission, a health care facility must have an organized, systematic, and ongoing method for documenting quality. Documentation must consistently meet Joint Commission standards because facilities are no longer notified about when the survey will take place. (See *Documenting to reflect Joint Commission standards,* page 44.)

Performance improvement

The Joint Commission defines performance improvement as a continuous process that measures the functioning of important processes or services. If issues or potential problems are identified, the organization must identify changes that enhance performance. To make sure that the changes to process, product, or services are incorporated, performance is monitored. The facility's leadership must establish a planned, systematic, organization-wide approach to their performance improvement activities. They set priorities, provide resources, and ensure collaboration among all disciplines. To improve performance, the health care organization must evaluate adverse outcomes to reduce system failures. Therefore, performance activities are part of all nurses' daily activities, ensuring high-quality patient care.

The Joint Commission requires use of a performance model to make sure the health care facility establishes a performance improvement program. Many such models are available. The Joint Commission doesn't currently recommend a specific one, but facility employees are expected to identify key performance activities for their specific work area. (See *Models for ensuring performance improvement,* page 45.)

Data are crucial to improvement efforts. The organization must identify national standards or benchmarks to compare the facility's level of performance. The Joint Commission requires that data be converted to information, which is shared throughout the organization. The facility needs to analyze its care by evaluating specific indicators or outcomes over time. (See *Transforming data into information,* page 46.)

Although an organization will choose most indicators for performance monitoring based on its mission and priorities, The Joint Commission requires all hospitals to collect data for specific high-risk processes: medication management, blood and blood product use, restraint use, seclusion use, behavior management and treatment, operative and invasive procedures, and resuscitation and its outcomes. Nurses must provide documentation any time they are involved in one of these high-risk processes, many of which are addressed in the National Patient Safety Goals. Compliance with these standards is evaluated during the survey process. It's important for nurses to understand that appropriate

Smarter charting

Documenting to reflect Joint Commission standards

When representatives of The Joint Commission review medical records, they look for indications that the health care facility provides quality care. Of particular interest is your documentation. As you document care, keep in mind that your documentation can prove beneficial or detrimental to your facility during Joint Commission surveys. Here are steps you can take to make sure you follow The Joint Commission standards when documenting patient care.

JOINT COMMISSION STANDARD	NURSING IMPLICATIONS
The hospital must have a complete and accurate medical record for the patient assessed, cared for, treated, or served.	▶ Date, time, and sign all notes; include your licensure with your signature. ▶ Make sure your notes reflect the care you gave and the patient response as well as the results of treatments, care, or services. ▶ Complete documentation within time frames identified in your facility's policy. ▶ Make sure your notes are legible, complete, and accurate.
The patient's medical record must contain patient-specific information that is appropriate to his care, treatment, and services.	▶ Complete and document your nursing assessment within the time frame specified in your facility policy. ▶ Make sure all orders are documented. ▶ Document medication administration including the dose, rate of administration, site and route of administration, and any devices used to administer the drug. ▶ Record allergies and adverse reactions; include treatment interventions and the patient's response to treatment.
The medical record contains documentation about operations, other high-risk procedures, and the use of moderate sedation, deep sedation, or anesthesia.	▶ Record postoperative vital signs, level of consciousness, and the administration of blood products, I.V. fluids, and medications. ▶ Document any complications, treatment interventions, and the patient's response. ▶ Use approved discharge criteria, and make sure documentation reflects the patient's readiness for discharge.
Only qualified personnel accept and transcribe verbal orders from authorized practitioners.	▶ Follow hospital policies that identify who is qualified to give and take verbal or telephone orders. ▶ Date, time, and identify the person giving you the verbal or telephone order. ▶ Verify the complete verbal or telephone order by reading back the complete order to the person who gave it to you. ▶ Record who implemented the telephone or verbal order. ▶ Verify a critical test result by reading back the test result to the person who gave it to you.
The hospital provides access to all relevant patient information as needed for patient care, treatment, and services.	▶ Make sure the medical record is organized according to facility policy, so other health care providers have access to required information. ▶ Help ensure the location of all portions of the medical record.

Models for ensuring performance improvement

A number of models have been developed to continuously evaluate and document the performance improvement process. The models listed below use mnemonics to show the steps in the process.

PDCA CYCLE
(Developed by Walter A. Shewart in the 1930s)
- ▶ **P**lan: Study a process by collecting data and evaluating results.
- ▶ **D**o: Carry out the plan on a small-scale pilot.
- ▶ **C**heck: Check results of the change. (Some now use "S" for "study.")
- ▶ **A**ct: Implement the change or abandon the plan and go through the cycle again.

FOCUS
(Developed by Hospital Corporation of America)
- ▶ **F**ind a process to improve.
- ▶ **O**rganize a team that knows the process.
- ▶ **C**larify current knowledge.
- ▶ **U**nderstand variation.
- ▶ **S**elect a potential process improvement.

FADE
(Developed by Organizational Dynamics, Inc.)
- ▶ **F**ocus: Narrow a list of problems to one.
- ▶ **A**nalyze: Collect data and determine influential factors.
- ▶ **D**evelop: Formulate a plan to solve the problem.
- ▶ **E**xecute: Gain an organizational commitment, put the plan into action, and monitor the effect.

IMPROVE
(Developed by Ernst and Young)
- ▶ **I**dentify and define the problem.
- ▶ **M**easure the impact on customers.
- ▶ **P**rioritize possible causes.
- ▶ **R**esearch and analyze root causes.
- ▶ **O**utline alternative solutions.
- ▶ **V**alidate that solutions will work.
- ▶ **E**xecute solutions and standardize.

documentation will support the facility's accreditation; incomplete or inaccurate documentation may put the facility's accreditation status in jeopardy.

PERFORMANCE IMPROVEMENT TEAM EFFORTS
One way an organization monitors and evaluates the quality and appropriateness of patient care is through performance improvement teams. Typically, such teams are convened to evaluate a specific issue, process, or event to improve patient outcomes. The team's functions are to evaluate processes and data and to recommend and implement changes. The team will identify and implement a monitoring process to make sure

that the changes improve outcomes. (See *Performance improvement activities report,* page 47.)

The types of data may include cost and length of stay information; patient outcomes, such as mortality rates, infection rates, or readmission rates; and chart abstraction of documented care or direct observation of a process or procedure.

Nurses at all levels in a facility may participate in these teams. The nurse may represent the expert-care provider or the "first-line" provider of an activity or process. She may assist in data collection, clarify current processes, or offer solutions to problematic situations. The nurse may be the administrative leader, driving change or providing resources to make sure that the

Transforming data into information

The Joint Commission requires that data be analyzed using appropriate statistical techniques. These data and their analysis should lead the organization to drive performance improvement processes leading to process change. Changes in data should indicate effectiveness of the process change.

COLLECTED DATA

	Jan-05	Feb-05	Mar-05	Apr-05	May-05	Jun-05	Jul-05	Aug-05	Sept-05
Length of stay in days	8.1	8.4	7.1	9.3	8.6	6.8	9.5	6.7	7.1

	Oct-05	Nov-05	Dec-05	Jan-06	Feb-06	Mar-06	Apr-06	May-06	Jun-06	Jul-06
Length of stay in days	6.4	7.8	6.5	6.3	7	6.6	8	6.7	6.6	7

DATA CONVERTED INTO INFORMATION

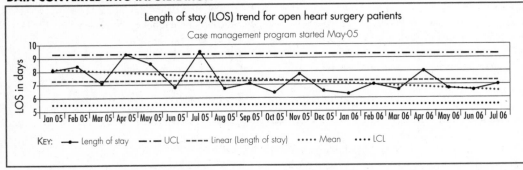

Length of stay (LOS) trend for open heart surgery patients

Case management program started May-05

KEY: —●— Length of stay   —·— UCL   ---- Linear (Length of stay)   ····· Mean   ···· LCL

team changes are implemented and evaluated. Any of these roles are activities within the performance improvement process.

Data collected during performance improvement activities can be used to assess a nurse's performance or competency and to support or eliminate services.

ORYX *initiative*

The ORYX initiative was implemented by The Joint Commission in 1995. The purpose was to use national standards to measure performance and the quality of care provided in hospitals. As the public became more concerned with health care reform, many other organizations began to evaluate hospitals using similar standards. The PROs assumed more performance measurement responsibilities as the monitoring body for the Centers for Medicare and Medicaid Services (CMS). Hospitals had to report data abstracted from medical records to The Joint Commission, the PROs, and individual state governments and departments of health. These data are available

ChartWizard

Performance improvement activities report

You can use different tools to help gather and report performance improvement activities. The form below uses the PDCA cycle model to guide the activity.

CLINICAL DEPARTMENT: *Telemetry unit*
DEPARTMENT: *Patient Care Services*
COMMITTEE: *Performance Improvement Council*
DATE: *November 2006*

Topic and description	*Compliance and completeness of discharge instruction documentation for patients with heart failure.*
Plan	*Data shows low rates for discharge instruction compliance and completeness of discharge instruction in 2004 and 2005 for patients with heart failure.*
Do	*1. Outcomes manager began a chart review—first quarter 2006* *2. Provided staff education about standard discharge instruction documentation—first quarter 2006* *3. Provided education to agency and per diem staff about standard discharge instruction documentation—first quarter 2006* *4. Revised patient-education booklets to include heart failure discharge instructions—third quarter 2006* *5. Provided a bulletin-board display with education included in discharge teaching—second quarter 2006* *6. Review of patient-education documentation completed by nurse-manager and staff members—second quarter 2006.*
Check	*Results show a significant improvement in completeness of discharge instruction documentation for patients with heart failure.*
Act	*1. Evaluate overall documentation of patient education in electronic medical record* *2. Continue to develop additional discharge instruction forms based on patient populations* *3. Evaluate patient satisfaction scores related to heart-failure discharge teaching.*

to the public through the Internet, allowing them to compare quality among hospitals.

In January 2004, The Joint Commission started to require hospitals to monitor three core measure sets from the following five measures: acute myocardial infarction, heart failure, pneumonia, pregnancy and related conditions, and surgical infection prevention. During the survey process, the reviewers evaluate and compare the hospital's performance against national standards for providing care to patients in these groups and also evaluate the hospital's process to improve their results.

Although the core measures are based on physician and professional organization standards, nursing documentation can support and drive performance improvement in these areas. The Joint Commission and other quality organizations are continuing to revise the indicators and develop new measures. Future core measures could include pediatric asthma indicators, sepsis indicators, and prevention of ventilator-acquired pneumonia.

DOCUMENTATION MODELS

Several models exist to document performance improvement. (See *Models for ensuring performance improvement,* page 45.)

PRO *focus*

Developed to assist in the utilization review process, PROs consist of groups of physicians and nurses required by the federal government to monitor and evaluate the quality and appropriateness of care given. In carrying out this task, PROs rely heavily on documentation in the medical record.

PROs evaluate a sample of a health care facility's medical records. They compare the data

with specific screening criteria to assess the need for and appropriateness of medical services. Their screening criteria include basic standards or conditions that a comparable group of health care facilities can reasonably be expected to meet. In studying a sample of the medical records, the PROs focus on the intensity of services and the severity of illnesses. (For more information on PROs, see chapter 1, Nursing Documentation and the Medical Record.)

Because a PRO's primary focus is quality patient care carried out within cost-containment guidelines, the reviewers also scrutinize documented care as a means for determining reimbursements. (See *How PROs screen specialized care.*)

Case management focus

Case management is a threefold process that consists of identifying individuals with specific health care needs, formulating and implementing a plan that efficiently uses health care resources, and measuring patient outcomes along a continuum of care.

A case management system provides an additional way for health care facilities to improve quality and contain costs. Case managers help to coordinate a patient's long-term care by using resources throughout the community. One of their primary goals is to control costs. In the process, they influence both the type of health care services a patient receives and where he receives them.

Case management began as an offshoot of the Medicare and Medicaid waiver-demonstration projects, which made exceptions to usual federal Medicare and Medicaid eligibility requirements. The exceptions (or waivers) extended health care coverage to certain patients who

How PROs screen specialized care

When reviewing medical records, peer review organizations (PROs) use special screening criteria to evaluate the intensity of services and the severity of illness. These factors have a direct impact on Medicare and Medicaid reimbursement.

Being familiar with a PRO's criteria can help you document appropriately to demonstrate that patient care complies with Medicare and Medicaid standards. That, in turn, maximizes reimbursement.

Below are the monitoring, medication, and treatment screening criteria that a PRO looks for when verifying that care given in an alcohol or drug detoxification unit meets Medicare and Medicaid standards.

MONITORING CRITERIA

A patient in an alcohol or drug detoxification unit should be monitored every 1 to 2 hours. Monitoring must be appropriate, needed, and ordered.

The caregiver needs to monitor:
► vital signs (pulse and respiratory rates and blood pressure every 1 to 2 hours; temperature at least every 4 hours)
► level of consciousness
► orientation to time and place
► fluid intake and output
► pupillary reaction to light and pupil size
► potential or actual signs and symptoms of withdrawal.

MEDICATION CRITERIA

Reimbursable medications include:
► I.V. medications (excluding vitamins and potassium unless potassium replacement was ordered and administered for documented hypokalemia)
► oral or I.M. medications to control acute withdrawal signs and symptoms (including chlordiazepoxide, magnesium sulfate, and thiamine).

TREATMENT CRITERIA

Besides medication administration, treatment may include:
► I.V. therapy to replace or maintain the patient's fluid volume (the flow rate needs to exceed a keep-vein-open rate and be appropriate for the patient's body mass and condition)
► initial need, continuing need, or both, as documented by the physician, for inpatient detoxification to stabilize the patient's mental and physical condition.

could use community and nursing services at home. The intent was to prevent unnecessary nursing home admissions; the result is an expanded role for many nurses.

NURSES AS CASE MANAGERS

Case managers direct patient care to the most cost-effective health care setting while still meeting quality standards. Today's case manager must make sure that the patient's care and reimbursement for care are appropriate for his diagnosis or diagnosis-related group (DRG).

The case management system forces health care facilities to deliver care economically without compromising quality. If you become a case manager, your role will change from giving hands-on nursing care to coordinating cost-effective health care in various settings. You'll manage a closely monitored and controlled system of multidisciplinary care. You'll be responsible for outcomes, length of stay, and use of resources throughout the patient's illness—not just during your shift. And you'll become an expert at scrutinizing and interpreting nursing documentation. These records play a key role in the effect case managers have on a facility.

Case managers scrutinize the medical record—especially the nursing documentation—to determine whether a patient's continued hospital and other health care costs and treatment are justified.

Case management is one of the services listed under the Comprehensive Omnibus Budget Reconciliation Act (COBRA). This federal law permits states to apply for waivers and offer community services for patients eligible for nursing home care.

Outside of the health care facility, case managers may be in private practice or employed by home care agencies, family service agencies, hospitals, area agencies on aging, and health maintenance organizations (HMOs).

Quality improvement organizations' focus

Quality improvement organizations are focused on improving health care quality. These organizations, funded by the CMS, are based at the state level and work with The Joint Commission, Hospital Quality Alliance, and other organizations to coordinate quality improvement activities. The majority of the quality improvement activities are focused on the core measures. Health care facilities aren't required by the CMS to report data collected on the core measures, but those that don't report receive a reduced Medicare reimbursement. Therefore, many facilities voluntarily report their findings. In the future, CMS plans to give financial rewards to top-performing facilities. Therefore, quality improvement could greatly influence the financial status of the facility.

Fiscal implications of documentation

What the nurse documents in the medical record—and how she documents it—has a direct impact not only on the quality of patient care but also on the health care facility's revenues. The nurse's progress notes, flow sheets, care plans, and medication administration records are scrutinized by Medicare, Medicaid, and insurance company reviewers in addition to peer reviewers, case managers, caregiving staff, and others.

The quality of care, the patient outcomes, and the need for continued treatment are judged according to the documentation. For example, vital signs, level of consciousness, infusion rates, and administration of injectable medications are all parameters used to determine whether the patient should continue his stay in a health care facility. Failure to provide sufficient documentation may result in denial of reimbursement or transfer of the patient to an alternative health care setting. Unsatisfactory but avoidable outcomes may result in denial of payment.

Specific and complete nursing records are the key to ensuring financial reimbursement. Your records must be clear and concise. They must validate not only care and treatment but also the items that are billed. For example, a bill for 20 suction catheters used in a 24-hour period is unlikely to be paid if nursing documentation indicates that the patient was suctioned as needed during that time.

Reimbursement structures

Today's health care system includes multiple, complex structures with multiple, complex requirements for receiving reimbursement. Caregivers and health care facilities must deal not only with internal performance improvement teams, case managers, and required reimbursement structures (such as DRGs and COBRA requirements) but also with federal and state agencies, HMOs, preferred provider organizations (PPOs), and independent practice associations (IPAs), among others.

Reviewers from these groups examine the medical record for discrepancies. They look for differences in the treatment ordered and the treatment provided. If a discrepancy can't be explained satisfactorily or reconciled reasonably, payment may be denied.

DRGs

The basis for federal health care reimbursements, the DRG system groups diseases and disorders into specific categories. A DRG includes information about the principal and secondary diagnoses, surgical procedures, and the patient's age, sex, and discharge status.

When Medicare adopted a prospective payment system (PPS), reimbursement regulations changed. Before PPS, Medicare reimbursed a health care provider according to a cost-per-case formula. After PPS, Medicare computed reimbursements prospectively, using a formula adjusted for diagnostic groups, signs and symptoms, health care facility, region, wage levels, and other relevant factors—the DRG system.

Today, health care facilities must ensure meticulous compliance with DRG preadmission and continued-stay criteria to ensure reimbursement. Likewise, they must adhere to the details of the DRG coding process.

The medical record must contain documentation verifying the DRG and supporting the appropriateness of care given in the health care facility. What's more, nursing documentation needs to support the diagnoses and indicate that appropriate patient and family teaching and discharge planning were provided.

COBRA

The federal law known as COBRA allows employees to temporarily be covered under their employer's health insurance when they would otherwise lose this benefit because of terminated employment or another qualifying event, such as a reduction in work hours or retirement.

Precise documentation is essential when providing care for patients insured under COBRA. The law requires health care facilities receiving federal funds to evaluate any patients admitted to the emergency department. Specifically, it states that a patient's condition must be stable before he's transferred to another health care facility. If the patient is in labor, her labor must be controlled before she's transferred to another health care facility.

To make sure that health care facilities comply with the law, COBRA and The Joint Commission require that all facilities thoroughly document their actions concerning patient transfers. This documentation must include the chronology of the event, measures taken or treatment implemented, the patient's response to treatment, and the results of the measures taken to prevent the patient's condition from worsening.

HMOs

An HMO is an organized system that provides an agreed-upon set of comprehensive inpatient and outpatient health services to a voluntarily enrolled population in exchange for a predetermined, fixed, and periodic payment.

An HMO may contract for beds and services and may build or buy hospitals. Many HMOs feature physicians who work for a salary or in a partnership arrangement. Or, the HMO may contract for medical services from individual physicians and may function as either a profit-making or a nonprofit organization.

IPAs

Consisting of an independent group of physicians, an IPA offers services to a specified group of patients. Many HMOs contract with IPAs for medical services.

PPOs

A PPO contracts with health care providers, including hospitals, physicians, therapists, pharmacies, and other professional services. The contracted fees are typically lower than customary, with the understanding that PPOs will channel patients into empty hospital beds and underutilized services.

MEDICARE AND MEDICAID PAYMENTS

Payments by Medicare and Medicaid are sources of operating revenue for hospitals. Both have specific requirements for participation and reimbursement.

Initially, a state agency determines whether a health care facility is eligible to participate in the Medicare program. In doing so, the state agency certifies that the facility:

▶ holds The Joint Commission or American Osteopathic Association accreditation
▶ uses an adequate utilization review plan that is, or will be, in effect on the first day of the facility's participation
▶ meets statutory requirements or, if not, proposes reasonable plans to correct deficiencies and demonstrates evidence of adequate patient care despite any shortcomings.

Medicare certifies hospitals for a 2-year period. Certification guidelines can be used to evaluate the function of all facility services. Medicare and Medicaid also examine compliance with state and local laws and The Joint Commission standards. Health care facilities can use the steps for Medicare certification as preparation for Joint Commission accreditation.

How documentation affects costs

Nursing documentation provides the data that examiners need to justify reimbursement for health care expenses. Besides studying the records to estimate revenues, examiners use the records to calculate nursing care costs.

CALCULATING NURSING CARE COSTS

Traditionally, the cost of nursing care was included in the patient's daily room rate. Now, however, health care facilities are applying standard cost-accounting techniques to nursing care.

First, nurses estimate the number of nursing hours required to provide a quality patient outcome. Then financial management personnel estimate the cost of that nursing time. A major component in providing patient care, the cost of nursing care is directly related to the type and level of care provided. Health care facilities typically factor nursing care costs into the financial and strategic planning process.

Some facilities bill patients separately for nursing care, using pricing systems that charge only for care the patient actually receives. Determining the cost of nursing time requires detailed documentation so that appropriate charges can be billed and validated. Nursing documentation then becomes a detailed financial record.

SKILLED NURSING CARE
Provided by registered nurses or by licensed practical nurses under a registered nurse's supervision, skilled nursing care involves continual use of the nursing process, technologically complex monitoring, and patient teaching. It also includes planning, organizing, and managing the care plan with the physician and other health care professionals.

Skilled nursing care requires specialized education and the ability to document competently. It differs from custodial care, which focuses on assistance with activities of daily living, such as eating, dressing, bathing, and walking, and which may be provided by nonskilled personnel.

Examples of skilled nursing care activities include:
▶ managing central venous lines
▶ administering I.M., subcutaneous, or I.V. fluids or medications
▶ treating infected or extensive pressure ulcers
▶ administering oxygen
▶ providing nasopharyngeal suctioning
▶ managing enteral feedings
▶ changing sterile dressings.

How documentation affects revenues

Medicare Part A provides coverage for skilled nursing care; Part B, for durable medical equipment and supplies. Payment for services to patients insured by Medicare is based on their documented need for skilled nursing care and covers supplies and equipment used during that care.

Continued payment depends on *daily* documentation demonstrating the patient's ongoing need for skilled care. The quality of documentation in this area directly affects the amount of Medicare payments and other insurance reimbursements.

Documentation must confirm that the nursing staff meets various care standards, such as:
▶ adhering to the nursing process
▶ recording changes in the patient's condition and care needs in a timely manner
▶ using medical equipment (such as bedpans, nebulizers, indwelling catheters, and walkers) judiciously and appropriately to meet the patient's needs
▶ adequately teaching the patient about his condition and treatment plan.

Finally, examiners search the documentation carefully for any inconsistencies that may hinder reimbursement. (See *Avoiding inconsistent documentation,* page 54.)

IMPORTANCE OF THE NURSING PROCESS
The nursing process involves the problem solving and decision making that nurses do to provide patient care. It's a simple, systematic process made up of five steps: assessment, nursing diagnosis, planning, implementation, and evaluation. The steps are always sequential, and the process is cyclical. The completion of the fifth step returns you to the first step for reassessment. The nursing process stops when the patient is discharged.

Correctly used, the nursing process permeates every aspect of nursing documentation. Every patient event and assessment is recorded. The five-step process ensures compliance with care plan requirements mandated by both acute care and long-term care standards. (For more information, see chapter 5, Documentation of the Nursing Process.)

Avoiding inconsistent documentation

Inconsistencies in documentation leave both you and your health care facility open to accusations of incompetence and fiscal irresponsibility. What's more, a medical record containing inconsistencies can be difficult or impossible to defend in court. To avoid inconsistencies, follow these guidelines.

BE PRECISE
For example, describing the exact size and location of a pressure ulcer (such as "2.5 cm × 2 cm × 3 cm deep, right elbow") minimizes guesswork when reviewing the patient's progress, whereas an approximation (such as "small, deep pressure ulcer on the patient's arm") may be judged inconsistent if previous or later descriptions differ.

BE SPECIFIC
For example, describing an object or process in quantifiable terms, such as "500 ml of tea-colored urine" clearly specifies characteristics, whereas "about 400 to 500 ml of discolored urine" leaves room for later misinterpretation and inconsistencies.

BE THOROUGH — AND AVOID SUMMARIZING
For example, a reviewer who encounters a complete outcome evaluation of teaching effectiveness, such as "Patient can correctly remove the colostomy bag, clean the ostomy site, and apply a new bag without assistance," is less likely to question your patient-teaching performance than a reviewer who encounters an evaluation stating "Patient handles his own colostomy care."

CHANGES IN CONDITION AND CARE
When a patient's condition changes, documentation becomes a quality, reimbursement, and legal issue. An improvement in the patient's condition may signal a successful outcome and the need for discharge. A deterioration demands concise, factual recording of events.

A baseline assessment is recorded when each patient is admitted to the facility. Later changes are evaluated against the presenting signs and symptoms, health history, physical examination, and ancillary test results.

Admission, transfer, and discharge notes must accurately reflect changes in the patient's condition. Condition changes justify changes in care and subsequent reimbursement. The appropriateness of admission, transfer, and discharge is also evaluated based on the patient's condition. The Joint Commission standards provide guidelines for recording changes in the patient's condition and care.

USE OF EQUIPMENT
Nursing documentation provides evidence that certain equipment is essential to patient care, verifies that the equipment has been used appropriately, and justifies reimbursement. For example, documentation of an order for bed rest supports a patient's need for a bedpan, and documentation of type 1 diabetes supports a patient's need for a blood glucose monitor. Examiners require this documentation before approving reimbursement.

PATIENT EDUCATION
The Joint Commission standards require comprehensive patient education. In addition to informing the patient about relevant tests, treatments, and procedures, patient teaching can verify that a patient is ready for discharge. Docu-

mented teaching outcomes can also protect a health care facility and its nurses from legal problems.

According to The Joint Commission guidelines, patient teaching is required for:
▶ medication use
▶ medical equipment use
▶ potential food and drug interactions
▶ rehabilitation techniques
▶ community resources
▶ further treatment.

Patient teaching must be interdisciplinary and related to the care plan. In addition, arrangements must be made to communicate all discharge instructions to the person or organization responsible for continuing the patient's care.

INCONSISTENCIES

Nursing documentation must be consistent to maximize reimbursement. Charting based on a central problem list or an interdisciplinary care plan produces uniform data. Inconsistencies occur when nurses use different baseline criteria or record imprecise information.

Keep in mind that Medicare and other insurance examiners will always request an explanation for conflicting data in the medical record and that accurate details may be difficult to obtain retrospectively. The result of inconsistent data could be denial of payment.

Selected references

Centers for Medicare and Medicaid Services. "Hospital Quality Initiatives: Overview." Available: *http://www.cms.hhs.gov/HospitalQualityInits* accessed June 13, 2006.

Health and Human Services. "Hospital Compare." Available: *http://www.hospitalcompare.hhs.gov* accessed June 14, 2006.

Jensen, S., and Teper, R. "Preparing for a deposition: The Case Manager's Role," *Lippincott's Case Management* 10(3):167-70 May-June 2005.

MedQIC. "Medicare Quality Improvement Organization Program Priorities." Available: *http://www.medqic.org/dcs* accessed June 23, 2006.

The Joint Commission. *2005 Comprehensive Accreditation Manual for Hospitals: the Official Handbook*. Oakbrook Terrace, Ill: The Joint Commission, 2005.

DOCUMENTATION SYSTEMS

4

Although each health care facility determines its own requirements for documentation and evaluation, those requirements must comply with legal, accreditation, and professional standards.

Similarly, a nursing department can select the documentation system it wants to use as long as the system demonstrates adherence to standards and care requirements. For example, the system known as charting by exception (CBE) requires you to document only significant or abnormal findings.

Regardless of the documentation system used, specific policies and procedures for documentation must be in place and known. Understanding these policies and procedures will help you document care accurately. It will also serve you well when evaluating or modifying your documentation system or selecting a new one.

System selection

As health care facilities strive for greater efficiency and quality of care, you may need to participate in the decision about whether your current documentation system needs a simple revision, a total overhaul, or no change at all. Your aim: a system that provides clear, concise communication and reflects not only the patient's response to care but also the quality of care (which must meet the profession's accepted standards).

Measuring up to standard
The committees that set up continuous performance improvement programs (mandated by state regulations, the Institute for Healthcare Improvements, and The Joint Commission)

choose well-defined, objective, and readily measurable indicators that help them assess the structure, process, and outcome of patient care. They use these indicators to monitor and evaluate the contents of a patient's medical record.

To verify that treatment was required and provided or that medical tests and supplies were used, third-party payers (the insurers) review nursing documentation carefully. As a result, nurses now document more than ever before, including such data as every I.V. catheter used to start an infusion, each use of an I.V. pump to deliver a specific volume of medication, and every test that the patient undergoes. (See chapter 1, Nursing Documentation and the Medical Record, and chapter 3, Performance Improvement and Reimbursement, for more information about standards and regulations concerning nursing documentation.)

Shorter hospital stays and the need to verify the use of supplies and equipment in patient care have placed greater emphasis on nursing documentation as a yardstick for measuring not only the provision of patient care but also its quality. As quality indicators change, facilities must change their documentation to remain in compliance. Therefore, documentation review must be ongoing.

Evaluating your current system

In evaluating your documentation system, ask the following questions:
▶ What are the specific positive features of the current documentation system?
▶ What are the specific problems or limitations of the current documentation system? Does it support regulatory requirements? How can these problems be solved?

▶ How much time will be needed to develop a new system, educate staff, and implement changes?
▶ How much will it cost to change the current system? (Consider the costs of time, staff education, and new equipment.) Will the result eventually save money?
▶ How will changing the documentation system affect other members of the health care team, including the business office, personnel, and medical staff? How will they handle resistance to the proposed changes? (See *Evaluating your documentation system,* page 58.)

Selecting a new system

If assessing your current system indicates the need for a new system, begin by organizing a committee (or task force) composed of members from all departments that the change will affect. Having interdisciplinary representatives on this committee will facilitate acceptance of the new system when it's put into effect. The committee should research all available systems; consult other health care facilities about systems that work or don't work for them; assess the change's likely costs, time commitment, and effects on staff members; and evaluate each system for how well it satisfies professional standards and regulation requirements. (See *Comparing charting systems,* pages 60 and 61.)

After the committee selects a new system, the next step is to initiate training sessions to familiarize staff members with it. Consider implementing change in one unit or area at a time.

Then select or design the appropriate forms, and allow enough time for the transition to take place. Participants should be encouraged to alert the committee to any problems that arise during implementation of the new system.

Evaluating your documentation system

When reviewing the usefulness of your current documentation system, consider the following questions. If you answer no to any of them, you might recommend a closer evaluation of your system.

DOCUMENTING INTERVENTIONS AND PATIENT PROGRESS

▶ Does your current system reflect the patient's condition and progress and the interventions based on recorded evaluations? Look for records that describe the patient's condition and progress, actual interventions, and evaluations of provided care.

▶ Does the record include evidence of the patient's response to nursing care? For example, does it report the effectiveness of analgesics or the patient's response to I.V. medications? Does it show that care was modified according to the patient's response to treatment? For example, does it show what action was taken if the patient tolerated only half of a prescribed tube feeding?

▶ Does the record note continuity of care or exhibit unexplained gaps? If gaps appear, are notes entered later that document previous happenings? If late entries appear in the nursing notes on subsequent days, do you have to check the entire record to validate care?

▶ Are activities of daily living documented? For example, do the notes include evidence that the patient bathed himself or indicate that the patient could independently transfer himself to a wheelchair?

DOCUMENTING THE HEALTH CARE TEAM'S ACTIONS

▶ Does the record portray the nursing process clearly? Look for actual nursing diagnoses, written assessments, interventions, and evaluation of the patient's responses to them.

▶ Does the current documentation system facilitate and show communication among health care team members through all levels of care? Check for evidence that telephone calls were made in a timely manner, that practitioners were paged and notified of critical laboratory values and changes in a patient's condition, and that actions reflected these communications.

▶ Does your documentation system contain a process for obtaining and documenting a complete list of the patient's current medications on admission to the facility? Is a complete list of the patient's medications communicated to the next health care provider when the patient is referred or transferred to another setting, service, practitioner, or level of care?

▶ Is discharge planning clearly documented? Do the records show evidence of interdisciplinary coordination, team conferences, completed patient teaching, and discharge instructions?

▶ Does the record reflect current standards of care? Does it indicate that caregivers and administrators follow facility policies and procedures? If not, does the system provide for explanations of why a policy wasn't implemented or was implemented in an alternative manner?

CHECKING FOR CLARITY AND COMPREHENSIVENESS

▶ Are all portions of the record complete? Are all flow sheets, checklists, and other forms completed according to facility policy? Are all necessary entries apparent on the medication forms? If not, does the record describe why a medication wasn't given as ordered and who was informed of the omission if necessary?

▶ Does the documentation make sense? Can you track the patient's care and hospital course on this record alone?

▶ Can you read your patient's record for the previous 24 hours of documentation and determine his problem, the interventions provided, and the outcomes obtained?

Revising an existing system

Altering a documentation system usually involves changing the way you collect, enter, and retrieve information, but it rarely affects the content of the information. If the content of your existing system is deficient in some way, changing formats probably won't solve the problem.

Content problems usually stem from sources outside the system—for example, inadequate objectives or guidelines or insufficient time to document properly. In such cases, it may be preferable to amend the existing system instead of selecting a new one.

Following the system format

Depending on the policies of your health care facility, you'll use one or more documentation formats to record your nursing interventions and evaluations and the patient's response.

Some health care facilities elect to use traditional narrative charting formats or newer narrative formats (such as assessment-intervention-response [AIR]). Others choose alternative formats, such as problem-oriented medical record (POMR), problem-intervention-evaluation (PIE), focus, CBE, flow sheets-assessment-concise-timely (FACT), and core documentation formats. In addition, many health care facilities are using electronic charting systems.

Of the many systems in current use, each has special features and distinct advantages and disadvantages.

Traditional narrative charting

Traditional narrative charting formats document ongoing assessment data, nursing interventions, and patient responses in chronological order. Today, few facilities rely on the narrative format alone; most combine it with other formats.

Format and components

Narrative charting consists of a straightforward chronological account of the patient's status, the nursing interventions performed, and the patient's response to those interventions. The nurse usually records the data on the progress notes, with flow sheets commonly supplementing the narrative notes.

Knowing when to document, what to document, and how to organize the data are the key elements of effective narrative notes. (See *Charting with the narrative format,* page 62.)

WHEN AND WHAT TO DOCUMENT

Current Joint Commission standards direct all health care facilities to establish policies about the frequency of patient reassessment. You must assess your patient as often as required by your facility's policy, if not more often, and then document your findings.

If you find yourself writing repetitious, meaningless notes, you may be documenting too often. In such a case, double-check your facility's written policy. You may find that you're following a time-consuming, unwritten standard initiated by staff members, not by your facility. To guard against this, review the policy at least every 6 months.

Besides documenting simply according to policy, be sure to record specific and descriptive narrative notes whenever you observe any of the following:

▶ a change in the patient's condition (progression, regression, or new problems). For

(Text continued on page 62.)

Comparing charting systems

This chart summarizes the main features of the most commonly used documentation systems, which are discussed later in this chapter.

SYSTEM	USEFUL SETTINGS	PARTS OF RECORD	ASSESSMENT
Narrative	▶ Acute care ▶ Long-term care ▶ Home care ▶ Ambulatory care	▶ Progress notes ▶ Flow sheets to supplement care plan	▶ Initial: history and admission form ▶ Ongoing: progress notes
POMR	▶ Acute care ▶ Long-term care ▶ Home care ▶ Rehabilitation ▶ Mental health facilities	▶ Database ▶ Care plan ▶ Problem list ▶ Progress notes ▶ Discharge summary	▶ Initial: database and care plan ▶ Ongoing: progress notes
PIE	▶ Acute care	▶ Assessment flow sheet ▶ Progress notes ▶ Problem list	▶ Initial: assessment form ▶ Ongoing: assessment form every shift
FOCUS	▶ Acute care ▶ Long-term care	▶ Progress notes ▶ Flow sheets ▶ Checklists	▶ Initial: patient history and admission assessment ▶ Ongoing: assessment form
CBE	▶ Acute care ▶ Long-term care	▶ Care plan ▶ Flow sheets, including patient-teaching records and patient discharge notes ▶ Graphic record ▶ Progress notes	▶ Initial: database assessment sheet ▶ Ongoing: nursing and medical order flow sheets
FACT	▶ Acute care ▶ Long-term care	▶ Assessment sheet ▶ Flow sheets ▶ Progress notes	▶ Initial: baseline assessment ▶ Ongoing: flow sheet and progress notes
AIR	▶ Acute care ▶ Long-term care	▶ Flow sheets ▶ Care plan ▶ Progress notes	▶ Initial: baseline assessment ▶ Ongoing: flow sheet and progress notes
Core (with DAE)	▶ Acute care ▶ Long-term care	▶ Kardex ▶ Flow sheets ▶ Progress notes	▶ Initial: baseline assessment ▶ Ongoing: progress notes

CARE PLAN	OUTCOMES AND EVALUATION	PROGRESS NOTES FORMAT
► Care plan	► Progress notes ► Discharge summaries	► Narration at time of entry
► Database ► Nursing care plan based on problem list	► Progress notes (section E of SOAPIE and SOAPIER)	► SOAP, SOAPIE, SOAPIER
► None; included in progress notes (section P)	► Progress notes (section E)	► Problem ► Intervention ► Evaluation
► Nursing care plan based on problems or nursing diagnoses	► Progress notes (section R)	► Data ► Action ► Response
► Nursing care plan based on nursing diagnoses	► Progress notes (section E)	► SOAPIE or SOAPIER
► Nursing care plan based on nursing diagnoses	► Flow sheet (section R)	► Data ► Action ► Response
► Nursing care plan	► Progress notes (section R)	► Assessment ► Intervention ► Response
► Care plan	► Progress notes (section E)	► Data ► Action ► Evaluation

ChartWizard

Charting with the narrative format

This progress note provides an example of the narrative documentation format.

Date	Time	Notes
2/18/07	1100	Removed three 4" x 4" gauze pads saturated with blood-tinged, nonodorous drainage from Ⓛ lower leg wound. Wound measures 6 cm x 6 cm wide x 1 cm deep. Surrounding skin reddened and tender. Redressed wound with four 4" x 4" dressings and one 4" x 8" dressing and hypoallergenic tape. Will check dressings q 1 hr to assess for continued drainage. Will monitor pt.'s T q 4 hr. T-98.8R; BP-122/84; P-86; R-22. Pt. reports pain in Ⓛ lower leg at 8 on scale of 0 to 10, with 10 being the worst he can imagine. Administered two Percocet tablets and repositioned pt. from back to Ⓛ side. Will give Percocet ½ hour before subsequent dressing changes. Instructed pt. in dressing change procedure. Pt. stated "I know that it's important to wash my hands before I do anything so I don't get germs in my wound." Pt. demonstrated sufficient manual dexterity to put on gloves and handle all dressing supplies. Instructed pt. in proper hand-washing technique, dressing removal and disposal, opening and positioning dressing supplies, and signs and symptoms of wound infection and the importance of reporting them. Pt. demonstrated acceptable hand-washing technique and ability to remove dressings but needed instruction on positioning the leg so he could reach the wound. —————————— Carol Witt, RN
2/18/07	1200	Ⓛ lower leg wound dressing dry and intact. Pt. reports pain in leg at 2 on scale of 0 to 10. —————————— Carol Witt, RN

example, write, "The patient can walk 300 feet assisted by one person."

▶ a patient's response to a treatment or medication. For example, write, "The patient states that right leg pain is unrelieved 1 hour after receiving medication. He's still grimacing and rubbing the site."

▶ a lack of improvement in the patient's condition. For example, write, "No change in size or condition of leg wound after 5 days of treatment. Dimensions and condition remain as stated in 4/4/07 note."

▶ a patient or family member's response to teaching. For example, write, "The patient performed a return demonstration of wound care and correctly stated that he should do it three times a day."

Document exactly what you hear, observe, inspect, do, or teach. Include as much specific, descriptive information as possible. For example, if your patient has lower leg edema, include ankle and midcalf measurements and skin characteristics. Always document how the patient responds to your care and the extent of his progression toward a desired outcome.

HOW TO WRITE MEANINGFUL NOTES

► Read the narrative notes written by other health care professionals before you write your own.
► Read the notes recorded by nurses on other shifts, and make additional comments on their findings. This demonstrates continuity of care.
► If policy permits, use flow sheets to document repetitive procedures or measurements and summarize the information in the narrative notes.
► Include specific information when you observe a change in your patient's condition, a lack of progress in his condition, or a response to treatment, medication, or patient teaching. Also record the exact time these events occurred and the exact time you notified the practitioner. (See *Using military time*.)
► When possible, document an event immediately after it occurs. If you wait until the end of your shift, you may forget some important information. If you can't document at the time of an event, make notes on a piece of paper to help you remember details.

HOW TO ORGANIZE YOUR NOTES

Before you write anything, organize your thoughts so your paragraphs will be coherent. If you have difficulty deciding what to write, refer to the patient's care plan to review unresolved problems, prescribed interventions, and expected outcomes. Then comment on the patient's progress in relation to these items.

If you still have trouble organizing your thoughts, use this sequence of questions to order your entry:

Smarter charting

Using military time

To promote accurate charting, many institutions use military time equivalents. Such use avoids confusion over a.m. and p.m. entries.

0100 = 1 a.m.	1300 = 1 p.m.
0200 = 2 a.m.	1400 = 2 p.m.
0300 = 3 a.m.	1500 = 3 p.m.
0400 = 4 a.m.	1600 = 4 p.m.
0500 = 5 a.m.	1700 = 5 p.m.
0600 = 6 a.m.	1800 = 6 p.m.
0700 = 7 a.m.	1900 = 7 p.m.
0800 = 8 a.m.	2000 = 8 p.m.
0900 = 9 a.m.	2100 = 9 p.m.
1000 = 10 a.m.	2200 = 10 p.m.
1100 = 11 a.m.	2300 = 11 p.m.
1200 = 12 p.m.	2400 = 12 a.m.

► How did I first become aware of the problem?
► What has the patient said about the problem that's significant?
► What have I observed that's related to the problem?
► What's my plan for dealing with the problem?
► What steps have I taken to intervene?
► How has the patient responded to my interventions?

To make your notes as coherent as possible, discuss each of the patient's problems in a separate paragraph.

Alternatively, you may use a head-to-toe approach to organize your information. Be sure to notify the practitioner of significant changes that you observe. Then document this communication, the practitioner's responses, any new orders

AIR: A narrative format

A charting format called AIR may help you organize and simplify your charting. The AIR format synthesizes major nursing events while avoiding repetition of information found elsewhere in the medical record. Combined with nursing flow sheets and the nursing care plan, the AIR format can document your care clearly and concisely.

Here's how it works:

ASSESSMENT

Summarize your physical assessment findings. Rather than simply describing the patient's current condition, document trends and record your impression of the problem. Begin by titling each specific issue that you address, such as nursing diagnosis, admission note, and discharge planning.

INTERVENTION

Summarize your actions and those of other caregivers in response to the assessment data. The summary may include a condensed nursing care plan or plans for additional patient monitoring.

RESPONSE

Summarize the outcome or the patient's response to the nursing interventions. Because a response may not be evident for hours or even days, this documentation may not immediately follow the entries. In fact, it may be recorded by another nurse, which is why titling each of your assessments and interventions is so important.

to be implemented, and the patient's response to the intervention.

Advantages

The most flexible of all the documentation systems, narrative charting suits any clinical setting and strongly conveys your nursing interventions and your patients' responses.

Because narration is the most common form of writing, the training time needed for new staff members is usually brief. Also, because narrative notes are in chronological order, other team members can review the patient's progress on a day-to-day basis.

The narrative format easily lends itself to presenting information collected over an extended period. Furthermore, the ease with which narrative notes combine with other documentation devices, such as flow sheets, helps to decrease charting time.

Disadvantages

Narrative charting can be weak when it comes to recording patient outcomes because you must read the entire record to arrive at the outcome. Even then, you may have trouble determining the outcome of a particular problem because the same information may not be consistently documented.

Tracking problems and identifying trends in the patient's progress can also be difficult and time-consuming for the same reason: You have to read the entire record to arrive at an overall impression of the patient's condition and a complete account of his treatment course.

Because the narrative format offers no inherent guide to what's important to document, the tendency is to document everything; the result is a long, rambling, repetitive, subjective, and time-consuming record. This system also makes it difficult to retrieve specific information, such as the patient's previous hospitalizations or surgeries, without reading the entire record.

The narrative format also lends itself to vague or inaccurate language, such as "appears to be bleeding" or "small amount." In addition, some problems may be documented briefly and others may be documented at length for no clear reason. (See *AIR: A narrative format.*)

Problem-oriented medical record system

Originally developed by physicians and later adapted by nurses, the POMR system (also called the *problem-oriented record*) focuses on specific patient problems. In this documentation system, you'll describe each problem on multidisciplinary patient progress notes, as well as in the nursing admission assessment form and nursing care plan. (See *Writing a problem-oriented progress note,* page 66.)

Format and components

The POMR has five components: database, problem list, initial plan, narrative progress notes, and discharge summary. You'll record your interventions and evaluations in the progress notes and the discharge summary only. To gain a full understanding of the POMR, briefly review all five components.

DATABASE

Usually completed by a nurse, the database (or initial assessment) is a collection of subjective and objective information about the patient that forms the foundation for the patient's care plan. This initial assessment includes the reason for hospitalization, medical history, allergies, medication regimen, physical and psychosocial findings, self-care ability, educational needs, and other discharge planning concerns. This information becomes the foundation for a problem list.

PROBLEM LIST

After analyzing the database, you, the practitioner, and other relevant health care team members will identify and list the patient's current problems in chronological order according to the date each was identified, not in order of acuteness or priority. Originally, this system called for one interdisciplinary problem list. You may still see this format used, but nurses and practitioners usually keep separate problem lists with problems stated as either nursing or medical diagnoses. This problem list provides an overview of the patient's health status.

Try to number each problem so you can use the numbers to refer to the problems in the rest of the POMR. Make sure that every entry on the patient's initial plan, progress notes, and discharge summary corresponds to a number, and file the numbered problem list at the front of the patient's chart. Keep the problem list current by adding new numbers as new problems arise.

As soon as a problem is resolved, draw a line through it, or show that it's inactive by retiring the problem number and highlighting the problem with a colored felt-tip pen. Don't use that problem number again for the same patient.

INITIAL PLAN

After constructing the problem list, write an initial plan for each problem. This plan should include the expected outcomes, plans for further data collection (if needed), and patient care and

ChartWizard

Writing a problem-oriented progress note

Here's the nursing portion of a problem-oriented progress note. The nurse used the SOAP framework in the sample below.

Date	Time	Notes
2/20/07	1000	#1 Ineffective tissue perfusion (cerebral) R/T transient decrease in blood flow.
		S: Pt.: "I can't remember from one minute to the next."
		O: Pt. states she has no idea what day or time it is.
		® pupil 3 mm and sluggish to react. Ⓛ pupil 3 mm and reacts briskly to light. Unsteady gait noted. Otherwise neurologic assessment normal.
		A: Pt. disoriented to time and has abnormal pupillary reaction in response to light.
		P: Notify the Doctor. Orient pt. to time, place, and person q hour. Assess the pt.'s ability to retain bilaterally equal motor function q hour. Assess the patient for sensory deficits q hour. Assess pupillary reaction to light q hour. Assess the pt.'s BP q hour. Assess pt.'s speech and memory for deficits q hour. ———— Marianne Evans, RN
		#2 Risk for injury R/T sensory and motor deficits.
		S: Pt.: "I feel dizzy and off balance."
		O: Pt.'s eyes fluttering; pt. holding onto bedside table.
		A: Pt. experiencing dizziness and loss of balance similar to previous episode of TIA.
		P: Assist pt. back to bed and place side rails up. Modify environment to prevent injury. ———— Marianne Evans, RN
		#3 Anxiety R/T possible stroke.
		S: Pt. reports being scared of what will happen to her if she has a stroke — who will take care of her?
		O: Pt. clutching onto siderails and hyperventilating.
		A: Pt. becoming increasingly anxious.
		P: Discuss pt.'s anxiety and feelings about her illness. Help pt. identify the source of her anxiety. Identify and use effective coping mechanisms with the pt. Assure pt. that she will be monitored closely. ——— Marianne Evans, RN

teaching plans. Mutual goal setting is essential to ensure patient compliance and the effectiveness of your interventions.

NARRATIVE PROGRESS NOTES

One of the most prominent features of the POMR system is the structured way in which all team members, using the SOAP, SOAPIE, or SOAPIER format, write narrative progress notes.

SOAP format

If you use the SOAP format, you'll document the following information for each problem:

▶ **S**ubjective data: information the patient or family members tell you, such as the chief complaint and other impressions

▶ **O**bjective data: factual, measurable data you gather during the assessment, such as observed signs and symptoms, vital signs, and laboratory test values

▶ **A**ssessment data: conclusions based on the collected subjective and objective data and formulated as patient problems or nursing diagnoses (this dynamic and ongoing process changes as more or different subjective and objective information becomes known)

▶ **P**lan: your strategy for relieving the patient's problem (including both immediate or short-term actions and long-term measures).

SOAPIE format

Some facilities use the SOAPIE format, adding:

▶ **I**ntervention: measures you've taken to achieve an expected outcome (as the patient's health status changes, you may need to modify these interventions; be sure to document the patient's understanding and acceptance of the initial plan in this section of your notes)

▶ **E**valuation: an analysis of the effectiveness of your interventions (if expected outcomes fall short, use the evaluation process as a basis for developing alternative interventions).

SOAPIER format

The SOAPIER format allows for the documentation of alternative interventions by including:

▶ **R**evision: any changes from the original care plan (interventions, outcomes, or target dates may need to be adjusted to reach a previous goal).

Typically, you must write a complete SOAP, SOAPIE, or SOAPIER note every 24 hours on any unresolved problem or whenever the patient's condition changes. When doing so, be sure to specify the appropriate number of the problem you're discussing. Keep in mind that you don't need to write an entry for each SOAP or SOAPIE component every time you document. If you have nothing to record for a component, either omit the letter from the note or leave a blank space after it, depending on your facility's policy.

If your facility uses the SOAP format, record your nursing interventions and evaluations on flow sheets. If you use the SOAPIE format, provide explanations as needed in your progress notes under I and E.

DISCHARGE SUMMARY

Completing the POMR format, the discharge summary covers each problem on the list and notes whether it was resolved. Discuss any unresolved problems in your SOAP or SOAPIE note, and specify your plan for dealing with the problem after discharge. Note communications with other facilities, home health care agencies, and the patient.

Advantages

POMR documentation organizes information about each problem into specific categories understandable to all health care team members, thereby promoting interdisciplinary communication and data retrieval. The problems serve as an index to the medical record.

POMR documentation also illustrates the continuity of care, unifying the care plan and progress notes into a full record of the care actually planned and delivered. This information is easily incorporated into care planning because the caregiver addresses each problem or nursing diagnosis in the nursing notes.

The POMR format also promotes documentation of the nursing process, facilitates more consistent documentation, and eliminates documentation of nonessential data, thereby eliminating the need for task documentation. It can also serve as a checklist that draws attention to problems requiring interventions. The POMR format is most effective in acute care or long-term care settings.

Disadvantages

A drawback of POMR documentation is its emphasis on the *chronology* of problems rather than their *priority*. Analyzing trends with this format can be difficult because information may be buried in the daily narrative.

The POMR format commonly produces repetitious charting of assessment findings and interventions, especially with the SOAPIE format, because your assessments and interventions commonly apply to more than one problem. The resulting overlap makes the POMR system time-consuming to perform and to read. In addition, because the format emphasizes problems, routine care may remain undocumented unless flow sheets are used.

Furthermore, difficulties may arise if teammates fail to update the problem list regularly or if they're confused about which problems should be listed. The considerable time and cost of training new personnel to use the SOAP, SOAPIE, or SOAPIER method may also be a disadvantage.

The POMR format isn't well suited for settings with rapid patient turnover, such as the postanesthesia care unit, short procedure unit, or emergency department.

Problem-intervention-evaluation system

The PIE documentation system was developed to simplify the documentation process. PIE charting organizes information according to patients' problems as defined by a group of nurses at Craven Hospital in New Bern, North Carolina, in 1985. As its name indicates, this problem-oriented documentation approach considers three categories: the problem, interventions, and evaluation. To follow this format, you'll need to keep a daily patient assessment flow sheet and progress notes.

By integrating the care plan into the nurses' progress notes, the PIE format eliminates the need for a separate care plan. The intention is to provide a concise, efficient record of patient care that has a nursing—rather than a medical—focus.

Format and components

To implement the PIE documentation system, first assess the patient and document your findings on a daily patient assessment flow sheet. This flow sheet lists defined assessment terms under major categories (such as respiration), along with routine care and monitoring (such as providing hygiene and monitoring breath sounds). The flow sheet typically includes space to record pertinent treatments.

Initial only the assessment terms on the flow sheet that apply to your patient, and mark abnormal findings with an asterisk. Record detailed information in your progress notes.

PROBLEM

After performing and documenting an initial assessment, use the collected data to identify

ChartWizard

Using the PIE format

This sample shows how to write progress notes using the problem-intervention-evaluation (PIE) format.

Date	Time	Notes
2/19/07	1600	P#1: Ineffective breathing pattern related to possible smoke inhalation. IP#1: Assessed respiratory rate and breath sounds q hour to R/O pulmonary edema and bronchospasm. Taught pt. how to perform deep-breathing and coughing exercises, and taught use of incentive spirometer. O_2 applied at 2 L/min via nasal cannula. EP#1: Pt. maintains patent airway and normal RR and depth. Pt. understands the importance of performing deep-breathing and coughing exercises q h. Pt. has normal ABG levels. —————— Deborah Ryan, RN
2/19/07	1615	P#2: Decreased cardiac output R/T reduced stroke volume as a result of fluid loss through burns. IP#2: Teach pt. to report any restlessness, diaphoresis, or light-headedness, which may indicate shock. Evaluate VS and hemodynamic readings at least q 2 hour. Monitor urine output q hour. Monitor ABG levels. Provide and monitor I.V. therapy. EP#2: Pt. maintains normal VS and stable hemodynamic status. ABGs WNL. Pt. has adequate urine output. Pt. verbalizes signs and symptoms of shock. Pt. receiving adequate replacement through I.V. therapy. —————— Deborah Ryan, RN
2/19/07	1630	P#3: Acute pain related to second-degree burns over 20% of body. IP#3: Assess pain q 2 hour and medicate q 3 to 4 hour with morphine, as ordered. EP#3: Pt. reports a decrease in pain rating from 8 to 2 on a scale of 0 to 10, with 10 being the worst pain imaginable. —————— Deborah Ryan, RN

pertinent nursing diagnoses. You can use the list of nursing diagnoses accepted by your facility, which usually corresponds to those approved by the North American Nursing Diagnosis Association, an international organization (NANDA-I).

If you can't find a nursing diagnosis on an approved list, write the problem statement yourself using accepted criteria. Document all nursing diagnoses or problems in the progress notes, labeling each as "P" with an identifying number (for example, P#1).

This labeling system allows you to refer later to a specific problem by label only, eliminating the need to redocument the problem statement. Some facilities also use a separate problem-list form to keep a convenient running account of the nursing diagnoses for a particular patient. (See *Using the PIE format*.)

INTERVENTION

In this step, document the nursing actions taken for each nursing diagnosis. Document each intervention on the progress sheet, labeling each as "I" followed by the assigned problem number. (To refer to an intervention for the first nursing diagnosis, for instance, you'd use IP#1.)

EVALUATION

After charting your interventions, document the related effects in your progress notes. Use the label "E" followed by the assigned problem number (for example, EP#1).

Make sure that you or another nurse evaluates each problem at least every 8 hours. After every three shifts, review the notes from the previous 24 hours to identify the patient's current problems and responses to interventions.

Document continuing problems daily, along with relevant interventions and evaluations. Cross out any resolved problems from the daily documentation.

Advantages

Using the PIE format ensures that your documentation includes nursing diagnoses, related interventions, and evaluations. This format also encourages you to meet The Joint Commission requirements, provides an organizing framework for your thoughts and writing, and simplifies documentation by incorporating your care plan into your progress notes.

The PIE format promotes continuity of care because it facilitates tracking the patient from admission to discharge. This method also improves the quality of progress notes by highlighting care interventions and requiring a written evaluation of the patient's response to those interventions.

Disadvantages

The PIE format may require in-depth training for staff members. The requirement that you reevaluate each problem during each shift is time-consuming and leads to repetitive entries; some problems simply don't need such frequent evaluation.

The PIE format omits documentation of the planning step in the nursing process. This step, which addresses expected outcomes, is essential to evaluating the patient's responses. Finally, PIE charting doesn't incorporate multidisciplinary charting.

FOCUS CHARTING

Developed by nurses at Eitel Hospital in Minneapolis who found the SOAP format awkward, FOCUS CHARTING encourages you to organize your thoughts into patient-centered topics, or foci of concern, and then to document precisely and concisely. This format encourages you to use assessment data to evaluate these patient care concerns. It also helps you identify necessary revisions to the care plan as you document each entry. FOCUS CHARTING works well in acute care settings and in areas where the same care and procedures are repeated frequently.

Format and components

To implement this format, use a progress sheet with categories for date, time, focus, and progress notes. (See *Using FOCUS CHARTING.*) Then identify the foci by reviewing your assessment data.

FOCI

Typically, you'll write each focus as a nursing diagnosis (such as decreased cardiac output or

ChartWizard

Using FOCUS CHARTING

This sample shows how to write progress notes using FOCUS CHARTING format.

Date	Time	Focus	Progress notes
02/08/07	0900	Ineffective breathing pattern R/T decreased energy.	D: Pt. dyspneic and diaphoretic after bathing at bedside. Skin reddened. T-99.0,R-26; P-94; BP-142/86. Pt. reports that the dyspnea disrupts her sleep and she has lost 20 lb in 3 months. Pt. states she feels hot and is having difficulty catching her breath. ——————————— A: Auscultation reveals decreased vesicular breath sounds, prolonged expiration, and scattered expiratory wheezes in both lung bases. O2 applied at 2 L/min via nasal cannula. Dr. Miller notified and will examine pt. within 10 min. Explained the purpose of patterned breathing to pt.; demonstrated correct breathing techniques and had the pt. demonstrate them. ———————— Ellen Grimes, RN
02/08/07	1630	Anxiety R/T difficulty in breathing.	D: Pt. shaking and grabbing my hand and stating she is scared. ——————————— A: Spent time with pt. providing support. Discussed importance of and demonstrated diaphragmatic pursed-lip breathing techniques. Allowed pt. to verbalize feelings when dyspnea improved. ——————————— R: Pt. states she feels less anxious and she appears calmer. ———————————— Adela Suarez, RN
02/08/07	2330	Deficient knowledge R/T disease process and its treatment.	D: Pt. reports smoking history of 40 pack years (2 packs x 20 years). Currently smokes one pack per day. Denies exposure to respiratory irritants. ——————————— A: Reviewed the most common signs and symptoms associated with the disease: dyspnea, especially with exertion; fatigue; cough; occasional mucus production; weight loss; rapid heart rate; irregular P and use of accessory muscles to help with breathing from limited diaphragm function. Provided information about smoking-cessation groups. Urged pt. to avoid fumes, temperature extremes, and people with infections. ——————— Marc Ponte, RN

deficient fluid volume). However, the focus may also refer to a sign or symptom (such as hypotension or chest pain), a patient behavior (such as inability to ambulate), a special need (such as a discharge need), an acute change in the patient's condition (such as loss of consciousness or increase in blood pressure), or a significant event (such as surgery).

PROGRESS NOTES
In the progress notes column, you'll organize information using three categories: data (D), action (A), and response (R). In the data category, include subjective and objective information that describes the focus.

In the action category, include immediate and future nursing actions based on your assessment of the patient's condition. This category also may encompass any changes to the care plan you deem necessary based on your evaluation.

In the response category, describe the patient's response to any aspect of nursing or medical care.

Using all three categories ensures complete documentation based on the nursing process. Be sure to record routine nursing tasks and assessment data on your flow sheets and checklists.

Advantages
FOCUS CHARTING is flexible and can be adapted to fit any clinical setting. It centers on the nursing process, and the data-action-response format provides cues that direct documentation in a process-oriented way.

By separating the focus statement from the narrative of the progress notes, this format makes it easy to find information on a particular problem, thereby saving time and promoting communication among health care team members.

The format also highlights the nursing process in the documentation of daily patient care, encourages regular documentation of patient responses to nursing and medical therapy, and ensures adherence to The Joint Commission

requirements for documenting patient responses and outcomes.

You can use this format to document many topics without being confined to those on the problem list or care plan. This format also helps you organize your thoughts and document succinctly and precisely.

Disadvantages
Learning the FOCUS CHARTING format may require in-depth training, especially for staff members familiar with other systems. Additionally, the system requires you to use many flow sheets and checklists, which can lead to inconsistent documentation and can cause difficulty in tracking a patient's problems.

▶ Charting by exception

The CBE documentation system was designed by nurses at St. Luke's Hospital in Milwaukee to overcome long-standing charting problems, such as lengthy and repetitive notes, poorly organized information, difficult-to-retrieve data, and a high risk of errors of omission. To avoid these pitfalls, the CBE format radically departs from traditional systems by requiring documentation of only significant or abnormal findings. These findings are documented in a narrative portion of the record. The CBE system also uses military time to help prevent misinterpretations.

Format and components
To use CBE documentation effectively, you must know and adhere to established guidelines for nursing assessments and interventions. The CBE nursing assessment format has printed

guidelines for each body system; this format relies on written standards of practice that identify
the nurse's basic responsibilities to patients.
For example, care standards for patient hygiene
might include your responsibility to ensure that
a patient has a complete linen change every 3
days or sooner if necessary.

Because the standards are clear and concise,
all charting related to routine nursing care—or
any other care outlined in the standards—is
eliminated. You document only deviations from
the standards, thereby omitting repetitive charting of routine procedures.

Intervention guidelines for the CBE system
stem from these sources:

▶ nursing diagnosis-based standardized care
plans—identification of patient problems,
desired outcomes, and interventions
▶ patient care guidelines—standardized interventions established for specific patient populations, such as patients with a nursing
diagnosis of pain, that outline the nursing
interventions, treatments, and time frame for
repeated assessments
▶ practitioner's orders—prescribed medical
interventions
▶ incidental orders—usually one-time, miscel-
laneous nursing or medical orders or interdependent interventions related to a protocol
or a piece of equipment
▶ standards of nursing practice—definition of
the acceptable level of routine nursing care
for all patients (the essential aspects of nursing practice for a specific unit or for all clinical areas).

The CBE format includes a nursing diagnosis-based standardized care plan and several
types of flow sheets, including the nursing care
flow sheet, graphic record, patient-teaching
record, and patient discharge note. In certain
cases, you may need to supplement your CBE
documentation by using nurses' progress notes.

NURSING DIAGNOSIS-BASED STANDARDIZED CARE PLANS

Use these preprinted care plans whenever you
identify a nursing diagnosis, and use a separate
form for each pertinent diagnosis. Keep in mind
that the forms have spaces that allow you to
individualize them as needed; for example, you
can include expected outcomes and major revisions to the care plan. Place the completed
forms in the nurses' progress notes section of the
clinical record.

NURSING CARE FLOW SHEET

Use this form to document your assessments
and interventions. Each flow sheet is designed
for a 24-hour period of care for one patient.

After completing an assessment, compare
your findings with the normal parameters defined in the printed guidelines on the form. If
the findings are within normal parameters, place
a check mark in the appropriate category box
and add your initials. If the findings aren't within
the normal range, put an asterisk in the category
box; then explain your findings in the comments
section on the form.

Remember, a finding that isn't defined in the
guidelines may be normal for a particular patient; for example, unclear speech may be a
normal finding in a patient with a long-standing
tracheostomy. If the patient's condition hasn't
changed from the last assessment, draw a horizontal arrow from the previous category box to
the current one.

After assessing your patient, review the previous nurse's note and symbol to determine
whether the patient's condition changed. Indicate significant findings or abnormal patient

responses with an asterisk, and write an explanation in the comments section. If the patient's response is unchanged, use an arrow.

After you document an entire column in the assessments and interventions section, initial it at the bottom. Also initial all of your entries in the comments section, and sign the form at the bottom of the page.

Some facilities use a nursing care flow sheet that combines all of the necessary sections, such as the graphic record, a daily nursing care activities checklist, and a patient care assessment section. (See *Using a combined nursing care flow sheet.*)

GRAPHIC RECORD
Use this flow sheet or section of a flow sheet to document trends in the patient's vital signs, weight, intake and output, and stool, urination, appetite, and activity levels. As with the nursing care flow sheet, use check marks to indicate expected findings and asterisks to indicate abnormal findings. Record information about abnormalities in the nurses' progress notes.

In the box labeled "Routine standards," check off the established nursing care interventions you performed such as providing hygiene. Don't rewrite these standards as orders on the nursing care flow sheet. Refer to the guidelines on the back of the graphic record for complete instructions.

PATIENT-TEACHING RECORD
Use this form or section on the form to identify the knowledge, psychomotor skills, and social or behavioral measures that your patient or his caregiver must learn by a predetermined date. The patient-teaching record includes teaching resources, dates of patient achievements, and other pertinent observations. You may use more than one form for a patient with multiple learning needs.

PATIENT DISCHARGE NOTE
Similar to other discharge forms, the patient discharge note is a flow sheet for documenting ongoing discharge planning. Follow the instructions printed on the back of the form.

PROGRESS NOTES
Another component of the CBE format, the progress notes are used to document revisions to the care plan and interventions that don't lend themselves to the nursing care flow sheet. Because the CBE format permits you to document most assessments and interventions on the nursing care flow sheet, the progress notes typically contain little assessment and intervention data.

Advantages
The CBE format has several advantages. By including only information that deviates from expected findings, it decreases the amount of documentation needed, eliminates redundancies, and clearly identifies abnormal data, thereby decreasing the time needed to document normal and abnormal findings. The use of well-defined guidelines and standards of care promotes uniform nursing practice. Also, the flow sheets let you easily track trends.

Guidelines, including normal findings, are printed on the forms for ready reference. Abnormal findings are highlighted to help you quickly pinpoint significant changes and trends in a patient's condition. Documentation of routine care is eliminated through the use of nursing care standards.

The fact that all flow sheets (which are part of the permanent record) are kept at the

(*Text continued on page 78.*)

ChartWizard

Using a combined nursing care flow sheet

This sample shows a portion of a nursing care flow sheet that combines a graphic record, a daily nursing care activities checklist, and a patient care assessment form.

Name	Alejandro Mendoza											
Date	02/28/07											

Hour		0700	0800	0900	1000	1100	1200	1300	1400	1500	1600	1700	1800
Temperature													
C°	F°												
40.4	105												
40.0	104												
39.4	103												
38.9	102												
38.3	101												
37.8	100												
37.2	99												
36.7	98												
36.1	97												
35.6	96												
Pulse		84	80	82	78	76	78	78	82	84	82	80	78
Respiration		16	20	20	22	24	24	18	20	22	20	18	24
BP	Lying												
	Sitting	136/82	130/80	126/74	132/82	132/80	140/82	136/74	130/70	138/78	140/80	132/78	136/76
	Standing												
Intake	Oral	400					300						100
	Tube												
	I.V.												
	Blood												
8-hour total		700											
Output	Urine	300					200						
	Other												
	Other												
8-hour total		500											
Teaching		Skin care, signs and symptoms of UT I, Safety											
Signature		Carol Witt, RN (0700-1530)								Donald Baron, RN (1500-2330)			

(continued)

Using a combined nursing care flow sheet (continued)

Hour		0700	0800	0900	1000	1100	1200	1300	1400	1500	1600	1700
ACTIVITY	Bed rest	CW ———————————————————→								DB ————————————→		
	OOB											
	Ambulate (assist)											
	Ambulatory											
	Sleeping											
	Bathroom privileges											
	HOB elevated	CW ———————————————————→								DB ————————————→		
	Cough, deep-breathe, turn		CW							DB		
	ROM: Active / Passive		CW							DB		
HYGIENE	Bath		CW									
	Shave		CW									
	Oral		CW									
	Skin care											
	Perianal care											
NUTRITION	Diet	Soft — no added salt										
	% Eating			90%				60%				90%
	Feeding											
	Supplemental											
	S=Self, A=Assist, F=Feed			S				S				S
BLADDER	Catheter											
	Incontinent											
	Voiding	clear, yellow urine										
	Intermittent cath.											
BOWEL	Stools (occult blood + or −)	negative (−) for occult blood										
	Incontinent											
	Normal	Small, soft, formed brown stool										
	Enema											
SPECIAL TREATMENTS	Special mattress	Low-pressure airflow mattress applied 0900										
	Special bed											
	Heel and elbow pads											
	Antiembolism stockings											
	Traction: + = on, − = off											
	Isolation type											

Using a combined nursing care flow sheet *(continued)*

ASSESSMENT FINDINGS

Key:
√ = normal findings
* = significant finding

	Day	Evening	Night	
Neurologic	√ CW	* DB		Limited ROM ① shoulder. Pt. states, "I have arthritis and my shoulder is always stiff." ——————— DB
Cardiovascular	√ CW	√ DB		
Respiratory	* CW	√ DB		Decreased breath sounds at ® base posteriorly at 0800. Lungs clear at 1200. ——————— CW
GI	√ CW	√ DB		
Genitourinary	√ CW	√ DB		
Surgical dressing and incision	N/A	N/A		
Skin integrity	* CW	* DB		Poor skin turgor; dry, flaky skin. ——————— CW 4 cm x 4 cm area of redness at sacral area. ——————— DB
Psychosocial	√ CW	√ DB		
Educational	√ CW	* DB		Taught pt. safety, skin care, and signs and symptoms of UTI —— CW
Peripheral vascular	√ CW	√ DB		

NORMAL ASSESSMENT FINDINGS

Neurologic
► Alert and oriented to time, place, and person
► Speech clear and understandable
► Memory intact
► Behavior appropriate to situation and accommodation
► Active range of motion (ROM) of all extremities; symmetrically equal strength
► No paresthesia

Cardiovascular
► Regular apical pulse
► Palpable bilateral peripheral pulses
► No peripheral edema
► No calf tenderness

Respiratory
► Resting respirations 10 to 20 per minute, quiet and regular
► Clear sputum
► Pink nail beds and mucous membranes

GI
► Abdomen soft and nondistended
► Tolerates prescribed diet without nausea or vomiting
► Bowel movements within own normal pattern and consistency

Genitourinary
► No indwelling catheter in use
► Urinates without pain
► Undistended bladder after urination
► Urine is clear yellow to amber color

Surgical dressing and incision
► Dressing dry and intact
► No evidence of redness, increased temperature, or tenderness in surrounding tissue
► Sutures, staples, Steri-Strips intact
► Sound edges well approximated
► No drainage present

Skin integrity
► Skin color normal
► Skin warm, dry, and intact
► Moist mucous membranes

Psychosocial
► Interacts and communicates in an appropriate manner with others (family, significant others, health care personnel)

Educational
► Patient or significant others communicate understanding of the patient's health status, plan of care, and expected response
► Patient or significant others demonstrate ability to perform health-related procedures and behaviors as taught
► Items taught and expected performance must be specifically described in significant findings section

Peripheral vascular
► Affected extremity pink, warm, and movable within average ROM
► Capillary refill time < 3 seconds
► Peripheral pulses palpable
► No edema: sensation intact without numbness or paresthesia
► No pain on passive stretch

patient's bedside, where they serve as a ready reference, encourages immediate documentation. Because patient data are written on the permanent record immediately, you don't have to keep temporary notes and later transcribe them to the patient's chart; in addition, other caregivers always have access to the most current data. Also, because assessments are standardized, all caregivers evaluate and document findings consistently.

Finally, information that has already been recorded isn't repeated; for instance, you don't have to write a long entry in a patient's chart each time you assess him if his condition remains the same.

Disadvantages

The chief drawback of the CBE format is the major time commitment needed to develop clear guidelines and standards of care. To ensure a legally sound patient record, these guidelines and standards must be in place and understood by all nursing staff members before the format can be implemented. This radical departure from traditional documentation systems takes time for people to learn, accept, and use correctly. Consistent use of the appropriate documenting procedures is vital.

If your health care facility uses multiple forms rather than one form that combines all the CBE components, the documenting process can be confusing and the records incomplete. Narrative notes may be too brief, and an evaluation of a patient's response may not be fully described.

CBE documentation doesn't accommodate integrated or multidisciplinary charting. Also, be aware that unexpected events or isolated occurrences may not be fully documented; these events will require a narrative note.

The CBE system was developed for registered nurses. If licensed practical nurses will be using the system, it must be evaluated and modified to meet their scope of practice. CBE charting complies with legal principles, but it may be questioned in court until the system becomes more widely known.

FACT system

Named for its individual elements, the FACT documentation system incorporates many CBE principles. It was designed to avoid the documentation of irrelevant data, repetitive notes, and inconsistencies among departments and to reduce the amount of time spent charting.

Format and components

The FACT system has four key elements:
▶ **F**low sheets individualized to specific services
▶ **A**ssessment features standardized with baseline parameters
▶ **C**oncise, integrated progress notes and flow sheets documenting the patient's condition and responses
▶ **T**imely entries recorded when care is given.

The FACT system requires that you document only exceptions to the norm or significant information about the patient. It eliminates the need to chart normal findings. It also incorporates each step of the nursing process. (See *Documenting with FACT.*)

FACT documentation begins with a complete initial baseline assessment on each patient using standardized parameters. This format uses an assessment-action flow sheet, a frequent assessment flow sheet, and progress notes. The content of the flow sheets and notes may be individualized to some extent. The flow sheets cover a

ChartWizard

Documenting with FACT

Developed in 1987 at Abbott Northwestern Hospital in Minneapolis, the FACT system records nursing assessment findings and interventions that are exceptions to the norm. This sample shows portions of an assessment flow sheet and a postoperative flow sheet using the FACT format.

ASSESSMENT AND ACTION RECORD

Patient: *Henry Aaron*
Medical Record Number: *026478*

	Date Time	02/04/07 1300	02/04/07 1800	02/04/07 2330
Neurologic Alert and oriented to time, place, and person. PERRLA. Symmetry of strength in extremities. No difficulty with coordination. Behavior appropriate to situation. Sensation intact without numbness or paresthesia.		✓	✓	✓
Orient patient.				
Refer to neurologic flow sheet.				
Pain No report of pain. If present, include patient statements about intensity (0 to 10 scale), location, description, duration, radiation, precipitating and alleviating factors.		*Abdominal incision pain 10 — "severe pain"*	✓	*4 — incision pain — "It hurts."*
Location		*RLQ*		*RLQ*
Relief measures		*Percocet 1 tablet by mouth*		*Percocet 1 tablet by mouth*
Pain relief: Y = Yes N = No		*y*		*y*
Cardiovascular Apical pulse 60 to 100. S_1 and S_2 present. Regular rhythm. Peripheral (radial, pedal) pulses present. No edema or calf tenderness. Extremities pink, warm, movable within patient's ROM.		✓	✓	✓
I.V. solution and rate		*D5½NSS at 125 ml/hr.*	*D5½NSS at 125 ml/hr.*	*D5½NSS at 125 ml/hr.*
Respiratory Respiratory rate 12 to 20 at rest, quiet, regular, and nonlabored. Lungs clear and aerated equally in all lobes. No abnormal breath sounds. Mucous membranes pink.		✓	*↓BS RUL*	✓
O_2 therapy				
Taught coughing, deep breathing/Incentive spirometer		✓	✓	✓
Musculoskeletal Extremities pink, warm, and without edema; sensation and motion present. Normal joint ROM, no swelling or tenderness. Steady gait without aids. Pedal, radial pulses present. Rapid capillary refill.		✓	✓	✓
Activity (describe)		*Bed rest*	*OOB in chair*	*Bed rest*
Nurse's signature and title		*Cindy Weir, RN*	*Dave Shaw, RN*	*Lynn Tate, RN*

Key: ✓ = Meets assessment criteria

(continued)

Documenting with FACT *(continued)*

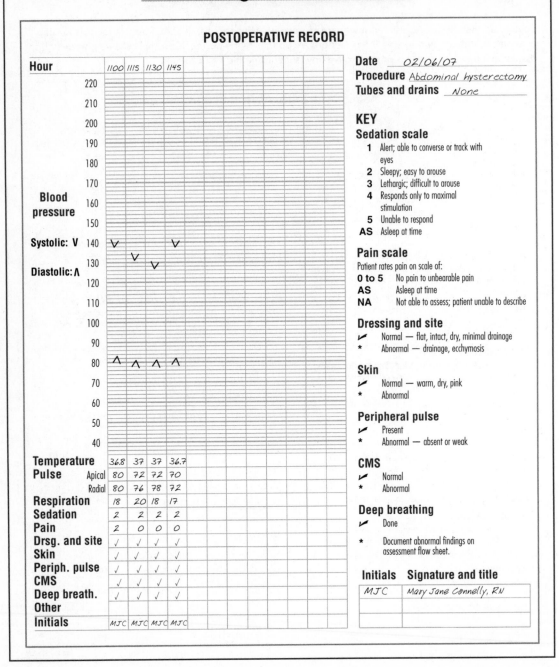

POSTOPERATIVE RECORD

Date 02/06/07
Procedure Abdominal hysterectomy
Tubes and drains None

Hour		1100	1115	1130	1145
Blood pressure	220				
	210				
	200				
	190				
	180				
	170				
	160				
	150				
Systolic: V	140	V			V
	130		V	V	
Diastolic: Λ	120				
	110				
	100				
	90				
	80	Λ	Λ	Λ	Λ
	70				
	60				
	50				
	40				
Temperature		36.8	37	37	36.7
Pulse	Apical	80	72	72	70
	Radial	80	76	78	72
Respiration		18	20	18	17
Sedation		2	2	2	2
Pain		2	0	0	0
Drsg. and site		✓	✓	✓	✓
Skin		✓	✓	✓	✓
Periph. pulse		✓	✓	✓	✓
CMS		✓	✓	✓	✓
Deep breath.		✓	✓	✓	✓
Other					
Initials		MJC	MJC	MJC	MJC

KEY

Sedation scale
- **1** Alert; able to converse or track with eyes
- **2** Sleepy; easy to arouse
- **3** Lethargic; difficult to arouse
- **4** Responds only to maximal stimulation
- **5** Unable to respond
- **AS** Asleep at time

Pain scale
Patient rates pain on scale of:
- **0 to 5** No pain to unbearable pain
- **AS** Asleep at time
- **NA** Not able to assess; patient unable to describe

Dressing and site
- ✔ Normal — flat, intact, dry, minimal drainage
- ✱ Abnormal — drainage, ecchymosis

Skin
- ✔ Normal — warm, dry, pink
- ✱ Abnormal

Peripheral pulse
- ✔ Present
- ✱ Abnormal — absent or weak

CMS
- ✔ Normal
- ✱ Abnormal

Deep breathing
- ✔ Done
- ✱ Document abnormal findings on assessment flow sheet.

Initials	Signature and title
MJC	Mary Jane Connelly, RN

24- to 72-hour period, and you'll need to date, time, and sign all entries.

ASSESSMENT-ACTION FLOW SHEET

Use this form to document ongoing assessments and interventions. Normal assessment parameters for each body system are printed on the form along with planned interventions. The flow sheet may be individualized according to the patient's needs.

FREQUENT ASSESSMENT FLOW SHEET

Use this form to chart vital signs and frequent assessments. On a surgical unit, for example, this form would include a postoperative assessment section.

PROGRESS NOTES

This form includes an integrated progress record where you'll use narrative notes to document the patient's progress and any significant incidents. As in focus charting, write narrative notes using the data-action-response method. Update progress notes related to patient outcomes every 48 hours.

Advantages

The computer-ready FACT charting system has several advantages. It eliminates repetition and encourages consistent language and structure. The system is outcome oriented and communicates patient progress to all health care team members. It permits immediate recording of current data and is readily accessible at the patient's bedside. The system also eliminates the need for many different forms and reduces the time spent writing narrative notes.

Disadvantages

FACT charting requires a major time commitment to develop standards and implement the system across all departments of the health care facility. Narrative notes may be too brief, and the nurse's perspective on the patient may be overlooked. The nursing process framework may be difficult to identify in this system as well.

Core system

The core documentation system focuses on the nursing process—the core, or most important part, of documentation.

Format and components

Consisting of a database, care plans, flow sheets, progress notes, and discharge summary, core charting requires you to assess and record a patient's functional and cognitive status within 8 hours of admission. (See *Using core charting*, pages 82 to 85.)

DATABASE AND CARE PLANS

This initial assessment focuses on the patient's body systems and activities of daily living and includes a summary of the patient's problems and appropriate nursing diagnoses. The completed database and care plan are then entered on the patient's medical record card (Kardex).

FLOW SHEETS

Use flow sheets to document the patient's activities and response to nursing interventions, diagnostic procedures, and patient teaching.

(Text continued on page 86.)

ChartWizard

Using core charting

Developed in 1986 by the nurses at St. Joseph's Hospital in Hamilton, Ontario, core charting focuses on the key elements of the nursing process. This sample shows the features of an initial assessment and care plan.

INITIAL ASSESSMENT

Patient: *Lawrence Meall*   **Medical record number:** *723465*

General appearance	Physical	*Immobile and severe headache*
	Skin	☑ Clear ☑ Dry ☑ Intact ☐ Other
	Hygiene	*Good*
Cardiopulmonary		*Tachycardia and tachypnea*
Mobility	*Unable to stand or walk*	Aided by *Wheelchair*
Vision	*Good*	Aided by
Hearing	*Good*	Aided by
Speech	Language *English*	
	Impediment *None*	Aided by
Appetite, diet	*Fair, regular*	
Dentures	☐ Upper ☐ Lower	☐ Partial ☑ None
Urination	*Good – voids freely*	Aided by *Urinal*
Bowel routine	*Daily*	Aided by *Laxatives*
Sleep and rest	*Poor, secondary to pain*	Aided by *Analgesics*
Pain and discomfort *Severe pain @ temporal area*		Aided by *Percocet*
Reproduction and sexuality *Normal*		
Mental status (orientation, memory) *Oriented x3*		
Emotional status (mood, attitude) *Agitated*		
Religion	*Catholic*	
Nationality	*Irish*	
Lifestyle habits ☑ Alcohol *occasional beer*		☐ Drugs *none*
☐ Tobacco *none*		☐ Other
Occupation	*Construction worker*	
Hobbies	*Sports*	

Patient's concerns for discharge   *Pt. states that he's concerned about when he will be able to return to work. States that if he requires surgery, no one will be home to help him because his wife works.*

Signature   *Pam Watts, RN*

Date and time   *02/16/07   0200*

Using core charting *(continued)*

VITAL SIGNS FLOW SHEET

Date		02/16/07						02/17/07						02/18/07		
Time		0200	0600	1000	1400	1800	2200	0200	0600	1000	1400	1800	2200	0200		
Temp	**Pulse**															
41	170															
	160															
40	150															
	140															
39	130															
	120			•												
38	110		X	X			•	X								
	100		•			•		•		•	X			•		
37	90				X	X					X	X		X		
	80	X			•		X		•	X	•		X			
36	70	•							X			•				
	60															
35	50															
	40															
Respirations		20	22	24	21	20	22	18	20	22	24	20	18	20		
Blood pressure																
	230															
	220															
	210															
	200															
	190															
	180															
	170															
	160															
	150		V	V				V								
	140	V			V	V		V			V			V		
	130									V		V				
	120															
	110															
	100															
	90												Λ			
	80		Λ	Λ	Λ	Λ		Λ	Λ	Λ	Λ	Λ		Λ		
	70	Λ														
	60															
	50															
Nurse's signature		Pam Watts, RN	Pam Watts, RN	Esther Blake, RN	Esther Blake, RN	Wendy Moss, RN	Wendy Moss, RN	Ann Jones, RN	Ann Jones, RN	Lisa Case, RN	Lisa Case, RN	John Smith, RN	John Smith, RN	Carol Davis, RN		

Key:
Temp = •
Pulse = X

Blood pressure, standing
Systolic = ∇
Diastolic = Δ

Blood pressure, lying
Systolic = V
Diastolic = Λ

(continued)

Using core charting (continued)

24-HOUR FLUID BALANCE FLOW SHEET

Date 02/16/07	INTAKE						OUTPUT						
	Oral or tube feeding	Intravenous DS1/2 NSS	TPN Travasol	TPN Lipid	Blood & blood products	Total	Urine	NG tube	Emesis	Stool	Drainage		Total
Time													
0800	250						500						
0900	100												
1000	250												
1100							500						
1200	400												
1300													
1400	250						1000						
1500													
Subtotal	1250	800				2050	2000						2000
1600							400						
1700	300												
1800													
1900	100						500						
2000													
2100													
2200							400						
2300													
Subtotal	400	800				1200	1300						1300
2400													
0100							200						
0200	100												
0300													
0400							400						
0500													
0600							400						
0700	100												
Subtotal	200	800				1000	1000						1000
Total	1850	2400				4250	4300						4300

Nurse's signature	Day 0800-1500	Pam Watts, RN		24-hour intake 0800-0700	4,250 ml
	Evening 1600-2300	Esther Blake, RN		24-hour output 0800-0700	4,300 ml
	Night 2400-0700	Wendy Moss, RN		Balance ±	–50 ml

Using core charting *(continued)*

PATIENT CARE PLAN

Date	Nurse's initials	NURSING DIAGNOSES	EXPECTED OUTCOMES	Deadline	Chart	NURSING INTERVENTIONS	Date resolved	Nurse's initials
						Monitor VS & neuro. VS q hour.		
						Monitor CSF output q hour.		
						Observe for signs of rebleeding.		
		Safety needs						
02/16/07	PW	Risk for injury related to altered LOC	Pt. will remain free from injury			Raise the bed side rails. Avoid using restraints, which may raise ICP.		
		Psychosocial needs						
		Fear related to unknown prognosis	Pt. will verbalize feelings of fear			Provide emotional support to pt. and family.	02/18/07	PW
		Spiritual, cultural needs						

PATIENT-TEACHING PLANS	DISCHARGE PLANNING
Teach pt. and family about condition.	Expected discharge date 02/20/07
Explain all tests, neurologic exams, treatments, and procedures to pt.	Home situation
	Discharge resources involved
Explain cerebral aneurysm precautions and their purpose.	Public health
Explain physical rehab. plan to pt. and family.	Home care
Provide nutrition guidelines to pt.	Social work
	Placement Cedar Crest Rehab.
	Other

Nurse's signature	Initials	Nurse's signature	Initials	Nurse's signature	Initials
Pam Watts, RN	PW				

PROGRESS NOTES

In the progress notes, record the following information (DAE) for each problem:
▶ **D**ata
▶ **A**ction
▶ **E**valuation or response.

DISCHARGE SUMMARY

This component of core documentation incorporates information related to nursing diagnoses and patient teaching. The discharge summary also includes recommended follow-up care.

Advantages

Core documentation incorporates the entire nursing process into one system. Complemented by the DAE component, this system groups nursing diagnoses and functional status assessments together, allowing various solutions to be considered. The system also promotes concise documentation with minimal repetition and encourages the daily recording of psychosocial information. Core charting is useful in acute care and long-term care facilities.

Disadvantages

Core documentation may require in-depth training for staff members who are familiar with other documenting systems. Developing forms may be costly and time-consuming. The DAE format doesn't always present information chronologically, making it difficult to perceive the patient's progress quickly. What's more, the progress notes may not always relate to the care plan, so you'll need to monitor your documentation carefully to ensure a record of quality care.

Electronic charting

Computerized, or electronic, charting can significantly reduce the amount of time you spend on documentation. Besides facilitating accurate and speedy documentation, computers can also help you complete nurse management reports, provide patient classification data, and make staffing projections. They can identify patient-teaching needs and supply data for nursing research and education. Some bedside terminals can track a patient's vital signs electronically. (For detailed information on computerized documentation systems, see chapter 13, Electronic Patient Records.)

Selected references

Chart Smart: The A-to-Z Guide to Better Nursing Documentation, 2nd ed. Philadelphia: Lippincott Williams & Wilkins, 2007.

Charting Made Incredibly Easy, 3rd ed. Philadelphia: Lippincott Williams & Wilkins, 2005.

Murphy, E.K. "Charting by Exception," *AORN Journal* 78(5):821-3, November 2003.

NANDA International. *Nursing Diagnoses: Definitions & Classification 2005-2006.* Philadelphia: NANDA International, 2005.

Resnick, B. "Malpractice in Geriatrics: Are We Surviving?" *Geriatric Nursing* 27(4):198-200, July-August 2006.

DOCUMENTATION OF THE NURSING PROCESS

5

Regardless of which documentation system you use, your documentation must reflect the nursing process, which is based on theories of nursing and other disciplines and follows the scientific method. This problem-solving process systematically organizes nursing activities to ensure the highest quality of care. It allows you to determine which problems you can help alleviate and which potential problems you can help prevent. The nursing process also helps you identify what kind and how much assistance a patient requires, who can best provide that assistance, which desired outcomes the patient can achieve, and whether he achieves them.

To get a complete picture of the patient's situation, you'll need to systematically follow the five steps of the nursing process—assessment, nursing diagnosis, planning, implementation, and evaluation—and document them effectively. (See *Five-step nursing process*, pages 88 and 89.)

Fundamentals of nursing documentation

To ensure clear communication and complete, accurate, and timely documentation of your nursing care, you must keep in mind the fundamentals of documentation. Follow these guidelines:

Write neatly and legibly

One important reason to document your nursing care is to communicate with other members of the health care team. Sloppy or illegible handwriting confuses people and wastes their time as they try to decipher it. More seriously, the patient might be injured if other caregivers can't understand crucial information.

Five-step nursing process

This flowchart shows the five steps of the nursing process and lists the forms you should use to document them.

Step 1
ASSESSMENT
Gather data from the patient's health history, physical examination, medical record, and diagnostic test results.
Documentation tools
Initial assessment form, flow sheets

Step 2
NURSING DIAGNOSIS
Make judgments based on assessment data.
Documentation tools
Nursing care plan, patient care guidelines, clinical pathway, progress notes, problem list

If you don't have room to chart something legibly, leave that section blank, put a bracket around it, and write "See progress notes." Then record the information fully and legibly in the notes.

Write in ink

Because it's a permanent document, the clinical record should be completed in ink or printed out from a computer. Use black ink because other colors may not photocopy well. Also, don't use felt-tipped pens on forms containing carbon paper; the pens may not produce sufficient pressure for copies.

Use correct spelling and grammar

Notes filled with misspelled words and incorrect grammar create the same negative impression as illegible handwriting. To avoid spelling and grammatical errors:

▶ keep a general and medical dictionary in documentation areas
▶ post a list of commonly misspelled words, especially terms and medications regularly used on the unit.

Use accepted abbreviations

The Joint Commission on Accreditation of Healthcare Organizations, now simply referred to as The Joint Commission, requires each organization to develop and standardize a list of abbreviations, symbols, acronyms, and dose designations that may not be used throughout the organization. The Joint Commission has developed a list of "Do Not Use" abbreviations that must be contained within each organization's standardized list. There are additional abbreviations in consideration for possible future inclusion in this list. (See *Abbreviations to avoid,* pages 90 and 91.)

Using unapproved abbreviations can result in misunderstanding or ambiguity, which may en-

Step 3
PLANNING
Establish care priorities, determine outcomes (goals), select interventions to accomplish expected outcomes, and develop a plan of care.
Documentation tools
Nursing care plan, patient care guidelines, clinical pathway

Step 4
IMPLEMENTATION
Carry out planned interventions.
Documentation tools
Progress notes, flow sheets

Step 5
EVALUATION
Use objective data to assess outcome.
Documentation tool
Progress notes

danger a patient's health. For example, if you use "o.d." for "once per day," another nurse may misinterpret it as "oculus dexter" (right eye) and mistakenly instill medication into the patient's eye instead of giving it once per day.

Write clear, concise sentences

Avoid using a long word when a short word will do. Clearly identify the subject of the sentence. Don't be afraid to use "I," as in "I contacted the patient's family at 1300 hours, and I explained the change in his condition." Doing so differentiates your actions from those of the patient, practitioner, or another staff member.

Say what you mean

Many nurses were taught that nurses don't make diagnoses, so you may sometimes qualify your observations with such words as "appears" or "apparently" when describing symptoms. How-

ever, if you use these inexact qualifiers, anyone reading the patient's chart may conclude that you weren't sure what you were describing or doing. The best approach is to state clearly and succinctly what you see, hear, and do. Don't sound tentative.

Chart promptly

Do your charting as soon as possible after you make an observation or provide care because that's when you'll recollect the circumstances most clearly. If you leave your charting until the end of the shift, you may forget important details.

Bedside flow sheets facilitate charting throughout the shift. Some facilities also place progress notes at the bedside. Of course, bedside computers also allow you to document promptly. All records must be kept in a secure place to maintain confidentiality.

Abbreviations to avoid

To reduce the risk of medical errors, The Joint Commission has created an official "Do Not Use" list of abbreviations. In addition, The Joint Commission offers suggestions for other abbreviations and symbols to avoid.

OFFICIAL "DO NOT USE" LIST[1]

ABBREVIATION	POTENTIAL PROBLEM	USE INSTEAD
U (unit)	Mistaken for "O" (zero), the number "4" (four), or "cc"	Write "unit"
IU (International Unit)	Mistaken for IV (intravenous) or the number 10 (ten)	Write "International Unit"
Q.D., QD, q.d., qd (daily) Q.O.D., QOD, q.o.d., qod (every other day)	Mistaken for each other Period after the Q mistaken for "I" and the "O" mistaken for "I"	Write "daily" Write "every other day"
Trailing zero (X.0 mg)* Lack of leading zero (.X mg)	Decimal point is missed	Write X mg Write 0.X mg
MS	Can mean morphine sulfate or magnesium sulfate	Write "morphine sulfate"
MSO_4 and $MgSO_4$	Confused for one another	Write "magnesium sulfate"

1 Applies to all orders and all medication-related documentation that is handwritten (including free-text computer entry) or on pre-printed forms.
* Exception: A "trailing zero" may be used only where required to demonstrate the level of precision of the value being reported, such as for laboratory results, imaging studies that report size of lesions, or catheter/tube sizes. It may not be used in medication orders or other medication-related documentation.

ADDITIONAL ABBREVIATIONS, ACRONYMS, AND SYMBOLS
(For possible future inclusion in the Official "Do Not Use" List)

ABBREVIATION	POTENTIAL PROBLEM	USE INSTEAD
> (greater than) < (less than)	Misinterpreted as the number "7" (seven) or the letter "L" Confused for one another	Write "greater than" Write "less than"
Abbreviations for drug names	Misinterpreted due to similar abbreviations for multiple drugs	Write drug names in full
Apothecary units	Unfamiliar to many practitioners Confused with metric units	Use metric units

Abbreviations to avoid *(continued)*

ABBREVIATION	POTENTIAL PROBLEM	USE INSTEAD
@	Mistaken for the number "2" (two)	Write "at"
cc	Mistaken for U (units) when poorly written	Write "ml" or "milliliters"
μg	Mistaken for mg (milligrams) resulting in one thousandfold overdose	Write "mcg" or "micrograms"

© The Joint Commission, 2006. Reprinted with permission.

If bedside flow sheets or computers aren't available, consider making notes on worksheets or pads that you keep in your pocket. Jot down key phrases and times; then transcribe the information into the chart later. Use these notes as a reminder, not as part of the medical record.

Note the time
Be specific about times in the chart. In particular, note the exact time of all sudden or significant changes in the patient's condition, significant events, and nursing actions. Avoid block charting such as "0700 to 1500." This sounds vague and implies inattention to the patient.

Chart in chronological order
Most assessments and observations are useful only as part of a pattern of assessments and observations. When isolated, most assessments tell us very little; in chronological order, they reveal a pattern of improvement or deterioration.

If you take the time to note your observations and assessments when you make them, they'll be recorded in chronological order. Too often, nurses wait until the end of the shift, then record groups of assessments that omit important variations.

Document accurately and completely
Record the facts, not opinions or assumptions. Although you don't need to chart routine tasks, such as changing bed linens, you do need to chart all relevant information relating to patient care and reflecting the nursing process.

Document objectively
Record exactly what you see, hear, and do. When you record a patient's statement, use his exact words. Avoid making subjective statements such as "Patient's level of cooperation has deteriorated since yesterday." Instead, include the

Smarter charting

Watch your charting language

At times, some of us may speak and write in a vague or judgmental manner without being aware of it. However, when you're charting, you should conscientiously avoid including ambiguous statements and subjective judgments.

AMBIGUOUS TIME PERIODS

"Mrs. Brown asks for pain medication *every so often*." How would you interpret "every so often"—once an hour, once per shift, or once per day? Although you can't time each and every interaction or occurrence precisely, you should document time relationships when appropriate. In this case, for example, you might chart, "Mrs. Brown asked for pain medication at 0800 and again at 1300."

AMBIGUOUS QUANTITIES

"A *large amount* of bloody drainage drained from the nasogastric tube" could mean 75 ml of fluid to you, 150 ml to the next nurse. Chart a specific measurement.

SUBJECTIVE JUDGMENTS

"Mr. Russo has a *good attitude*." How do you know? Support your judgment with an objective rationale—for example, "Mr. Russo states, 'I am going to learn insulin injection techniques before discharge.'"

Don't be afraid to give your impressions of the patient; just make sure that you support your observations—for example, "Leslie was frustrated, voicing dismay at being unable to walk around the room without help." Avoid using words such as "seems" or "appears"—they make you sound unsure of your observations.

---

facts that led you to this conclusion. For example, write "The patient stated, 'I don't want to learn how to inject insulin. I tried yesterday, but I'm not going to do it today.'" In some cases, you may include your conclusion, as long as you record the objective assessment data that supports it.

Remember to document only data you witness yourself or data from a reliable source—such as the patient or another nurse. When you include information reported by someone else, cite your source. (See *Watch your charting language*.)

Sign each entry

Legibly sign each entry you make in your progress notes with your first name or initial, full last name, and professional licensure (such as RN or LPN). If you find the last entry unsigned, immediately contact the nurse who made the entry and have her sign her name. If you can't locate her, simply write and sign your progress notes. The different times and handwriting on the chart should dispel confusion as to the author. (See *Signing nurses' notes*.)

Assessment

Your assessment of a patient begins when you first encounter him and continues throughout

ChartWizard

Signing nurses' notes

To discourage others from adding information to the nurses' notes, draw a line through any blank spaces and sign your name at the far right of the column.

1/5/07	1200	Will continue plan and request enterostomal therapist to assess patient's knowledge and acceptance of colostomy on the 2nd postop day. ——————————— Nora Martin, RN

If you don't have enough room to sign your name after the last word of your entry, draw a line from the last word to the end of the line. Then go to the next line and draw a line from the left margin toward the right margin, leaving room to sign your name on the far right side.

1/5/07	0900	Pt.'s respiratory status markedly improved after diuretic and O_2 therapy. Continue to monitor ABGs, urine output, weight, and breath sounds. Continue diuretic therapy as prescribed. ——————— ————————————— Nora Martin, RN

If you want to record a lot of information but think you'll run out of room on the page, leave space at the bottom of the page to write "Continued on next page," and add your signature. Start the next page with "Continued from previous page." Then finish your notes and sign the second page as usual.

		Medication effective. Patient drowsy and (continued on next page) ——— Nora Martin, RN

1/5/07	1500	(continued from previous page) relaxed. States that pain is now 2 on a scale of 1 to 10. ——————— Nora Martin, RN

his hospitalization as you obtain more information about his changing condition. The first step of the nursing process, assessment, includes collecting relevant information from various sources and analyzing it to form a complete picture of your patient.

As you obtain assessment information, you need to document it accurately for several reasons. First of all, accurately recorded assessment information helps guide you through the rest of the nursing process. Using reliable assessment documentation, you can formulate nursing diagnoses, create patient problem lists, and write nursing care plans. Properly documented assessment information also serves as a vital communication tool for other health care team members, forming a baseline from which to evaluate a patient's progress.

You also need to document your assessments accurately to meet the requirements of The Joint Commission and other regulatory agencies. Good documentation provides a means of indicating that quality care has been given. Peer review organizations and other quality assurance reviewers often look to the nursing assessment data as proof of quality care. Finally, in case of litigation, your record of your assessments can be used as evidence in court.

Initial assessment

You'll perform your initial assessment when you first meet a patient. Before getting started, consider two questions:
▶ Which information will be most relevant for this patient?
▶ How much time do I have to gather the information?

Your answers will help you collect meaningful information during your assessment. This, in turn, makes comprehensive, goal-directed nursing interventions possible.

COLLECTING RELEVANT INFORMATION
Your initial assessment of a patient may begin with his signs and symptoms, chief complaint, or medical diagnosis. It also may focus on the type of care he received in another unit, such as the intensive care unit (ICU) or the emergency department (ED).

Start by finding out some basic information: Why has the patient sought health care? What are his immediate problems? Are these problems life-threatening? Does a potential for injury exist? What other influences—such as advanced age, fear, cultural differences, or lack of understanding—might affect treatment outcomes? What medications does he take? Does he have a latex allergy? (See *Handling latex allergy.*)

COMPLYING WITH THE TIME FRAME
Your time limit for completing the initial assessment depends on the policy of your health care facility. The Joint Commission requires facilities to establish an assessment time frame for each type of patient they serve. However, a registered nurse must complete a nursing assessment within 24 hours of admission. Typically, depending on the unit where you work, the time frame for starting the first assessment may range from 15 minutes to 8 hours. On medical-surgical units, for example, the initial assessment should usually be completed within 1 hour of the patient's arrival on the unit.

Because many facilities offer a wide variety of care, they must establish individual assessment time frames for units or groups of units that share similar patient populations. Thus, a nurse on an ICU or a trauma emergency unit would have a much shorter time frame for completing an initial assessment than a nurse on an elective surgical unit.

CATEGORIZING ASSESSMENT DATA

When you collect and analyze assessment information, you need to distinguish between two types—subjective and objective. Subjective information represents the patient's perception of his problem. A patient's complaint of chest pain, for example, is subjective information. Objective information, on the other hand, is something you can observe and verify—such as a patient's blood pressure reading or laboratory test results. During your assessment, you'll gather both types of information from primary and secondary sources.

Subjective data

Subjective data collected during the patient history generally include the patient's chief complaint or concern, current health status, health history, family history, psychosocial history, medication history, activities of daily living (ADLs), and a review of body systems.

The patient's history, embodying his perception of his problems, is your most important source of assessment information. However, it's also subjective, so you must interpret it carefully.

Suppose, for instance, that a patient complains of frequent stomach pain. To find out what he considers "frequent," ask if the pain occurs once per week, once per day, twice per day, or all day. To find out what he means by "stomach," have him point to the specific area affected. This also tells you if the pain is localized or generalized. To find out how he defines "pain," have him describe the sensation. Is it stabbing or dull, twisting or nagging? How does he rate its severity on a scale of 0 to 10?

When documenting subjective data, be sure to record it as such. Whenever possible, write

---

Handling latex allergy

Allergy to latex, a material derived from natural rubber, is a large and growing problem in the United States. Reactions range from mild dermatitis to anaphylactic shock. As part of the initial patient evaluation, you should ask each patient if he has an allergy to latex or natural rubber.

When caring for a patient with a known or suspected latex allergy, clearly document the allergy in the computer and Kardex, and document latex precautions in the body of the chart, including precautions you've taken to create a latex-safe environment for the patient. Also, place a "Latex allergy" label across the front of the patient's chart, place latex allergy signs over the patient's bed and at the door to the room, and apply a latex allergy identification bracelet to the patient's wrist.

Latex allergy policies may vary from one institution to another, so follow your facility's protocol. If your facility has a latex-free supply cart, be sure to document that it was placed in or outside the patient's room, according to your facility's protocol.

---

the patient's own words in quotation marks. Introduce patient statements with a phrase such as "Patient states." For instance, you would document the previous example like this: "Patient states, 'I have frequent stomach pain.' He describes pain as dull and nagging. Patient rates pain as 4 on a scale of 0 to 10. The pain occurs after eating, is relieved by antacids, and is located in the left lower quadrant."

If the patient uses unfamiliar words or phrases, such as slang words, ask him to define them. For clarity, record both the phrase and the patient's definition of it.

Objective data

Unlike subjective data, objective data involve no interpretation. If another practitioner were to make the same observations under the same circumstances, he would obtain the same information. That's why it's important to be specific and avoid using subjective descriptions, such as "large," "small," or "moderate," when documenting your findings.

Whenever possible, use measurements to record data clearly. Specify color, size, and location when appropriate. For instance, "small amount of abdominal wound drainage" could be more specifically described as "serosanguineous nonodorous abdominal wound drainage that completely saturated three 4″ × 4″ gauze pads."

Also, avoid interpreting the data and reflecting your opinion. For example, don't write "Patient is in shock." Instead, document the findings: "Pale skin, pulse rate of 140 beats/minuute, blood pressure of 90/60 mm Hg."

Sources of data

Usually, information gathered directly from the patient (primary source data) is the most valuable because it reflects his situation most accurately. Additional data about a patient can be obtained from secondary sources, including family members, friends, and other members of the health care team. Written records—past clinical records, transfer summaries, and personal documents such as a living will—also provide important information about the patient.

Information from secondary sources often gives you alternative viewpoints to the patient's. In addition, because of a patient's condition or age, secondary sources may be essential to establish a complete profile. For example, a child or a patient who is profoundly confused may be able to answer only the simplest questions.

Besides providing essential data, family members and friends give important indications of family dynamics, educational needs, and available support systems. Also, including people close to the patient helps alleviate their feelings of helplessness during the hospitalization. Remember to cite your source when documenting information obtained from someone other than the patient.

Performing the initial assessment

An initial assessment consists of your general observations, the health history, and the physical examination.

GENERAL OBSERVATIONS

You can obtain a wealth of information simply by observing the patient. These observations can begin as soon as you meet him. You may, for instance, observe him while taking him to his room or helping him change into a hospital gown.

Continue to make general observations during the interview and physical examination as well as throughout the patient's hospitalization. By looking critically at the patient, you can collect valuable information about his emotional state, immediate comfort level, mobility status, and general physical condition. (See *Observing the patient.*)

Keep your observations objective and don't draw conclusions. Just document the facts. Remember, initial conclusions are frequently wrong because they're based on too little evidence.

Suppose, for example, that your patient is a middle-aged man who is brought to the ED by ambulance after being found lying in a deserted alley. His clothes are soiled and torn, and he smells of urine and feces. He babbles inco-

Observing the patient

A patient's behavior and appearance can offer subtle clues about his health. Carefully observe him for unusual behavior or signs of illness. Use this mnemonic checklist—SOME TEAMS—to help you remember what to look for.

 Symmetry—Are his face and body symmetrical?

 Old—Does he look his age?

 Mental acuity—Is he alert, confused, agitated, or inattentive?

 Expression—Does he appear ill, in pain, or anxious?

 Trunk—Is he lean, stocky, obese, or barrel-chested?

 Extremities—Are his fingers clubbed? Does he have joint abnormalities or edema?

 Appearance—Is he clean and appropriately dressed?

 Movement—Are his posture, gait, and coordination normal? Does he move around in a normal fashion?

 Speech—Is his speech relaxed, clear, strong, understandable, and appropriate? Does it sound stressed?

herently, although obscenities are clearly discernible.

To document properly, you should record these facts, but you shouldn't conclude that the patient is intoxicated. He may have diabetes mellitus and be suffering from acute hypoglycemia.

HEALTH HISTORY

A guide to subsequent physical assessment, the health history organizes pertinent physiologic, psychological, cultural, spiritual, and psychosocial information. It consists of subjective data about the patient's current health status and provides clues that point to actual or potential health problems. It also reveals the patient's ability to comply with health care interventions and his expectations for treatment outcomes. Finally, the health history yields details about the patient's lifestyle, family relationships, and cultural influences—all of which may affect his health care needs.

Use the health history to identify patient problems that your nursing interventions can help resolve. Then formulate your nursing diagnoses and subsequent care plans based on these problems.

Preparing to take the health history

Obtain the patient's health history by interviewing him in a comfortable environment and recording his answers to your questions. If appropriate, also interview the patient's family members and close friends.

Before the interview, consider the patient's ability and readiness to participate. For example, if he's sedated or confused, hostile or angry, or experiencing pain or dyspnea, ask only the most essential questions. You can perform a more in-depth interview later, when his condition improves. In the meantime, secondary sources can often provide much of the needed information.

Try to alleviate as much of the patient's discomfort and anxiety as possible. Also, attempt to create a quiet, private environment. Avoid interruptions by arranging for another nurse to cover your other patients during the interview. Your efforts let your patient know that you're interested in what he tells you and that you respect the confidentiality of the information he shares.

Tell the patient how long the interview will last—usually from 15 to 30 minutes for a medical-surgical patient. Explain the purpose of the history, so he understands why you'll be asking him personal questions. Finally, be calm, relaxed, and unhurried. Your actions will convey to the patient the importance of the health history interview.

Conducting the interview

You'll need to show empathy, compassion, self-awareness, and objectivity to promote a trusting relationship with your patient—the first step toward a successful interview. To obtain a comprehensive health history, you'll also need to use a variety of interviewing techniques. Here are some examples:

Use general leads. Broad opening questions allow the patient to relate information that he deems essential. Asking such questions as "What brought you to the hospital?" or "What concerns do you have?" encourages the patient to discuss what's most important to him.

Restate information. To help clarify the patient's meaning, restate, or summarize, the essence of his comments. For instance, suppose a patient says, "I have pain after I eat," and you respond, "So, you have pain about three times per day." This might prompt the patient to reply, "Oh no, I eat only breakfast, and then the pain is so severe that I don't eat for the rest of the day."

Use reflection. Asking a question in a different way offers the patient an opportunity to reconsider his response. A patient might say, "I've told you everything about my home life." Using reflection, you might respond, "Do you have any other concerns about your situation after you leave the hospital?"

State the implied meaning. A patient may hint at difficulties or problems. By stating what he has left unspoken, you give him an opportunity to clarify his thoughts and accurately interpret the meaning of his statements. For example, a patient's remark, "I'm sure my wife is glad that I'm in the hospital," may imply several things. To clarify this statement, you might respond, "By saying your wife is glad, do you mean she has been concerned about your condition, or do you feel you've been a burden to her at home?"

Focus the discussion. Patients often stray from the topic at hand to relate other information they feel you should know. You need to get the conversation back on track without insulting the patient or making him feel that the information isn't important. To help him refocus the conversation, you might say, "That's very interesting, but first I'd like to get back to our discussion about your last hospitalization."

Ask open-ended questions. Questions that encourage the patient to express himself elicit more information than questions that call for a one-word response. If you ask, "Do you take your medications?" the patient may respond with a simple "Yes." But if you say, "Please explain how you take your medications," you might discover that the patient takes his antihypertensive pills sporadically because they make him feel dizzy.

Techniques to avoid

To avoid alienating the patient during the interview and thus hindering communication, don't use the following techniques:

Judgmental or threatening questions. A patient shouldn't have to justify his feelings or actions. Questions such as "Why did you do that?" or demanding statements such as "Explain your behavior" may be perceived as a threat or challenge. They force the patient to defend himself. Furthermore, when a patient doesn't have a specific answer to this type of question, he may invent an appropriate response merely to satisfy you.

Probing and persistent questions. This style of questioning can make the patient feel manipulated and defensive. Make only one or two attempts to obtain information about a particular subject. If the patient seems to be avoiding the topic or is reluctant to answer, reevaluate the relevance of the information. Respect his right to privacy.

Inappropriate language. Don't use technical terms or jargon when interviewing the patient. Questions such as "Do you take that med q.i.d. or p.r.n.?" can intimidate or alienate the patient and his family. Using unfamiliar language can make the patient feel that you're unwilling to share information about his condition or to converse on his level.

Advice. Giving advice implies that you know what's best for the patient. Instead, you should encourage the patient and family members to participate in health care decisions. If the patient asks for advice, inform him about available options and then help him explore his own opinions about them.

False reassurances. Statements such as "You'll be all right" or "Everything will work out fine" tend to devalue a person's feelings. By recognizing those feelings, you can open communication channels. Saying something such as "You seem worried or frightened" encourages the patient to speak candidly. Always try to be honest and sensitive. Even when a patient asks, "Am I going to die?" you can honestly state, "I don't know. Tell me what makes you ask that."

Timesaving measures

Although increased patient acuity and staff shortages sometimes make conducting a thor-

When interview time is limited

When you're pressed for time, the following tips will help you obtain a health history more quickly.

► Before the interview, fill in as much of the health history information as you can from secondary sources, such as admission forms, transfer summaries, and the medical history. This avoids duplication of effort and reduces interview time. If some of this information needs clarification, you can ask the patient to give you a fuller explanation. For instance, you might say something such as "You told Dr. Smith that you have periodic dizzy spells. Can you tell me more about those spells?"

► Check your facility's policy regarding who can gather assessment data. You may be able to have a nursing assistant collect routine information, such as allergies and past hospitalizations. Remember, however, that you must review the information and verify it, as necessary.

► Begin by introducing yourself and explaining the purpose of the health history. Ask about the patient's chief complaint and the reason for his hospitalization. Then, if the interview is interrupted, you'll have some initial information on which to base a care plan.

► Use your facility's nursing assessment documentation form only as a guide to organize information. Ask your patient only pertinent questions from the form.

► Take only brief notes during the interview to avoid interrupting the flow of conversation. Write a longer summation or expand on information as soon as possible after the interview. You can always go back to the patient if you need to clarify or verify information.

► Record your findings using concise, specific phrases and approved abbreviations.

ough patient interview difficult, certain strategies can help you make the most of the time you have without compromising quality. For example, in some cases, you can ask the patient to complete a questionnaire about his past and present health status instead of conducting a patient interview. Then you can quickly and easily document his health history by reviewing the information on the questionnaire. This method tends to be most successful in short procedure units and before admission for elective procedures. Unfortunately, although it saves time, this method doesn't give you an opportunity to develop a positive relationship with the patient. (See *When interview time is limited.*)

PHYSICAL EXAMINATION

Perform the physical examination by using the assessment techniques of inspection, palpation, percussion, and auscultation. During this phase of the assessment, you'll obtain objective data that may confirm or rule out suspicions raised during the health history interview. Your findings will enable you to plan care and start teaching your patient about his condition. For example, an elevated blood pressure reading tells you that a patient may need a sodium-restricted diet and, possibly, patient teaching on how to control hypertension.

The scope of the physical examination depends on the patient's condition, the clinical setting, and the policies and procedures established by your health care facility. A routine neurologic examination on a medical-surgical unit, for example, may include assessments of level of consciousness (LOC), orientation, muscle strength, and pupillary response. Abnormal findings would then call for you to perform a more in-depth assessment—an assessment that would be routine on a neurologic unit or ICU.

The major components of the physical examination include height, weight, vital signs, and a review of the major body systems. A routine review for an adult patient on a medical-surgical unit includes the following body systems:

Respiratory system

Note the rate, rhythm, and effort of respirations, and auscultate the lung fields. Inspect the lips, mucous membranes, and nail beds. Also inspect any sputum, noting color, consistency, and other characteristics.

Cardiovascular system

Auscultate for heart sounds. Note heart rate and rhythm. Document the color and temperature of the extremities, and assess the peripheral pulses. Also, check for edema. Inspect the neck veins, noting their appearance—for example, flat or distended.

Neurologic system

Inspect the patient's head for evidence of trauma. Then assess his LOC, noting his orientation to time, place, and person and his ability to follow commands. Also assess his pupillary reactions and cranial nerve function. Check his extremities for movement and sensation.

Eyes, ears, nose, and throat

Assess the patient's ability to see objects with or without corrective lenses as appropriate, and note the condition of these lenses. Also assess his ability to hear spoken words clearly, and note the effectiveness and condition of hearing aids, if applicable. Inspect the eyes and ears for discharge; the nasal mucous membranes for dryness, irritation, and the presence of blood; and the teeth for cleanliness.

If appropriate, note how well the patient's dentures fit. Observe the condition of the oral mucous membranes, and palpate the lymph nodes in the neck.

GI system

Auscultate for bowel sounds in all quadrants. Note any abdominal distention or ascites. Palpate the abdomen to assess for tenderness.

Musculoskeletal system

Assess the range of motion of major joints. Look for any swelling at the joints as well as for any contractures, muscular atrophy, or obvious deformity.

Genitourinary system

Check for any bladder distention or incontinence. If indicated, inspect the genitalia for rashes, edema, or deformity. (Inspection of the genitalia may be waived at the patient's request or if no dysfunction was reported during the interview.)

Reproductive system

If indicated, inspect the genitalia for sexual maturity. Also, obtain patient permission to perform a breast examination, if appropriate, noting any abnormalities.

Integumentary system

Note any sores, lesions, scars, wounds, pressure ulcers, rashes, bruises, or petechiae. Also note the patient's skin turgor.

Meeting The Joint Commission requirements

The Joint Commission requires that health care professionals in accredited facilities meet certain standards for performing patient assessments. By reviewing the documentation of patient assessments, The Joint Commission determines whether these standards have been met. (See chapter 3, Performance Improvement and Reimbursement, for more information on The Joint Commission requirements.)

One key Joint Commission requirement is that you obtain assessment information from the patient's family or friends when appropriate. When you interview someone close to the patient who isn't part of his family, make sure that you note the nature of the relationship and the length of time the person has known the patient. For instance, in your documentation, you might write something such as "Information supplied by Daniel Rosenberger, a friend who has lived with the patient for 3 years."

ASSESSMENT REQUIREMENTS

Current Joint Commission standards mandate that each patient's initial assessment include three key categories: physical, psychological, and social factors. The standards go on to state that the scope and intensity of any further assessments are based on the patient's diagnosis, the care setting, the patient's desire for care, and his response to previous care. If appropriate, the patient's nutritional status and functional status should be assessed as well. If the patient is receiving end-of-life care, spiritual and cultural factors that influence how the patient, family, and significant others perceive and express grief should also be explored. The patient's learning needs and discharge planning needs should be assessed early in the admission process.

Physical factors

Physical factors include physical examination findings from your review of the major body systems. All patients also should be assessed for pain.

Psychological factors

Psychological factors include the patient's fears, anxieties, and other concerns related to his hospitalization. To find out what support systems the patient has, you might ask something such as "How does being in the hospital affect your home situation?" or "How is your family coping while you're hospitalized?" A patient's concerns about these matters may impair his willingness or ability to comply with health care interventions.

Social factors

Social factors include family structure and the patient's role or roles within that structure. Questions regarding work status, income level, and socioeconomic concerns may also be included, as indicated. The patient's home environment also affects care needs during hospitalization and after discharge. Factors to ask about may include where he lives (whether it's a house or an apartment); whether he has adequate heat, ventilation, hot water, and bathroom facilities; how many flights of stairs he has to climb and whether the layout of his home poses any hazards; and whether his home is convenient to stores and practitioners' offices. In addition, ask if he uses equipment that isn't available in the hospital when he performs ADLs at home. Tailor your questions to his condition.

Nutritional status

Questions regarding food and fluid intake, use of nutritional supplements or vitamins (or both), elimination patterns, and any recent weight gain or loss are included. A registered dietitian should be consulted as warranted by the patient's needs or condition.

Functional status

Because a patient's ability to perform ADLs affects how well he complies with his treatment regimen both before and after discharge, you must assess his ability to eat, wash, dress, use the bathroom, turn in bed, get out of bed, and get around. At some health care facilities, you'll use a checklist to indicate if a patient can perform these tasks independently or if he needs partial or total assistance. The use of any assistive devices should be noted.

Learning needs

An early assessment of what the patient needs to know about his condition leads to effective patient teaching. During the initial assessment, evaluate your patient's knowledge of the disease process, self-care, diet, medications, lifestyle changes, treatment measures, and any limitations resulting from the disease or its treatment.

One way to evaluate your patient's educational needs is to ask open-ended questions such as "What do you know about the medicine you take?" His response will tell you if he understands and complies with his medication regimen or if he needs more teaching.

You should also assess factors that may hinder learning. These include the nature of the patient's illness or injury as well as his health beliefs, religious beliefs, educational level, sensory deficits (such as hearing difficulties), language barriers, stress level, age, and any pain or discomfort he may be experiencing.

Discharge planning needs

As with patient teaching, discharge planning should begin as soon as possible. You must identify the discharge planning needs of every patient—especially those who are most likely to require help after discharge.

Find out where the patient will go after discharge. Will follow-up care be accessible? Are community resources, such as visiting nurse services and Meals On Wheels, available where the patient lives? Answers to such questions will help you plan effectively for your patient's discharge.

Documenting the initial assessment

Depending on where you work, you may hear the initial assessment information referred to by any of several names, including the "nursing admission assessment" and the "nursing database." Some facilities have adopted initial assessment forms that include information gathered from different members of the health care team, such as physicians, nurses, advanced practitioners, social workers, physical or occupational therapists, nutritionists, and pastoral care workers. These forms may be called "integrated," "interdisciplinary," or "multidisciplinary" care team assessment forms. (See *Integrated admission database form,* pages 104 to 107.)

Documentation styles and formats vary, depending on the facility's policy and the patient population. Furthermore, health care facilities have different policies for documenting learning needs, discharge planning, and incomplete initial assessment data. You must be familiar with your facility's standards to document your initial assessment findings appropriately.

DOCUMENTATION STYLES

Initial assessment findings are documented in one of three basic styles: narrative notes, standardized open-ended style, and standardized closed-ended style. Many assessment forms use a combination of all three styles.

Narrative notes

Narrative notes consist of handwritten accounts in paragraph form, summarizing information ob-

(*Text continues on page 108.*)

ChartWizard

Integrated admission database form

Most health care facilities use a multidisciplinary admission form. The sample form below has spaces that can be filled in by the nurse, physician, and other health care providers.

Name _Beatrice Perry_
Medical Record Number _556705_
Address _2 Clayton Street Dallas, Texas_
Admission Date _2/26/07_   Time _1345_
Admitted per: _____ Ambulatory
  ✔ Stretcher _____ Wheelchair
T _97_ P _92_ R _24_ BP _98/52_
Ht. _5'2"_   Wt. _225 lb_
  (estimated (actual))
SECTION COMPLETED BY: _P. Lippman, CST_

ORIENTATION TO ROOM/UNIT POLICIES EXPLAINED
✔ Call light
✔ Bed oper.
✔ Phone
✔ Television
✔ Meals
___ Advance directive explained
___ Living will
___ Living will on chart
___ Valuables form completed
✔ Elec.
✔ Smoking
___ Side rails
✔ ID bracelet on
___ Visiting hours

TIME: _1350_

Name and phone numbers of two people to call if necessary:

Name	Relationship	Phone#
Mary Ryan	_daughter_	_665-2190_
Thomas Perry	_son_	_630-4785_

REASON FOR HOSPITALIZATION (patient quote:) _I go numb in my rt. arm and leg_
ANTICIPATED DATE OF DISCHARGE: _2/28/07_
PREVIOUS HOSPITALIZATIONS: SURGERY/ILLNESS
  TIA   DATE _1/15/07_

INITIAL PAIN ASSESSMENT
Does patient have complaint of or admitting diagnosis of pain? ___ Yes ✔ No   Intensity (0-10 scale) ____
Location: ☐ Head ☐ Chest ☐ Back ☐ Abdomen ☐ Upper extremity ☐ R ☐ L ☐ Lower extremity ☐ R ☐ L
  ☐ Other ____
Description: ☐ Constant ☐ Intermittent ☐ Sharp ☐ Stabbing ☐ Burning ☐ Other ____
Onset/Duration of pain ____   What aggravates/alleviates pain? ____
Impact of ADLs: ☐ Decreased activity/Self care   ☐ Decreased appetite/Nausea/Vomiting ☐ Other ____

HEALTH PROBLEM	Yes	No	?
Arthritis		✔	
Blood problem (anemia, sickle cell, clotting, bleeding)		✔	
Cancer		✔	
Diabetes	✔		
Eye problems (cataracts, glaucoma)		✔	
Heart problem		✔	
Liver problem		✔	
Hiatal hernia		✔	
High blood pressure	✔		
HIV/AIDS		✔	
Kidney problem		✔	
Comments:			

HEALTH PROBLEM	Yes	No	?
Lung problem ((emphysema,) asthma, bronchitis, TB, pneumonia, shortness of breath)	✔		
Stroke		✔	
Ulcers		✔	
Thyroid problem		✔	
Psychological disorder		✔	
Alcohol abuse		✔	
Drug abuse			
Drug(s) ____		✔	
Smoking	✔		
Other			

ALLERGIES: (circle (Drug)/Food/Dyes/Latex/Tape ☐ None known
Allergy: _Penicillin_   Reaction: _Rash_
Allergy: ____   Reaction: ____
Allergy: ____   Reaction: ____

Complete medication reconciliation form for all medications

Vaccines
☐ Influenza date: ____   ☐ Pneumonia date: ____
☑ Doesn't remember

ADVANCE DIRECTIVES: ☐ NA (Patient < 18 years old) ☐ Unable to Assess
Does the patent have an advance directive? ☑ Yes
☐ Refer to old records   ☑ Copy to current chart
☐ Patient/Family to obtain copy for record
☐ Patient to formulate another advance directive
☐ Substance as stated by patient: ____

☐ No
☐ Information given   ☐ Information declined
☐ Patient declines stating content
☐ Patient/Family declines to bring, and/or complete advance directive information
☐ Refer to Social Worker

Information received from:
☑ Patient ☐ Relative ____ ☐ Friend ____ ☐ Other ____

Section completed by:
Jill O'Brien, RN Date _2/26/07_ Time _1405_

Integrated admission database form (continued)

All assessment sections are to be completed
by a professional nurse. Date _2/26/07_

Patient name _Beatrice Perry_
Medical record number _556705_

GENERAL PHYSICAL APPEARANCE

✔ Clean _____ Disheveled

SKIN INTEGRITY: Indicate the location of any of the following on the chart to the right using the designated letter: a = rashes, b = lesions, c = significant bruises/abrasions, d = burns, e = pressure sores, f = recent scars, g = presence of tubes/appliances, h = other

Comments: _b: ischemic leg ulcer (2 cm – healing)_

CULTURAL/RELIGIOUS/SPIRITUAL

Religious Preference: _Lutheran_ ☐ NA

Would like to see:
☐ Hospital Chaplain/Representative
☑ Personal Religious Leader
   (Name) _Rev. William Lacy_
   (Phone #) _726-8039_
☐ No visits

Any cultural, spiritual or religious requests while in the hospital?
☑ No ☐ Yes Specify:_____

PRESSURE SORE POTENTIAL ASSESSMENT

PARAMETERS	0	1	2	3	Score
Mental status	(Alert)	Lethargic	Semi-comatose	Comatose	0
			Count these conditions as double		
Activity	Ambulatory	(Needs help)	Chairfast	Bedfast	1
Mobility	Full	(Limited)	Very limited	Immobile	1
Incontinence	(None)	Occasional	Usually of urine	Total of urine and feces	0
Oral nutrition intake	Good	(Fair)	Poor	None	1
Oral fluid intake	(Good)	Fair	Poor	None	0
Predisposing diseases (diabetes, neuropathies, vascular disease, anemias)	Absent	Slight	Moderate	(Severe)	6

Patients with scores of 10 or above should be considered at risk. **Total** 9

_b_ (label on body chart)

FALL-RISK

Impaired:
___ Sensory function   ___ Mental status   ✔ History of recent falls/dizziness/blackouts
___ Urinary/GI function   ___ General debility/weakness   (automatically designates patient as prone-to-fall)
___ Mobility function   ✔ Prone-to-fall risk (indicated on nursing Kardex ✔)

NEUROLOGICAL ASSESSMENT

___ Dizziness   ___ Syncope   ___ Headache   ___ Blurred vision
___ Recent seizure   ✔ Numbness/tingling location:_ Rt. arm and rt. leg_

LOC: ✔ Alert ___ Lethargic ___ Semi-comatose ___ Comatose
Mental Status: ✔ Oriented ___ Confused ___ Disoriented
Speech: ✔ Clear ___ Slurred ___ Garbled ___ Aphasic

CODE
Pupils (mm):
Pupil Reaction
+ Reactive
− Nonreactive
D Dilated
C Constricted
> Greater than
< Less than
= Equal
S Sluggish

Neurological Checklist

	Right Arm	Right Leg	R. Pupil	Pupil Reaction	Eyes Open	Best Verbal Response	Best Motor Response	Total
	Left Arm	Left Leg	L. Pupil					
	+2/+4	+2/+4	5/6	+	4	5	6	15

Coma Scale

Response	1	2	3	4	5	6
EYES OPEN	Never	To Sound	To Pain	Spontaneously		
VERBAL	None	Incomprehensible Sounds	Inappropriate Words	Confused Conversation	Oriented	
MOTOR	None	Extension	Flexion Abnormal	Flexion Withdrawal	Localizes Pain	Obeys commands

COMA SCALE CODE

+1: cannot move   +3: move against gravity
+2: cannot move against gravity   +4: move strongly against gravity

Comments: _numbness transient_   Signature: _T. Jones, MD_

(continued)

Integrated admission database form (continued)

Patient name _Beatrice Perry_
Medical record number _556705_

Date _2/26/07_

CARDIOVASCULAR

Skin color: ___ Normal ___ Flushed ___ Pale ✔ Cyanotic
Apical pulse: ___ Regular ✔ Irregular ___ Pacemaker: Type ___ Rate ___
Peripheral pulses: ✔ Present ___ Equal ✔ Weak ___ Absent
Comments: _bilat. weak lower extremities_
Specify: R ___ radial ___ pedal L ___ radial ___ pedal
Comments: ___
Edema: ___ No ✔ Yes _+1 bilat. pretibial_ Numbness: ___ No ✔ Yes Site: _Rt. arm and rt. leg_
Chest pain: ✔ No ___ Yes P ___ Q ___ R ___ S ___ T ___
Family cardiac history: ___ No ✔ Yes Telemetry Monitor: ___ No ✔ Yes Rhythm _normal sinus_
Comments: ___

RESPIRATORY

Respirations: ✔ Regular ___ Irregular ___ Shortness of breath ___ Dyspnea on exertion
O$_2$ use at home? ___ Yes ✔ No
Chest expansion: ✔ Symmetrical ___ Asymmetrical (explain: ___)
Breath sounds: ___ Clear ___ Crackles ___ Rhonchi ✔ Wheezing Location _bilat upper lobe, inspiratory_
Cough: None ✔ Nonproductive ___ Productive ___ Describe ___
Comments: _pulse oximetry 98% on 2 L; sleeps with 2 pillows_

GASTROINTESTINAL

Stool: ✔ Formed ___ Loose ___ Liquid ___ Mucus ___ Ostomy ___ Incontinent
Color: ✔ Brown ___ Black ___ Red tinged ___ Bloody

___ Diarrhea ___ Constipation
Abdomen: ✔ Soft ✔ Rigid ✔ Nontender ___ Tender ___ (Location)
Bowel sounds ✔ Present ___ Absent ___ Hypoactive ___ Hyperactive

Obese ✔
Thin ___
Emaciated ___
Nourished ___

*NUTRITION:
✔ Special Diet
1800 ADA
___ Tube feeding
___ Chewing problem
___ Swallowing problems
___ Nausea/vomiting
___ Poor appetite
___ Wt. loss/gain ___ lb

*Refer to dietitian if any ✔

GENITOURINARY/REPRODUCTIVE

Color of urine: ✔ Yellow ___ Amber ___ Pink/Red tinged ___ Brown ___ Orange ___ Clear ___ Cloudy
___ Ileo-conduit ___ Incontinent ___ Catheter in place ___ Frequency ___ Urgency
___ Difficulty in initiating stream ___ Pain ___ Burning ___ Oliguria ___ Anuria
___ Dialysis ___ Access site: ___ Date of last dialysis: ___
Comments: ___
Date of LMP _1980_ Date of last PAP _5/00_ Breast self-exam ___ Yes ✔ No
Use of contraceptives: ___ Yes (type ___) ___ No ✔ N/A
Vaginal discharge: ___ Yes (describe ___) ✔ No
Bleeding: ___ Yes (amount ___) ✔ No
Pregnancies: Pregnant ___ Yes ___ Weeks ___ Gravida ___ Para ✔ No
Date of last prostate exam ___ Testicular self-exam ___ Yes ___ No
Comments: ___

MUSCULOSKELETAL/MOBILITY

___ Ambulates independently ___ Full ROM ___ Limited ROM (explain: ___)
✔ Ambulates with assistance (explain: ___) ✔ cane ___ walker ___ crutches
___ Gait steady/unsteady ___ Mobility in bed (ability to turn self) ___
Musculoskeletal ___ Pain ___ Weakness ___ Contracture ___ Joint swelling ___ Arthritis/DJD ___ Osteoporosis
___ Paralysis ___ Deformity ___ Joint stiffness ___ Cast ___ Amputation ___ Joint replacement
Describe: ___
Comments: ___

REST/SLEEP PATTERNS

___ Use of sleeping aids ___ Sleeps _6_ hr/day
Comments: ___

Additional assessment comment: _On arrival, diaphoretic and Ⓛ hand tremors. Vital signs stable. glucose 56 mg/dl_
Orange juice and lunch given to patient. 2 hr postprandial glucose 204. Symptoms subsided with juice. Nutrition
and diabetes educator consulted. ——————————————————— _Jill O'Brien, RN_
MRI shows no cerebral lesions. Carotid doppler ultrasound pending. ——————— _B. Mayer MD_

Integrated admission database form (continued)

EDUCATION/DISCHARGE SECTION
Instructions: Assessment sections must be completed within 8 hours of admission. Discharge planning and summary must be completed by day of discharge.

Patient name _Beatrice Perry_
Medical record number _556705_

EDUCATIONAL ASSESSMENT

Yes	No	
✔		Patient understands current diagnosis
✔		Family/significant other understands diagnosis
✔		Patient able to read English
✔		Patient able to write English
✔		Patient able to communicate
	✔	Patient/family understands pre-hospital medication/treatment regimen

Yes	No	**Emotional factors:**
✔		Patient appears to be coping
✔		Family appears to be coping
	✔	Any suspicion of family violence
	✔	Any suspicion of family abuse
	✔	Any suspicion of family neglect

Comment: _diabetic teaching_

Language spoken, written, and read (other than English): _____
Interpreter services needed: ✔ No ___ Yes
Are there any barriers to learning (e.g., emotional, physical, cognitive)? _NO_
Religious or cultural practices that may alter care or teaching needs? ___ Yes ✔ No Describe: _____
Is pt/family motivated to learn? ✔ Yes ___ No Describe: _____

DISCHARGE ASSESSMENT

Living arrangements/caregiver (relationship): _lives alone_
Type of dwelling: ___ Apartment ✔ House ___ Nursing home ___ More than 1 floor? ✔ Yes ___ No Describe: _____
___ Boarding home ___ Other _____
Physical barriers in home: ✔ No ___ Yes (explain: _____
Access to follow-up medical care: ✔ Yes ___ No (explain: _____)
Ability to carry out ADL: ___ Self-care ✔ Partial assistance ___ Total assistance
Needs help with: ✔ Bathing ___ Feeding ___ Ambulation ___ Other _____
Anticipated discharge destination: ✔ Home ___ Rehab. ___ Nursing home ___ SNF ___ Boarding home
___ Other _____
Currently receiving services from a community agency? ___ Yes ✔ No
If yes, check which one ___ Visiting nurses ___ Meals on Wheels
Concerned about returning home? ___ Being alone ___ Financial problems ___ Homemaking ___ Meal prep.
___ Managing ADLs ___ Other _____

Assessment completed by: _J. O'Brien, RN_ Date _2/26/07_ Time _1430_
Assessment completed by: _B. Mayer, MD_ Date _2/26/07_ Time _1445_

DISCHARGE PLANNING

Resources notified	Name	Date	Time	Signature
Social worker				
Home care coordinator	M. Murphy, RN	2/28/07	0900	
Other_____				

Equipment/supplies needed: _stair chair_
Arranged for by: _M. Murphy, RN_ Date _2/28/07_ Time _0930_
Comment: _Daughter to stay with pt at home_

DISCHARGE SUMMARY

Alterations in patterns (If yes, explain.)	Yes	No	Explanation
Nutrition	✔		adherence to ADA diet regimen
Elimination		✔	
Self-care		✔	
Skin integrity		✔	
Mobility	✔		needs help with stairs
Comfort pain		✔	
Mental status/behavior		✔	
Vision/hearing/speech		✔	

Discharge instructions given (specify): _standard hosp. discharge instruction sheet_
Effects of illness on employment/lifestyle: _____
Central venous line removed: _N/A_ By whom: _____
Belongings sent with patient: ✔ clothes ✔ dentures ✔ eyeglasses ___ hearing aid ___ prosthesis ___ valuables
✔ prescriptions ✔ other _cane_
Follow-up medical supervision to be provided by: _Dr. Schneider_
✔ Patient/family instructed to call for follow-up appointment Discharge destination: _pt's home with daughter_
Section completed by: _C. Rafferty, RN_ Date _2/28/07_ Time _1130_

tained by general observation, interview, and physical examination.

Although narrative notes allow you to list your findings in order of importance, they also pose problems. In many cases, the notes mimic the medical model by focusing on a review of body systems. They're also time-consuming—both to write and to read. Plus, narrative notes require you to remember and record all significant information in a detailed, logical sequence—often an unrealistic goal in today's hectic world of health care. Finally, difficulty in interpreting handwriting can easily lead to misinterpretation of findings.

Narrative notes are most practical for independent practitioners. Within health care institutions, however, exclusive use of narrative notes wastes time and may jeopardize quality monitoring.

Standardized open-ended style

The typical "fill-in-the-blanks" assessment form comes with preprinted headings and questions. This form saves you time in a couple of ways. Information is categorized under specific headings, so you can easily record and retrieve it. And the form can be completed using partial phrases and approved abbreviations. (See *Documenting assessment on an open-ended form.*)

Unfortunately, however, open-ended forms don't always provide enough space or instructions to encourage thorough descriptions. Thus, under the heading *type of dwelling,* one nurse may write "apartment" whereas another may write "apartment in four-flight walk-up, without heat or hot water."

Nonspecific responses can lead to misinterpretation. For instance, a nurse may write that a patient performs a task "within normal limits." But unless normal limits have been defined, this notation is neither clear nor legally sound.

Standardized closed-ended style

Standardized closed-ended assessment forms provide preprinted headings, checklists, and questions with specific responses. You simply check off the appropriate response. (See *Documenting assessment on a closed-ended form,* page 110.)

In addition to saving time, the closed-ended form eliminates the problem of illegible handwriting and makes checking documented information easy. In addition, the form can be easily incorporated into most computerized systems.

This kind of form also clearly establishes the type and amount of information required by the health care facility. And even though the closed-ended forms usually use nonspecific terminology, such as "within normal limits" or "no alteration," guidelines clearly define these responses.

Closed-ended forms also have some disadvantages. For instance, many of them don't provide a place to record relevant information that doesn't fit the preprinted choices. In addition, the forms tend to be lengthy, especially when a facility's policy calls for recording in-depth physical assessment data.

DOCUMENTATION FORMATS

Historically, nursing assessment has followed a medical format, emphasizing the patient's initial symptoms and a comprehensive review of body systems. Although many health care facilities still use a medical format to organize their nursing assessment forms, some facilities have adopted formats that more readily reflect the nursing process.

Most facilities that use a nursing format for assessment base it on either human response patterns or functional health care patterns. Other documentation formats are modeled on specific conceptual frameworks based on published nursing theories.

ChartWizard

Documenting assessment on an open-ended form

At some health care facilities, you may use a standardized open-ended form to document initial assessment information. Below you'll find a portion of such a form.

Reason for hospitalization *"My blood sugar is high"*
Expected outcomes *By discharge, the patient and his family will understand the disease process of diabetes mellitus, demonstrate correct insulin administration techniques, and identify signs and symptoms of hyperglycemia and hypoglycemia.*

Last hospitalization
Date *3/01/05* Reason *high blood pressure*

Medical history *hypertension, diabetes mellitus*

Medications and allergies

Drug	Dose	Date and time of last dose	Patient's statement of drug's purpose
Humulin N	*30 units*	*2/10/07 0730*	*for sugar*
Humulin R	*5 units*	*2/10/07 0730*	*for sugar*
furosemide	*20 mg*	*2/10/07 1000*	*water pill*
atenolol	*50 mg*	*2/10/07 0800*	*for BP*

Allergy	Reaction
shellfish	*hives*

Human response patterns

The North American Nursing Diagnosis Association-International (NANDA-I), has developed a classification system for nursing diagnoses based on human response patterns. These patterns relate directly to actual or potential health problems, as indicated by assessment data.

Thus, when you use an assessment form organized by these patterns, you can easily establish appropriate diagnoses while you record assessment data—especially if a listing of diagnoses is included with the form. The main drawback is that these forms tend to be lengthy.

Functional health care patterns

Some health care facilities organize their assessment data according to functional health care patterns. Developed by Marjory Gordon, this system classifies nursing data according to the

ChartWizard

Documenting assessment on a closed-ended form

At some health care facilities, you may use a standardized closed-ended form to document initial assessment information. Below you'll find a portion of such a form.

SELF-CARE ABILITY

Activity	1	2	3	4	5	6
Bathing		✔				
Cleaning		✔				
Climbing stairs			✔			
Cooking	✔					
Dressing and grooming		✔				
Eating and drinking	✔					
Moving in bed	✔					
Shopping					✔	
Toileting			✔			
Transferring			✔			
Walking		✔				
Other home functions			✔			

Key
1 = Independent
2 = Requires assistive device
3 = Requires personal assistance
4 = Requires personal assistance and assistive device
5 = Dependent
6 = Experienced change in last week

Assistive devices
- ☑ Bedside commode
- ☐ Brace or splint
- ☐ Cane
- ☐ Crutches
- ☐ Feeding device
- ☐ Trapeze
- ☑ Walker
- ☐ Wheelchair
- ☐ Other
- ☐ None

Activity tolerance
- ☐ Normal
- ☑ Weakness
- ☐ Dizziness
- ☑ Exertional dyspnea
- ☐ Dyspnea at rest
- ☐ Angina
- ☐ Pain at rest
- ☐ Oxygen needed
- ☐ Intermittent claudication
- ☐ Unsteady gait
- ☐ Other

Rest pattern
Sleep habits
- ☑ Less than 8 hours
- ☐ 8 hours
- ☐ More than 8 hours
- ☐ Morning nap
- ☑ Afternoon nap

Sleep difficulties
- ☐ Insomnia
- ☑ Early awakening
- ☐ Unrefreshing sleep
- ☐ Nightmares
- ☐ None

patient's ability to function independently. Many nurses consider functional health care patterns easier to understand and remember than human response patterns.

Conceptual frameworks

At some health care facilities, assessment forms have been modeled on the nursing philosophies that the nursing departments follow. Some examples include Dorothea Orem's self-care model, Imogene King's theory of goal attainment, and Sister Callista Roy's adaptation model. Assessment forms based on these nursing philosophies reflect the individual theory's approach to nursing care.

DOCUMENTING LEARNING NEEDS

Most initial assessment forms have a separate section for documenting a patient's learning needs. When you reassess your patient's learning needs, you can document your findings in the progress notes, on an open-ended patient education flow sheet, or on a structured patient education flow sheet designed for a specific problem such as diabetes mellitus.

DOCUMENTING DISCHARGE PLANNING NEEDS

Effective discharge planning begins when you identify and document the patient's needs during the initial assessment. Depending on the policy at your health care facility, you'll record the patient's discharge needs on the initial assessment form (in a designated section), on a specially designed discharge planning form, in a separate section on the patient care card file, in the progress notes, or on a discharge planning flow sheet. (See *Documenting discharge planning needs,* page 112.)

DOCUMENTING INCOMPLETE INITIAL DATA

No matter which assessment tool you use, you may not always be able to obtain a complete health history during the initial assessment. For instance, the patient may be too ill to participate, and secondary sources may be unavailable.

When this occurs, base your initial assessment on your observations and physical examination of the patient. When documenting your findings, be sure to write a comment such as

"Unable to obtain complete data at this time." Otherwise, it might appear that you failed to perform a complete assessment.

Try to obtain missing information as soon as possible, either when the patient is able to provide the information or when family members or other secondary sources are available. Be sure to record how and when you obtained the missing data. Depending on your facility's policy, you may record the information on the progress notes, or you may return to the initial assessment form and add the new information along with the date and your signature. Both methods have advantages and disadvantages.

Adding to the initial assessment form makes it easy to retrieve the data when it's needed—either during the patient's hospitalization or after discharge for quality assurance. Putting the information into the nursing progress notes aids in the day-to-day communication with others who read the notes but makes it difficult to retrieve the data later.

Remember, when you add information to complete an initial assessment, be sure to revise your nursing care plan accordingly.

Ongoing assessment

Your assessment of a patient, of course, is a continuous process. Reassessment lets you evaluate the effectiveness of your nursing interventions and determine your patient's progress toward the desired outcomes. Effective documentation of your assessment findings facilitates communication with other health care practitioners, allowing you to plan the most appropriate patient care.

How often should you reassess a patient? That depends primarily on his condition. However, The Joint Commission requires that each patient be reassessed at appropriate intervals, as

ChartWizard

Documenting
discharge planning needs

How and where you document your discharge planning will depend on the policy at the health care facility where you work. Here's one way to document this information:

DISCHARGE PLANNING NEEDS

Occupation _Retired college professor_   **Language spoken** _English_

Patient lives with _Wife_

Self-care capabilities _Needs extensive assistance_

Assistance available

☐ Cooking   ☐ Cleaning   ☑ Shopping

☑ Dressing changes/treatments _Irrigate @ lower leg wound b.i.d. with 1/2 strength H_2O_2, fol-_
lowed by rinse with normal saline solution. Pack with 1/2" iodoform gauze. Apply dry sterile
dressing.

Medication administration routes

☑ P.O.   ☐ I.M.   ☐ Other: _____

☐ I.V.   ☐ Subcutaneous

Dwelling

☐ Apartment   ☑ Inside steps   ☑ Bathrooms (number) _2_

☑ Private home   (number) _12_   (location) _one upstairs, one_

☐ Single room   ☑ Kitchen   _downstairs_

☐ Institution   (gas stove)   ☑ Telephones (number) _1_

☐ Elevator   electric stove   (location) _kitchen_

☑ Outside steps   wood stove

(number) _6_   ☐ other _____

Transportation

☐ Drives own car   ☐ Takes public trans-   ☑ Relies on family member or friend

     portation   Name: _____

     Phone: _____

After discharge, patient will be:

☐ Home alone   ☑ Home with family   ☐ Other: _____

Patient has had help from:

☑ Visiting nurse   ☑ Housekeeper   ☑ Other: _social worker_

Anticipated needs _Nurse for dressing changes, transportation for groceries, etc._

Social service requests _VNA_

Date contacted _2/16/07_   **Reason** _Contacted VNA for dressing changes and transportation needs._

designated by the institution's policy. You need to be aware of your facility's policy on reassessing patients and plan your care accordingly. (See *The Joint Commission reassessment guidelines*.)

PLANNED REASSESSMENT

A planned reassessment provides the routine data you need to evaluate a patient on a daily basis. On a medical-surgical unit, this may include reviewing the patient's mental status, respiratory status, vital signs, skin integrity, self-care capabilities, appetite, and fluid balance as well as psychosocial factors. You'll also need to regularly reassess environmental factors and his learning and discharge needs. Based on the patient's condition, your nursing care plan may specify other reassessments as well.

At some facilities, health care team members must meet every 2 or 3 days during a patient's hospital stay to discuss and update discharge plans. At these meetings, staff representatives from various departments—including nursing, medicine, social services, physical therapy, and dietary—evaluate the patient's progress toward established goals and revise the care plan as needed. Records of these meetings are maintained in the medical record to ensure communication with other team members.

UNPLANNED REASSESSMENT

An unplanned reassessment occurs whenever the patient's condition, circumstances, or diagnosis changes unexpectedly. For example, suppose a patient with no previous cardiac dysfunction suddenly develops severe chest pain and shortness of breath. You would perform a complete assessment and schedule future cardiac reassessments according to the revised care plan.

Or suppose you're caring for an elderly patient whose wife is his primary home caregiver. If his wife suddenly becomes incapacitated, you

---

The Joint Commission reassessment guidelines

- ▶ Reassessment occurs at regular intervals in the course of care, according to facility policy.
- ▶ Reassessment evaluates a patient's response to care.
- ▶ Significant change in a patient's condition requires reassessment.
- ▶ Significant change in a patient's diagnosis results in reassessment.

---

would need to perform an unplanned reassessment of the patient's discharge needs to accommodate this change.

Documenting ongoing assessment

You'll usually document ongoing assessment data on flow sheets or in narrative notes on the patient's progress report. Ideally, you should use flow sheets to document all routine assessment data and nursing interventions. That way, you can shorten the narrative notes to include only information regarding the patient's progress toward achieving desired outcomes as well as any unplanned assessments.

Flow sheets come in many varieties, including temperature graphs and intake and output forms. When used to record routine assessment data, flow sheets are a quick and consistent way to highlight trends in the patient's condition. A flow sheet for documenting information about a patient's skin integrity, for instance, will clearly show the progression of any pressure ulcers or reddened areas.

Because flow sheets are legally accepted components of the patient's medical record, they must be documented correctly. Give yourself enough time to evaluate each piece of information on the flow sheet. And keep in mind that it must accurately reflect the patient's current clinical status.

In some cases, you'll find that recording only the information requested on a flow sheet may not be sufficient to give a complete picture of the patient's status. When this occurs, record additional information in the space provided on the flow sheet. If additional information isn't necessary, draw a line through the space. Doing so indicates that, in your judgment, further information isn't required. If your flow sheet doesn't have additional space, and you need to record more information, use the progress notes.

Nursing diagnosis and care plan

When you formulate nursing diagnoses and write a care plan for a patient, you're playing a key role in his recovery. To build a solid foundation for your care plan, you need to identify nursing diagnoses carefully. Then you must write a plan that not only fits your nursing diagnoses, but also fits your patient—taking into account his needs, age, developmental level, culture, strengths and weaknesses, and willingness and ability to take part in his care.

Your plan should help the patient reach his highest functional level with minimal risk and without new problems. If a complete recovery is unlikely or impossible, your care plan should help him cope physically and emotionally with his impaired or declining health. And, of course, you need to document all of this—carefully and completely.

That's a tall order, but part of this chapter will help you by explaining the nursing diagnosis and planning processes, and by showing you how to document them most effectively. The first section discusses how to formulate nursing diagnoses, the second step of the nursing process. The subsequent sections focus on the third step of the nursing process, planning, beginning with prioritizing diagnoses. Ranking the diagnoses will help you to address your patient's most urgent needs first.

Next comes a review of how to develop realistic expected outcomes—goals your patient should reach by or before discharge, so he can function as effectively as possible. In the following section, you'll learn how to choose the nursing interventions that will help your patient reach those expected outcomes.

The subsequent section explains how to write care plans, including how to use practice guidelines to make planning and documentation more efficient and how to document your patient teaching and discharge planning. The final section looks at case management, a comprehensive way of caring for a patient that attempts to meet both clinical and financial goals.

Formulating nursing diagnoses

Unlike a medical diagnosis, which focuses on the patient's pathophysiology or illness, a nursing diagnosis focuses on the patient's responses to illness. (See *Nursing diagnoses: Avoiding the pitfalls.*)

TYPES OF NURSING DIAGNOSES

Depending on the policy of your health care facility, you'll either use standardized diagnoses or formulate your own diagnoses.

Using standardized diagnoses

To make nursing diagnoses consistent, several organizations have developed standardized lists, which are used by a growing number of health care facilities. NANDA-I has developed the most widely accepted taxonomy of nursing diagnoses. This taxonomy, which has been revised several times, is known as the Taxonomy II. Its code structure consists of three levels: domains, classes, and diagnoses. This structure is compliant with recommendations concerning health care terminology codes set forth by the National Library of Medicine. NANDA-I publishes a classifications and definitions book for their diagnoses every other year. The 2007-2008 edition contains 187 diagnoses.

NANDA-I diagnoses are now contained within the NNN *Taxonomy of Nursing Practice,* which was published in 2003 and developed through the NNN Alliance. The Alliance is formed by NANDA-I, Nursing Interventions Classification (NIC), and the Nursing Outcomes Classification (NOC)—NNN—which contribute their diagnoses, interventions, and outcomes (respectively) in standardized languages that are recognized by the American Nurses Association.

Diagnoses can also be categorized according to nursing models, such as the one developed by Marjory Gordon, in which nursing diagnoses correspond to functional health patterns. Other ways of categorizing diagnoses—for instance, according to Orem's self-care model—may also be used. Or your health care facility or unit can establish its own list of nursing diagnoses, categorizing them according to medical diagnoses and surgical procedures, for example.

No accrediting organization requires the use of standardized diagnoses. By using nationally accepted nursing diagnoses such as the NANDA-I taxonomy, however, health care facili-

---

Nursing diagnoses: Avoiding the pitfalls

To avoid making common mistakes when formulating your nursing diagnoses, follow these guidelines.

USE NURSING DIAGNOSES
Don't use medical diagnoses or interventions. Terms such as angioplasty and coronary artery disease belong in a medical diagnosis—not in a nursing diagnosis.

USE ALL RELEVANT ASSESSMENT DATA
If you focus only on the physical assessment, for instance, you might miss psychosocial or cultural information relevant to your diagnoses.

TAKE YOUR TIME
Take enough time to analyze the assessment data. If you rush, you might easily miss something important.

INTERPRET THE ASSESSMENT DATA ACCURATELY
Make sure that you follow established norms, professional standards, and interdisciplinary expectations in interpreting the assessment data. In addition, don't permit your biases to interfere with your interpretation of information.

For instance, don't assume your patient is exaggerating if he states that he feels pain during what you would consider a painless procedure. If possible, have the patient verify your interpretation.

KEEP DATA UP-TO-DATE
Don't stop assessing and updating your diagnoses after the initial examination. As the patient's condition changes, so should your evaluation.

ties help establish a common language for nursing diagnoses—making communication easier and diagnoses more precise.

Formulating your own nursing diagnoses

Developing your own diagnoses takes more effort than using standardized ones. Even so, some nurses prefer this approach because they find the standardized diagnoses incomplete or their language overly formal or abstract. Such an approach can also help you characterize a problem that standardized diagnoses don't readily address.

DECIDING ON A DIAGNOSIS

Before developing or using nursing diagnoses, you must evaluate relevant assessment data. You'll usually find this data on a standardized assessment form that groups related information into categories. Looking at the data in these groupings lets you determine which patient needs require nursing intervention. (See *Evaluating assessment data*.) Some assessment forms list relevant nursing diagnoses next to specific assessment findings. (See *Relating assessment data to nursing diagnoses*.)

Components of the diagnosis

Once you've examined the assessment data, you're ready to formulate your nursing diagnoses. A diagnosis usually has three components: the human response or problem, related factors, and signs and symptoms.

Human response or problem. The first part of the diagnosis, the human response, identifies an actual or a potential problem that can be affected by nursing care. For instance, if assessment information on a patient with osteoarthritis shows that he has trouble moving, you might turn to the NANDA-I taxonomy, look under the human response pattern of moving, and identify the problem as impaired physical mobility. If the NANDA-I taxonomy doesn't provide a label that fits a patient's problem or if your facility doesn't use standardized diagnoses, create your own label for the patient's condition.

Related factors. The second part of the nursing diagnosis identifies related factors. Such factors may precede, contribute to, or simply be associated with the human response. But no matter how they relate, these factors make your diagnosis more closely fit the particular patient

ChartWizard

Relating assessment data to nursing diagnoses

Some assessment forms group assessment information and relevant nursing diagnoses together so that you can immediately relate one to the other. This saves you from looking back through the form for assessment data when determining the nursing diagnosis. Here's a section of this type of form.

Patient *Michael Ramsey*   **Age** *72*
Medical record number *110676*
Medical diagnosis: *Heart failure*

ASSESSMENT FINDINGS

NURSING DIAGNOSES

Cardiopulmonary

Breath sounds	*crackles, bilateral bases*
Breathing pattern	☑ cough *dry* ☐ smoker
Dyspnea	☐ on exertion ☐ nocturnal
Sputum	color _____
	consistency _____
Heart sounds	*S₃ and S₄ present*
Peripheral pulses	*all peripheral pulses +1*
Edema	☑ Extremities *ankles*
	☐ Other _____
Cyanosis	☑ Extremities *nail beds*
	☑ Other *lips*

☑ Impaired gas exchange
☐ Ineffective airway clearance
☐ Impaired spontaneous ventilation
☑ Ineffective breathing pattern
☑ Decreased cardiac output
☐ Ineffective tissue perfusion (peripheral)
☐ Ineffective tissue perfusion (cardiopul-
monary)

Nutrition

Diet *2G Na, low cholesterol*

Appetite
☐ normal   ☐ increased   ☑ decreased
☐ vomiting   ☐ nausea

☑ Imbalanced nutrition: Less than body requirements
☐ Imbalanced nutrition: More than body
requirements
☐ Risk for imbalanced nutrition: More than
body requirements

---

and help you choose the most effective interventions.

For example, for your patient with osteoarthritis, you could write "Impaired physical mobility related to stiff knees" or "Impaired physical mobility related to depression." Depending on

these related factors, your interventions would probably differ.

When you can't determine the related factors, write "related to unknown etiology" and modify your diagnosis as you obtain more information. To save charting time, use the standard abbreviation "R/T" for "related to" when writing your nursing diagnoses.

Signs and symptoms. Finally, a complete nursing diagnosis includes the signs and symptoms that led you to the diagnosis—what NANDA-I calls the "defining characteristics." You'll draw these from the assessment data. Not all nurses include signs and symptoms in their diagnoses but, like related factors, they help tailor the nursing diagnosis to the particular patient.

To help keep the nursing diagnosis brief, choose only the key characteristics. You can list them after the human response and related factors. For instance, you might write "Disturbed thought processes R/T uncompensated perceptual or cognitive impairment. Defining characteristics: short attention span during conversation; minimal speech; confused, oriented to person."

Alternatively, you can join the signs and symptoms to the first part of the nursing diagnosis with the words "as evidenced by," abbreviated "AEB." For example, you would write "Excess fluid volume R/T increased sodium intake AEB edema, weight gain, shortness of breath, and an S_3."

Setting priorities

Once you've determined your nursing diagnoses, you'll move on to the third step in the nursing process, planning, in which you'll need to rank the diagnoses based on which problems require immediate attention. Whenever possible, you should include the patient in this process. Maslow's hierarchy of needs is generally accepted as the basis for setting priorities. (See *Maslow's hierarchy of needs.*)

Typically, the first nursing diagnosis will stem from the primary medical diagnosis or from the patient's chief complaint. This nursing diagnosis points out a threat to the patient's physical well-being—sometimes to his life. For a patient who has a primary medical diagnosis of heart failure, for instance, you would give first priority to the nursing diagnosis of "Decreased cardiac output R/T decreased contractility and altered heart rhythm."

Related nursing diagnoses come next. These define problems that pose less immediate threats to the patient's well-being. For instance, you may have also selected for the heart failure patient the nursing diagnosis of "Excess fluid volume R/T compromised regulatory mechanism."

Then you'll usually list nursing diagnoses that pertain to the patient's psychosocial, emotional, or spiritual needs. For the heart failure patient, a nursing diagnosis of "Anxiety R/T possible loss of employment" doesn't carry the same urgency as the previous two nursing diagnoses.

Even though a nursing diagnosis may have a lower priority, you shouldn't necessarily wait to intervene until you've resolved all the higher-priority problems. Helping the heart failure patient cope with anxiety about losing his job, for example, may speed his recovery because psychological problems can have an impact on physical well-being.

Developing expected outcomes

After you've established and ranked nursing diagnoses, you're ready to develop relevant expected outcomes. Based on the nursing diagnoses, expected outcomes are goals that the patient should reach as a result of planned nursing interventions. (Once achieved, an expected outcome is called a patient outcome.) You may find that one nursing diagnosis requires more than one expected outcome.

Maslow's hierarchy of needs

Abraham Maslow's hierarchy of needs, shown below, is a system for classifying human needs that may prove useful when establishing priorities for your patient's care, especially if he has several nursing diagnoses. According to Maslow, a person's lower-level physiologic needs must be met before higher-level needs—those less crucial to survival—can be addressed. In fact, higher-level needs may not become apparent until lower-level needs are at least partially met.

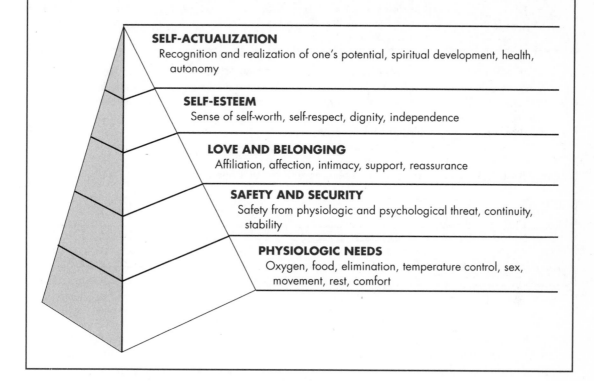

SELF-ACTUALIZATION
Recognition and realization of one's potential, spiritual development, health, autonomy

SELF-ESTEEM
Sense of self-worth, self-respect, dignity, independence

LOVE AND BELONGING
Affiliation, affection, intimacy, support, reassurance

SAFETY AND SECURITY
Safety from physiologic and psychological threat, continuity, stability

PHYSIOLOGIC NEEDS
Oxygen, food, elimination, temperature control, sex, movement, rest, comfort

An outcome can specify an improvement in the patient's ability to function, such as an increase in the distance he can walk, or an amelioration of a problem, such as a reduction of pain. Each outcome should call for the maximum realistic improvement for a particular patient.

Now linked to the NANDA-I nursing diagnoses, NOC is the standardized classification of patient outcomes. The most recent (third) edition, published in 2004, contains 330 outcomes grouped into 31 classes and 7 domains. These outcomes help establish the criteria for determining whether nursing interventions have been successful, and whether progress has been made in the patient's care.

WRITING OUTCOME STATEMENTS
Ideally, an outcome statement should include four components: the specific behavior that will demonstrate the patient has reached his goal,

Writing an outcome statement

An outcome statement should consist of four components:

B	**M**	**C**	**T**
BEHAVIOR A desired behavior for the patient. This behavior must be observable.	**MEASURE** Criteria for measuring the behavior. The criteria should specify how much, how long, how far, and so on.	**CONDITION** The conditions under which the behavior should occur.	**TIME** The time by which the behavior should occur.

As indicated, the two outcome statements below have these four components.

Limit sodium intake	2 g/day	using hospital menu	by 2/21/07
Eat	50% of all meals	unassisted	by 2/21/07

criteria for measuring the behavior, the conditions under which the behavior should occur, and the time by which the behavior should occur. (See *Writing an outcome statement.*)

When you're writing outcome statements, follow the guidelines listed below.

Make your statements specific

Use action verbs, such as *walks, demonstrates, consumes,* and *expresses.* A vague statement, such as "Patient improves nutritional intake," gives you and your colleagues little to go on. Instead, clearly state which behaviors you expect the patient to exhibit and when—for example, "Patient will consume 1,200 calories daily by 3/10/07."

Focus on the patient

Make sure that the outcome statement reflects the patient's behavior—not your intervention. The statement "Medication brings chest pain relief" doesn't say anything about the patient's behavior. A proper statement would be "Patient will express relief of chest pain within 1 hour of receiving medication."

Let the patient help you

A patient who takes part in developing outcome statements is more motivated to achieve his goals. His input—and the input of family members—can help you set realistic goals.

Take medical orders into account

Make sure that you don't write outcome statements that ignore or contradict medical orders. For example, before writing the outcome statement "Patient will ambulate 10 feet unassisted twice per day by 1/10/07," make sure that the medical orders don't call for more restricted activity such as bed rest.

Adapt the outcome to the circumstances

Consider the patient's coping ability, age, educational level, cultural influences, support systems, living conditions, and socioeconomic status. Also consider his anticipated length of stay when you're deciding on time limits for achieving goals. In some cases, you'll need to consider the health care setting itself. For instance, an outcome statement such as "Patient will ambulate outdoors with assistance for 20 minutes t.i.d. by 2/15/07" may be unrealistic in a large city hospital.

Change your statements as necessary

Sometimes, you may need to revise even the most carefully written outcome statements. For example, if the patient has trouble reaching his goal, you may have to choose a later target date or change the goal to one the patient can reach more easily.

Use shortcuts

You can save charting time by including only the essentials in your outcome statements. For example, in many cases, you can omit the words "Patient will" from your outcomes because "patient" is understood. Thus, rather than writing "Patient will demonstrate insulin self-administration by 1/18/07," you can simply write "Demonstrate insulin self-administration by 1/18/07."

Many facilities also use abbreviations for target dates, such as "HD2" for "hospital day 2" and "POD3" for "postoperative day 3."

Selecting interventions

Now you're ready to select interventions—nursing actions that you and your patient agree will help him reach the expected outcomes. Base these interventions on the second part of your nursing diagnosis, the related factors. With a nursing diagnosis of "Impaired physical mobility R/T arthritic morning stiffness," for example, you would select interventions that reduce or eliminate the patient's stiffness, such as mild stretching exercises. You'll need to write at least one intervention for each outcome statement.

As mentioned earlier, the NIC is the standardized classification for nursing interventions. The most recent (fourth) edition, published in 2004, contains 514 interventions grouped into 30 classes and 7 domains. Each NIC intervention has a label name, a definition, and a list of about 10 to 30 nursing activities. The label names and definitions themselves are standardized, but the activities aren't. Nurses may choose appropriate activities from these lists, or they may modify or add activities as long as they are consistent with the definition of that intervention.

You also can determine interventions in other ways. Start by considering ones that your patient or you have successfully tried before. Consider a patient who's having difficulty sleeping. He knows he sleeps better at home if he has a glass of warm milk at bedtime. That could work as an intervention for the expected outcome "Patient will sleep through the night without medication by 1/16/07."

You also can select interventions from standardized care plans, talk with your colleagues about interventions they have used successfully, or check nursing journals that discuss interventions for standardized nursing diagnoses.

WRITING INTERVENTION STATEMENTS
Your intervention statements must communicate your ideas clearly to other staff members. When writing your interventions, follow the guidelines listed below.

List assessment as an intervention
One of the first interventions in your care plan must include an assessment intervention to allow for reevaluation of the problem in the nursing diagnosis. For example, with a nursing diagnosis of excess fluid volume, one of the first interventions should be to assess breath sounds, since crackles can be a sign or complication of excess fluid volume.

Clearly state the necessary action
To ensure continuity of care, include as much specific detail as possible in your interventions. Note how and when to perform the intervention as well as any special instructions. An intervention such as "Promote comfort" doesn't tell another nurse what specific actions she should take. However, "Administer ordered analgesic ½ hr before dressing change" lets her know exactly what to do and when to do it.

Tailor the intervention to the patient
Keep in mind the patient's age, condition, developmental level, environment, and value system when writing your interventions. For instance, if your patient is a vegetarian, you shouldn't write an intervention that requires him to eat lean meat to gain extra protein for healing. Instead, your intervention could call for him to eat legumes and dairy products.

Keep the patient's safety in mind
Take into account the patient's physical and mental limitations so that your interventions don't worsen existing problems or create new ones. For example, if the patient needs the support of two nurses during ambulation, include that information in your intervention. If you're teaching a patient how to perform a new exercise, make sure that he's physically capable of doing it without hurting or straining himself.

Follow the rules of your health care facility
If your facility has a rule that only nurses may administer medications, you obviously wouldn't write an intervention calling for the patient to "administer hemorrhoidal suppositories as needed."

Take other health care activities into account
Sometimes, other necessary activities may interfere with interventions you want to use. For example, you may want your patient to get plenty of rest on a day he has several diagnostic tests scheduled. In this case, you would need to adjust your interventions.

Include available resources
To help carry out interventions effectively, be sure to make full use of your facility's resources and outside sources. For example, if your patient needs to learn about his cardiac problem, provide him with literature from your facility's education department, brochures and videotapes from the American Heart Association, and referrals to local support groups. Then write the intervention to reflect the use of these resources. In this example, you also would be sure to document appropriately all patient teaching and resources provided.

Writing your care plan

A good care plan is the blueprint for concise, meaningful charting. If you write a good care plan, your nurses' notes will practically write themselves. A good plan consists of the following:
▶ prioritized patient problems identified during the admission interview and hospitalization
▶ realistic, measurable expected outcomes and target dates
▶ nursing interventions that will help the patient or his family achieve these outcomes
▶ an evaluation of the patient's responses to intervention and progress toward outcome achievement.

To document your nursing diagnoses, expected outcomes, interventions, and evaluations, you can use either a traditional or a standardized care plan. You may also decide to use protocols along with one of these plans. In some cases, you can use protocols alone to demonstrate planned care. The care plan will also include your patient-teaching and discharge plans.

TYPES OF NURSING CARE PLANS

Two basic types of care plans exist: traditional and standardized. No matter which you use, your plan should cover all nursing care from admission to discharge and should be a permanent part of the patient's medical record. Be sure to write the care plan and put it into action as soon as possible after the initial assessment. Then you can revise and update it throughout the patient's hospitalization.

Traditional care plan

Also called the individually developed care plan, the traditional care plan is written from scratch for each patient. After analyzing the assessment data, you'll either write the plan or enter it into a computer. Although the traditional care plan is now rarely used because of the time required to write one for each patient, it's worthwhile to understand how it's developed.

The basic form can vary, depending on the needs of the health care facility or department. Most forms have four main columns: one for nursing diagnoses, another for expected outcomes, a third for interventions, and a fourth for outcome evaluation. Other columns allow you to enter the date you initiated the care plan, the target dates for expected outcomes, and the dates for review, revisions, and resolution. Most forms also have a place for you to sign or initial when you make an entry or a revision.

What you must include on these forms also varies. With shorter stays brought on by the advent of diagnosis-related groups (DRGs), most facilities require you to write only short-term outcomes that the patient should reach by or before discharge. However, some facilities—particularly long-term care facilities—also want you to include long-term outcomes that reflect the maximum functional level the patient can reach. Such facilities frequently use forms that provide separate places for short- and long-term outcomes. (See *Using a traditional care plan,* page 124.)

Standardized care plan

Developed to save documentation time and improve the quality of care, standardized care plans provide a series of standard interventions for patients with similar diagnoses. These standardized care plans can be computer-generated or preprinted, and become a part of the permanent patient record. Most standardized plans also supply root outcome statements. Some of these plans are classified by medical diagnoses or DRGs; others, by nursing diagnoses.

The early versions of standardized care plans made no allowances for differences in patient

ChartWizard

Using a traditional care plan

Here's an example of a traditional care plan. It shows how these forms are typically organized. Remember that a traditional plan is written from scratch for each patient.

DATE	NURSING DIAGNOSIS	EXPECTED OUTCOMES	INTERVENTIONS	OUTCOME EVALUATION (INITIALS AND DATE)
1/8/07	Decreased cardiac output R/T reduced stroke volume secondary to fluid volume overload	Lungs clear on auscultation by 1/10/07. BP will return to baseline by 1/10/07.	Monitor for signs and symptoms of hypoxemia, such as dyspnea, confusion, arrhythmias, restlessness, and cyanosis. Ensure adequate oxygenation by placing patient in semi-Fowler's position and administering supplemental O₂ as ordered. Monitor breath sounds q 4 hr. Administer cardiac medications as ordered and document pt's response, drugs' effectiveness, and any adverse reactions. Monitor and document heart rate and rhythm, heart sounds, and BP. Note the presence or absence of peripheral pulses. ———————— ———————— KK	

REVIEW DATES

Date	Signature	Initials
1/8/07	Karen Kramer, RN	KK

needs. But current versions allow you to customize the plan to fit your patient's specific needs. In fact, they require you to explain how you have individualized the care plan. To use such a plan, you'll usually fill in:

▶ related factors and signs and symptoms for a nursing diagnosis. For instance, the form will provide a root diagnosis such as "Acute pain R/T...." You might fill in "inflammation as exhibited by grimacing, expressions of pain."

▶ time limits for the outcomes. To a root outcome statement of "Perform postural drainage without assistance," you might add "for 15 minutes immediately upon awakening in the morning by 2/8/07."

▶ frequency of interventions. You can complete an intervention such as "Perform passive range-of-motion exercises" with "twice per day: 1 x in the morning and 1 x in the evening."

▶ specific instructions for interventions. For a standard intervention of "Elevate patient's head," you might specify "Before sleep, elevate the patient's head on three pillows."

When a patient has more than one diagnosis, the resulting combination of standardized care plans can be long and cumbersome; computerized documentation can help. With computerized plans, you can pull only what you need from each one and combine them to make one manageable plan. Some computer programs simply provide a checklist of interventions you can use to build your own plan.

Keep in mind that standardized plans usually include only essential information. However, most provide space for you to add further nursing diagnoses, expected outcomes, interventions, and evaluations. (See *Using a standardized care plan*, page 126.)

PRACTICE GUIDELINES

A newer documentation tool, practice guidelines (also referred to as protocols) give specific sequential instructions for treating patients with particular problems. Developed to help nurses manage equipment and provide specific treatments, practice guidelines are now also used to manage patients with specific nursing diagnoses. (See *Managing ineffective breathing pattern,* page 127.)

Practice guidelines offer several advantages. Because they spell out the steps to follow for a patient with a particular nursing diagnosis, they can help you provide thorough care and ensure that the patient receives consistent care from all caregivers. Many detailed practice guidelines even specify what to teach the patient and what to document, and they include a reference section that lets you quickly determine how up-to-date they are.

Some practice guidelines also spell out the role of other health care professionals, helping all team members coordinate their efforts. By supplying such comprehensive instruction, practice guidelines also help teach inexperienced staff members. Used in conjunction with other care plans or alone, practice guidelines can also save documentation time.

Using practice guidelines

Use the practice guidelines that best fit your patient. You'll probably use some practice guidelines, such as the generic one for pain, for many patients and others rarely. For example, the practice guideline *Risk for self-directed violence* applies mainly to patients in psychiatric settings. If you find that a practice guideline doesn't exist for a patient problem, you can help develop a new one.

ChartWizard

Using a standardized care plan

The standardized care plan below is for a patient with a nursing diagnosis of *Impaired tissue integrity*. To customize it to your patient, complete the diagnosis—including signs and symptoms—and fill in the expected outcomes. Also modify, add, or delete interventions as necessary.

Date _2/15/01_

Nursing diagnosis
Impaired tissue integrity related to arterial insufficiency

Target date _2/17/01_

Expected outcomes
Attains relief from immediate symptoms: _pain, ulcers, edema_
Voices intent to change aggravating behavior: _will stop smoking immediately_
Maintains collateral circulation: _palpable peripheral pulses, extremities warm and pink with good capillary refill_
Voices intent to follow specific management routines after discharge: _foot care guidelines, exercise regimen as specified by physical therapy department_

Date _2/15/01_

Interventions
• Provide foot care. Administer and monitor treatments according to facility protocols.
• Encourage adherence to an exercise regimen as tolerated.
• Educate the patient about risk factors and prevention of injury. Refer the patient to a stop-smoking program.
• Maintain adequate hydration. Monitor I/O _q 8h_
• To increase arterial blood supply to the extremities, elevate head of bed _6" to 8"_
• Additional interventions: _inspect skin integrity q 8h_

Date _____

Outcomes evaluation
Attained relief of immediate symptoms: _____
Voiced intent to change aggravating behavior: _____
Maintained collateral circulation: _____

Voiced intent to follow specific management routines after discharge:
_____

Managing ineffective breathing pattern

Below you'll find a portion of a practice guideline for a patient who has chronic obstructive pulmonary disease (COPD) and a nursing diagnosis of ineffective breathing pattern.

NURSING DIAGNOSIS AND PATIENT OUTCOME	IMPLEMENTATION	EVALUATION
Ineffective breathing pattern related to decreased lung compliance and air trapping By _3/10/07_ the patient will: ▶ demonstrate a respiratory rate within 5 breaths/minute of baseline ▶ maintain arterial blood gas (ABG) levels within acceptable ranges ▶ verbalize his understanding of the disease process, including its causes and risk factors ▶ demonstrate diaphragmatic pursed-lip breathing ▶ take all medication as prescribed ▶ use oxygen as prescribed.	▶ Monitor respiratory function. Auscultate for breath sounds, noting improvement or deterioration. ▶ Obtain ABG levels and pulmonary function tests as ordered. ▶ Explain lung anatomy and physiology, using illustrated teaching materials, if possible. ▶ Explain COPD, its physiologic effects, and its complications. ▶ Review the most common signs and symptoms associated with the disease: dyspnea, especially with exertion; fatigue; cough; occasional mucus production; weight loss; rapid heart rate; irregular pulse; and use of accessory muscles to help with breathing because of limited diaphragm function. ▶ Explain the purpose of diaphragmatic pursed-lip breathing for patients with COPD; demonstrate the correct technique and have the patient perform a return demonstration. ▶ If the patient smokes, provide information about smoking cessation groups in the community. ▶ Explain the importance of avoiding fumes, respiratory irritants, temperature extremes, and exposure to upper respiratory tract infections. ▶ Review the patient's medications and explain the rationale for their use, their dosages, and possible adverse effects. Advise him to report any adverse reactions to the practitioner immediately. ▶ For the patient receiving oxygen, explain the rationale for therapy and the safe use of equipment. Explain that the oxygen flow rate should never be increased above the prescribed target.	▶ Patient's respiratory rate remains within 5 breaths/minute of baseline. ▶ ABG levels remain within established limits. ▶ Patient verbalizes an understanding of his disease. ▶ Patient properly demonstrates diaphragmatic pursed-lip breathing. ▶ Patient takes all medication as prescribed. ▶ Patient demonstrates the appropriate use of oxygen as prescribed.

When you've selected a practice guideline, make sure that you tailor it to fit your patient's needs. Record any modifications you made on the patient's care plan.

Documenting practice guidelines

To document a practice guideline on a care plan, note in the interventions section that you'll follow the guideline—for instance, "Follow impaired gas exchange guideline." Or list the practice guidelines you plan to use on a flow sheet. Be sure to document any modifications you'll need to make.

After you intervene, simply write in your progress notes that you followed the practice guidelines, or check off the practice guidelines box on your flow sheet and initial it. The guidelines themselves usually remain at the nurses' station.

CORE MEASURES AND CARE BUNDLES
In an effort to measure and improve patient care, The Joint Commission developed a process to identify, test, specify, and implement a set of core performance measures known as Core Measures. There are currently five focus areas, or *measure sets*, each containing numerous measures. Participating hospitals are now required to collect data on three of these five measure sets: acute myocardial infarction (AMI), heart failure (HF), pneumonia (PN), pregnancy and related conditions (PRC), and surgical infection prevention (SIP). Several core performance measure sets are planned for future inclusion, such as pain management and children's asthma care.

Hospitals began collecting core measure data in July 2002. In 2004, the data became available for public viewing. The Joint Commission is working with other organizations to continue identifying additional core measure sets. One example is an agreement reached between The Joint Commission and the Centers for Medicare and Medicaid Services to align common performance measures, thereby easing the data collection burden on hospitals.

The Institute for Healthcare Improvement (IHI) is another organization dedicated to the improvement of patient care. IHI has initiated the term *bundle* to refer to a grouping of three

to five evidence-based, scientifically proven practices that grouped together, cause significantly improved patient care. The IHI has created several bundles, including the ventilator care bundle, sepsis bundle, and central line bundle.

The IHI has incorporated these bundles into the *100,000 Lives Campaign*, which aims to implement six changes in patient care that have been proven to prevent avoidable deaths. The IHI and many other participating organizations are asking thousands of hospitals in the American health care system to commit to this campaign by implementing the following six changes: (1) deploy rapid response teams; (2) deliver reliable, evidence-based care for acute myocardial infarction; (3) prevent adverse drug events; (4) prevent central line infections; (5) prevent surgical site infections; and (6) prevent ventilator-associated pneumonia.

CLINICAL PATHWAYS
One of the newest documentation tools is the clinical pathway, also known as a critical pathway or care map. (See *Take the clinical pathway*, pages 130 and 131.) This tool uses input from all disciplines involved in caring for a group of similar patients (usually those with the same diagnosis) and defines the care to be provided on each anticipated day of stay. For a more detailed explanation of clinical pathways, see "Case management," page 135.

PATIENT-TEACHING PLAN
You'll also need to include a patient-teaching plan as part of your care plan. You may include this on your main plan or write a separate plan. Today, many health care facilities require a separate plan because of the emphasis placed on patient teaching by accrediting and regulatory organizations. The need to control costs and the

current practice of discharging patients earlier also calls for more extensive teaching plans.

Besides identifying what the patient needs to learn and how he'll be taught, a teaching plan sets criteria for evaluating how well he learns. The plan also helps all the patient's educators coordinate their teaching. Plus, it serves as legal proof that the patient received appropriate instruction and satisfies the requirements of regulatory agencies such as The Joint Commission.

To make sure that your teaching plan does all that it should, carefully organize what the patient needs to learn and how you'll provide the instruction and measure the results. Work closely with other health care team members as well as with the patient and his family to make the plan's content realistic and attainable during his stay. Include provisions for follow-up teaching at home.

Also, keep your patient-teaching plan flexible. Take into account such variables as the patient's being unreceptive because of a poor night's sleep as well as your own daily time limits.

Components of the plan

Although the scope of each teaching plan differs, all should contain the same elements:
▶ patient-learning needs
▶ expected learning outcomes
▶ teaching content, organized from the simplest concepts to the most complex
▶ teaching methods and tools
▶ barriers to learning and readiness to learn.

Patient-learning needs. Identifying learning needs helps you decide which outcomes you should establish for your patient. Be sure to consider not only what you, the practitioner, and other health care team members want the patient to learn, but also what he wants to learn.

Expected learning outcomes. As with your other expected outcomes, expected learning outcomes should focus on the patient and be readily measurable.

Your patient's learning behaviors and the outcomes you develop fall into three categories:
▶ cognitive, relating to understanding
▶ psychomotor, covering manual skills
▶ affective, dealing with attitudes.

For a patient learning to give himself subcutaneous injections, identifying an injection site would be the cognitive outcome; giving the injection, the psychomotor outcome; and coping with the need for injections, the affective outcome. (See *Writing clear learning outcomes,* page 132.)

To help formulate precise, measurable outcomes, decide which evaluation techniques will best reveal the patient's progress. For cognitive learning, you might use questions and answers; for psychomotor learning, you might use return demonstration. To measure affective learning, which can be difficult because changes in attitudes develop slowly, you can use several evaluation techniques. For example, to determine whether a patient has overcome his anxiety about giving himself an injection, you can ask him if he still feels anxious, you can assess his willingness to perform the procedure, and you can observe whether he hesitates or shows other signs of stress while doing it.

Teaching content. Next, you'll need to select what to teach the patient to help him achieve the expected outcomes. As you make these decisions, be sure to include family members and other caregivers in your plan. Even if a patient will learn to care for himself, you can teach a family member how to provide physical and emotional support or how to serve as a

(Text continues on page 132.)

ChartWizard

Take the clinical pathway

At any point in a treatment course, a glance at the clinical pathway allows you to compare the patient's progress and your performance as a caregiver through the use of standards. Below is a sample pathway.

CLINICAL PATHWAY: COLON RESECTION WITHOUT COLOSTOMY

	Patient visit	Preoperative Day 1	Day 0 O.R. day	Postoperative Day 1
Assessments	History and physical with breast, rectal, and pelvic exam Nursing assessment	Nursing admission assessment	Nursing admission assessment on patients in holding area Postoperative review of systems assessment*	Review of systems assessment*
Consults	Social service consult Physical therapy consult	Notify referring physician of impending admission		
Labs and diagnostics	CBC PT/PTT Electrocardiogram Chest X-ray (CXR) Chemistry profile CT scan ABD w/wo contrast CT scan pelvis Urinalysis Barium enema & flexible sigmoidoscopy or colono-scopy Biopsy report	Type and screen for patients with hemoglobin (Hg) level <10	Type and screen for patients in holding area with Hg level <10	CBC
Interventions	Many or all of the above labs and diagnostics will have already been done. Check all results and fax to the surgeon's office.	Admit by 0800 Check for bowel prep orders Bowel preparation* Antiembolism stockings Incentive spirometry Ankle exercises* I.V. access* Routine vital signs (VS)* Pneumatic inflation boots	Shave and prepare in operating room NG tube maintenance.* Intake and output (I/O) VS per routine* Foley care* Incentive spirometry* Ankle exercises* I.V. site care* Head of bed (HOB) 30°* Safety measures* Wound care* Mouth care*	NG tube maintenance* I/O* VS per routine* Foley care* Incentive spirometry* Ankle exercises* I.V. site care* HOB 30°* Safety measures* Wound care* Mouth care* Antiembolism stockings
I.V.s		I.V. fluids, $D_5\frac{1}{2}$ NSS	I.V. fluids, D_5LR	I.V. fluids, D_5LR
Medication	Prescribe GoLYTELY or NuLYTELY 1000-1400 Neomycin @ 1400, 1500, and 2200 Erythromycin @ 1400, 1500, and 2200	GoLYTELY or NuLYTELY 1000-1400 Erythromycin @ 1400, 1500, and 2200 Neomycin @ 1400, 1500 and 2200	Preoperative antibiotics (ABX) in holding area Postoperative ABX × 2 doses PCA (basal rate 0.5 mg) subQ heparin	PCA (basal rate 0.5 mg) SubQ heparin
Diet/GI	Clear fluids	Clear fluids NPO after midnight	NPO/NG tube	NPO/NG tube
Activity			4 hours after surgery, ambulate with abdominal binder* D/C pneumatic inflation boots once patient ambulates	Ambulate t.i.d. with abdominal binder* May shower Physical therapy b.i.d.
KEY: *NSG activities **V = Variance** **N = No variance**	1. V/N 2. V/N 3. V/N	1. V/N 2. V/N 3. V/N	1. V/N 2. V/N 3. V/N	1. V/N 2. V/N 3. V/N
Signatures:	1. C. Molloy, RN 2. _____ 3. _____	1. M. Connel, RN 2. C. Roy, RN 3. J. Kane, RN	1. L. Singer, RN 2. J. Smith, RN 3. P. Joseph, RN	1. L. Singer, RN 2. J. Smith, RN 3. P. Joseph, RN

Take the clinical pathway (continued)

CLINICAL PATHWAY: COLON RESECTION WITHOUT COLOSTOMY

	Postoperative Day 2	Postoperative Day 3	Postoperative Day 4	Postoperative Day 5
Assessments	Review of systems assessment*	Review of systems assessment*	Review of systems assessment*	Review of systems assessment*
Consults		Dietary consult		Oncology consult if indicated (Dukes B2 or C or high-risk lesion (or to be done as outpatient)
Labs and diagnostics	Electrolyte 7 (EL-7) CXR	CBC EL-7	Pathology results on chart	CBC EL-7
Interventions	Discontinue NG tube if possible* (per guidelines) I/O* VS per routine* Discontinue Foley* Ambulating* Incentive spirometry* Ankle exercises* I.V. site care* HOB 30°* Safety measures* Wound care* Mouth care* Antiembolism stockings	I/O* VS per routine* Incentive spirometry* Ankle exercises* I.V. site care* Safety measures* Wound care* Antiembolism stockings	I/O* VS per routine* Incentive spirometry* Ankle exercises* I.V. site care* Safety measures* Wound care* Antiembolism stockings	Consider staple removal Replace with Steri-Strips Assess that patient has met discharge criteria*
I.V.s	I.V. fluids $D_5\frac{1}{2}$ NSS+ MVI	I.V. convert to saline lock	Continue saline lock	D/C saline lock
Medication	PCA (0.5 mg basal rate)	D/C PCA P.O. analgesia Resume routine home meds	P.O. analgesia Preoperative meds	P.O. analgesia Preoperative meds
Diet/GI	D/C NG tube per guidelines: (Clamp tube at 0800 if no N/V and residual <200 ml, D/C tube @ 1200)* (Check with doctor first)	Clears if + BM/flatus Advance to postoperative diet if tolerating clears (at least one tray of clears)*	House	House
Activity	Ambulate q.i.d. with abdominal binder* May shower Physical therapy b.i.d.	Ambulate at least q.i.d. with abdominal binder* May shower Physical therapy b.i.d.	Ambulate at least q.i.d. with abdominal binder* May shower Physical therapy b.i.d.	
Teaching	Reinforce preoperative teaching* Patient and family education p.r.n.* Re: family screening	Reinforce preoperative teaching* Patient and family education p.r.n.* Re: family screening Begin discharge teaching	Reinforce preoperative teaching* Patient and family education p.r.n.* Discharge teaching re: reportable s/s, follow-up and wound care*	Review all discharge instructions and Rx including* follow-up appointments: with surgeon within 3 weeks, with oncologist within 1 month if indicated
KEY: *NSG activities **V = Variance** **N = No variance**	1. 2. 3. Ⓝ Ⓝ Ⓝ	1. 2. 3. Ⓝ Ⓝ Ⓝ	1. 2. 3. Ⓝ Ⓝ Ⓝ	1. 2. 3. Ⓝ Ⓝ N
Signatures:	1. _A. McCarthy, RN_ 2. _R. Moyer, RN_ 3. _P. Drake, RN_	1. _A. McCarthy, RN_ 2. _R. Moyer, RN_ 3. _P. Drake, RN_	1. _L. Singer, RN_ 2. _J. Smith, RN_ 3. _P. Joseph, RN_	1. _L. Singer, RN_ 2. _J. Smith, RN_ 3.

Smarter charting

Writing clear learning outcomes

The patient's learning behaviors fall into three categories: cognitive, psychomotor, and affective. With these categories in mind, you can write clear, concise, expected learning outcomes. Remember, your outcomes should clarify what you're going to teach, indicate the behavior you expect to see, and set criteria for evaluating what the patient has learned.

Review the two sets of sample learning outcomes for a patient with chronic renal failure. Notice that the outcomes in the well-phrased set start with a precise action verb, confine themselves to one task, and describe measurable and observable learning. In contrast, the poorly phrased outcomes may encompass many tasks and describe learning that's difficult or even impossible to measure.

WELL-PHRASED LEARNING OUTCOMES	**POORLY PHRASED LEARNING OUTCOMES**
Cognitive domain The patient with chronic renal failure will be able to: ▶ state when to take each prescribed drug ▶ describe symptoms of elevated blood pressure ▶ list permitted and prohibited foods on his diet.	▶ know his medication schedule ▶ know when his blood pressure is elevated ▶ know his dietary restrictions.
Psychomotor domain The patient with chronic renal failure will be able to: ▶ take his blood pressure accurately, using a stethoscope and a sphygmomanometer ▶ read a thermometer correctly ▶ collect a urine specimen, using sterile technique.	▶ take his blood pressure ▶ use a thermometer ▶ bring in a urine specimen for laboratory studies.
Affective domain The patient with chronic renal failure will be able to: ▶ comply with dietary restrictions to maintain normal electrolyte values ▶ verbally express his feelings about adjustments to be made in the home environment ▶ keep scheduled practitioners' appointments.	▶ appreciate the relationship of diet to renal failure ▶ adjust successfully to limitations imposed by chronic renal failure ▶ understand the importance of seeing his practitioner.

source of information in case the patient forgets some aspect of his care.

Once you've decided what to teach, carefully organize the content. Start with the simplest concepts and work toward the more complex ones. You'll find this especially helpful for teaching a patient with little education or one who doesn't learn well by listening.

Teaching methods. You'll also need to select the appropriate teaching method for your patient. You can probably plan to do most of your teaching on a one-on-one basis. This method gives you a chance to learn about your patient, build a relationship with him, and tailor your teaching to his learning needs.

However, you can use other methods too—either in place of or in conjunction with one-on-

one teaching. For instance, you may want to incorporate demonstration, practice, and return demonstration in your teaching plan. Role playing can help involve your patient in learning, as can case studies, which call for him to evaluate how someone else with his disorder responds to different situations. Self-monitoring also involves the patient because he must assess his situation and determine which aspects of his environment or behavior need correction. If you have several patients who need similar instruction, you can also try group teaching or lecturing.

Teaching tools. Teaching tools—ranging from printed pamphlets to closed-circuit television programs—can help familiarize the patient with a specific topic.

When choosing your tools, focus on what will work best for the particular patient. For instance, if your patient likes to watch how something is done, he may respond best to a videotape of a procedure, a closed-circuit television demonstration, or a slide show. For a patient who prefers a hands-on approach, you might use a working model or let him handle the equipment he'll use. A computerized patient-teaching program may be best for a patient who likes to work interactively at his own pace. And some patients may simply want to read about a treatment or procedure.

Keep your patient's abilities and limitations in mind as you choose teaching tools. For instance, if you plan to provide written materials to reinforce your instructions, make sure that he can understand them. (The average adult has only a seventh-grade reading level.)

To get the tools you need, consult the staff-development instructors on your unit, the health care facility's librarian, or staff specialists. If your facility doesn't have what you need, you might try pharmaceutical and medical supply compa-

nies in your community. Don't overlook national associations and foundations such as the American Cancer Society. These organizations usually have large supplies of patient-teaching materials written specifically for laymen.

Barriers to learning and readiness to learn. Another important aspect of the teaching plan is assessing any barriers to learning and the patient's readiness to learn. The patient's physical condition may impede the learning process—he may be experiencing fatigue, pain, physical disability, communication problems, cognitive or sensory impairment, or lack of motivation. Initially the patient may be unwilling or unable to learn because he's overwhelmed by his illness, frightened, in denial, or all three. That's why it's important to assess your patient's response to teaching. If the patient isn't receptive to the information you're giving him, wait, if possible, until he's ready. In any event, always document the presence of any learning barriers as well as the patient's willingness to learn.

Documenting the patient-teaching plan

Several forms are available for documenting your patient-teaching plan. Many of them include the phases of the nursing process as they relate to patient education. (See *Documenting patient teaching,* page 134.) Health care facilities are also being encouraged to create systematic interdisciplinary approaches to patient teaching.

Patient-teaching plans come in two basic types that are similar to traditional and standardized care plans. The traditional type begins with the nursing diagnosis statement *Deficient knowledge* and an individualized *related-to* statement—for example, *Deficient knowledge related to low-sodium diet.* It provides the format and requires you to come up with the plan. When a patient

ChartWizard

Documenting patient teaching

Below, you'll find the first page of a patient-teaching flow sheet. Such flow sheets let you quickly and easily tailor your teaching plan to fit your patient's needs.

PATIENT-TEACHING FLOW SHEET

DIABETES MELLITUS

Problems affecting learning
- ☐ None
- ☑ Fatigue or pain
- ☐ Communication problem
- ☐ Cognitive or sensory impairment
- ☐ Physical disability
- ☐ Lack of motivation
- ☐ Other _____

LEARNING OUTCOMES	INITIAL TEACHING						REINFORCEMENT					
	Date	Time	Learner	Techniques and tools	Evaluation	Initials	Date	Time	Learner	Techniques and tools	Evaluation	Initials
Basic knowledge												
▪ Define diabetes mellitus (DM).	2/10/07	1000	P	E,W	S	JM	2/11/07	1000	P	E,W	S	JM
▪ List four symptoms of DM.	2/10/07	1000	P	E,W	S	JM	2/11/07	1000	P	E,W	S	JM
Medication												
▪ State the action of insulin and its effects on the body.	2/10/07	1000	P	E,W	S	JM						
▪ List the three major classifications of insulin. Give their onsets, peaks, and durations.	2/10/07	1000	P	E,W	S	JM						
▪ Demonstrate the ability to draw up insulin in a syringe and mix the correct amount.	2/10/07	1000	P	D,V	Dp	JM						

KEY

Learner
- P = patient
- S = spouse
- M = mother
- F = father
- D1 = daughter 1 _____
- D2 = daughter 2 _____
- S1 = son 1 _____
- S2 = son 2 _____
- O = other _____

Teaching techniques
- D = demonstration
- E = explanation
- R = role-playing

Teaching tools
- F = filmstrip
- P = physical model
- S = slide
- V = videotape
- W = written material

Evaluation
- S = states understanding
- D = demonstrates understanding
- Dp = demonstrates understanding with physical coaching
- Dv = demonstrates understanding with verbal coaching
- T = passes written test
- N = no indication of learning
- NE = not evaluated

requires extensive teaching, you may be able to use a standardized plan instead, checking off or dating steps as you complete them and adding or deleting information.

Depending on the plan's format, it may include space for problems that may hinder learning, comments and evaluations, and dates and signatures. You may also be instructed to include this information in the progress notes. Whichever plan you use becomes a permanent part of the medical record.

DISCHARGE PLANNING

The final part of the planning process, the discharge plan, has gained importance recently because of the trend toward shorter hospital stays. To help avert problems, start your discharge planning the day your patient is admitted—or sooner, for a planned admission.

Responsibility for discharge planning

In some health care facilities, the social services department carries the major responsibility for discharge planning. Larger organizations may hire a nurse discharge planner to facilitate home care planning. However, staff nurses still play a major role in preparing patients and caregivers to assume responsibility for ongoing care.

Even if you don't have the primary responsibility for discharge planning, you still play an important part. You and other health care team members need to coordinate your efforts with the discharge planners or social services department. Typically, you'll do this at a multidisciplinary discharge conference, in which team members evaluate the patient's discharge needs, discuss appropriate plans, and evaluate his progress.

Components of the plan

A discharge plan should note the anticipated length of stay and specify what the patient needs to learn, including:

▶ diet
▶ medications
▶ treatments
▶ physical activity limitations
▶ signs and symptoms to report to the physician
▶ follow-up medical care
▶ equipment
▶ appropriate community resources.

As part of your plan, make sure that the patient receives an instruction sheet to reinforce what he learns and what he needs to remember about follow-up care. The discharge plan should also spell out future care, including the setting for it, the patient's intended caregiver and support systems, actual or potential barriers to care, and any referrals.

Documenting the discharge plan

How you document the discharge plan will depend on the policy at your health care facility. Some policies require you to include your assessment of discharge needs on the initial assessment form, then document the discharge plan itself on a separate form. At many facilities, you must include the discharge plan as a component of the discharge summary. Some forms used for discharge planning allow several members of the health care team to include information.

Case management

A method of delivering health care that controls costs while still ensuring quality care, case management goes a step beyond planned care to managed care. It came into being after the federal government introduced the prospective payment system in 1983. Under this system, Medicare pays the facility based on the patient's diagnosis—not on his length of stay or the number or types of services he receives. Thus, the facility loses money if the patient has a lengthy stay or develops complications.

Such a system forces health care facilities to deliver cost-effective care—without compromising the quality of care. And the case management system proposes to help them do that by managing each patient's care to meet both clinical and financial goals.

YOUR ROLE IN CASE MANAGEMENT

If you become a case manager, your role will expand beyond giving nursing care. You'll learn to manage a closely controlled system of multidisciplinary care. You'll also take on responsibility for outcomes, length of stay, and use of resources throughout the patient's illness—not just during your shift.

HOW THE SYSTEM WORKS

When a patient is assigned a particular DRG, he's also assigned a case manager. (In some facilities, a patient isn't assigned a DRG until after discharge—in which case, you'll need to make an educated guess about which DRG will be assigned to him.) Each DRG case management plan has standard outcome criteria and includes medical and nursing interventions as well as interventions from other disciplines.

As the case manager for a patient, you'll discuss the outcomes with the patient and his family, using the established time line for the patient's DRG. This time line should cover all the processes that must occur in order for the patient to reach the expected outcome—including tests, procedures, and patient teaching—and the resources the patient will need, such as social services. If it doesn't, you'll adapt it as necessary to fit the patient's needs. If possible, you should do all this before the patient is even admitted, but you must complete these steps within the time limit set by your facility—usually 24 hours.

Once the patient is admitted, the multidisciplinary team evaluates his progress and suggests any necessary revisions, keeping in mind the need for continuity of care and the best use of resources. You'll document any variations in the time line, processes, or outcomes, along with the reasons for the changes. Plus, you'll keep a lookout for duplication of services and medical orders.

You must also start discharge planning, beginning an assessment of the patient's discharge needs at or before admission. You're also responsible for activating home health care services—including obtaining personnel and equipment—well before discharge.

TYPES OF CASE MANAGEMENT SYSTEMS

Several case management systems and various adaptations exist, and health care facilities continue to create new systems. But most facilities pattern their systems after the one developed at the New England Medical Center (NEMC), one of the first centers to use case management in an acute care setting. Facilities typically adapt this system to meet their own needs and philosophy of care.

TOOLS FOR CASE MANAGEMENT

Most facilities also pattern their case management tools after those of the NEMC system. Called the *case management plan* and the *clinical pathway,* they allow you to direct, evaluate, and revise patient progress and outcomes.

Case management plan

The basic tool of case management systems, the case management plan spells out the standardized care that a patient with a specific DRG should receive. The plan covers:

▶ nursing-related problems

▶ patient outcomes

▶ intermediate patient outcomes

▶ nursing interventions

▶ medical interventions

▶ target times.

Each subsection of the plan covers a care unit to which the patient may be admitted during his illness. For instance, a patient with a myocardial infarction may go to both the intensive care and medical-surgical units.

Clinical pathway

Because of the length of case management plans, you probably won't use them on a daily basis. Instead, you'll turn to an abbreviated form of the plan: the clinical pathway. The clinical pathway (also known as the health care map) covers only the key events that must occur in order for the patient to be discharged by the target date. Such events include consultations, diagnostic tests, physical activities the patient must perform, treatments, diet, medications, discharge planning, and patient teaching. (For more details, see chapter 6, Documentation in Acute Care.)

Once you've established a pathway, you must note any variances from it, grouping them by cause. Variances may result from the system, the caregivers, or a problem the patient develops, and they can be justifiable or not. For instance, you may have a patient who doesn't walk in the hall as scheduled. If he has a secondary infection that prevents him from walking, you'll list the variance as justifiable. However, if the patient simply prefers to stay in bed watching television, you'll need to list the variance as unjustifiable and take steps to correct the problem.

At shift report each day, you should review the clinical pathways with the other nurses. Before you go off duty, note any changes in the expected length of stay and point out critical events scheduled for the next shift to the nurses coming on duty. Also, discuss any variances that may have occurred during your shift.

DRAWBACKS OF CASE MANAGEMENT

The case management system usually works well for a patient with one primary diagnosis, no secondary diagnoses, and few complications. However, for some patients, you'll have trouble even establishing a time line. For example, you can't easily predict when treatment will succeed for a patient with a seizure disorder. For a patient with several variances, the expected course of treatment and length of stay will likely change, and documentation can become lengthy and complicated.

Implementation

Documenting nursing interventions has long been standard practice. However, documentation methods have changed dramatically over the years, mainly because of frustration with tedious traditional methods and the urgent economic need to streamline hospital operations. No longer must you always write lengthy narrative notes. In many cases, you can use flow sheets or refer to practice guidelines instead.

This section will help you keep pace with these changes by explaining how to implement and document your interventions, including patient teaching and the discharge summary.

Performing interventions

Implementing nursing interventions represents a crucial step in the nursing process. When you carry out your interventions, you're putting your carefully constructed care plan into action.

Once you've established and recorded your care plan, you'll begin to implement it. You'll find that your interventions fall into two general categories: interdependent and independent. Before performing either type, you'll need to make a brief reassessment.

NEED FOR REASSESSMENT

Just before performing a particular intervention, quickly reassess the patient to ensure that your care plan remains appropriate. For example, what if the plan calls for helping the patient walk every 2 hours throughout the day, but your reassessment reveals that he recently returned from a physical therapy session and feels fatigued? In this case, making the patient walk would be inappropriate—despite the care plan.

TYPES OF INTERVENTIONS

Interdependent interventions include those you perform in collaboration with other health care professionals to help achieve a patient outcome. For example, if the outcome calls for the patient to walk independently on level surfaces, you would support the physical therapist's regimen by reinforcing positioning and ambulation techniques between therapy sessions.

Interdependent interventions also include activities you perform at a practitioner's request to help implement the medical regimen. These activities include administering medications and performing invasive procedures, such as indwelling urinary catheter insertion and venipuncture.

Independent interventions are measures you take at your own discretion, independent of other health care team members. Such interven-

tions include instituting common comfort measures and teaching routine self-care techniques.

Documenting interventions

You need to record the fact that you performed an intervention, the time you performed it, the patient's response to it, and any additional interventions that you took based on his response (including your reasons for these additional interventions). Recording all this information makes your documentation outcome-oriented.

You can document interventions on graphic records, a patient care flow sheet that integrates all nurses' notes for a 1-day period, integrated or separate nurses' progress notes, and other specialized documentation forms, such as the medication administration record (MAR). Your facility's policies will dictate the exact style, format, and location of your documentation. You'll record interventions when you give routine care, observe changes in the patient's condition, provide emergency care, and administer medications. (See chapter 10, Documentation of Everyday Events, and chapter 12, Legally Perilous Charting Practices, for more information on charting specific interventions.)

ROUTINE CARE

For years, The Joint Commission has encouraged health care facilities to use flow sheets for documenting routine care measures. In response, many facilities have developed these forms for such measures as making basic assessments, giving wound care, and providing hygiene. In many facilities, you may also use flow sheets to document vital signs checks, I.V. monitoring, equipment checks, patient education, and discharge summaries. Some flow sheets are simple patient care checklists; others provide space for you to record specific care given. (See chapter 4, Documentation Systems, for more information on flow sheets and samples of different types.)

Because of their brevity, flow sheets make documenting and reviewing documented material quick and easy. Specifically, they allow you to evaluate patient trends at a glance. However, keep in mind that overusing flow sheets can lead to fragmented documentation that may obscure the patient's clinical picture.

CHANGES IN CONDITION

In your progress notes, you'll need to document any changes in your patient's condition. Suppose, for instance, that you observe a sudden increase in your patient's wound drainage. In a narrative format, your progress note describing this observation should look something like the sample note below.

2/5/07	1100	Left arm wound drainage has saturated six 4" x 4" gauze pads and one 4" x 8" dressing since last dressing check at 1000. Wound dimensions remain as on 2/4/07 note, but drainage now dark yellow and foul-smelling. Obtained specimens for culture and sensitivity testing and sent to the lab per impaired skin integrity practice guidelines. Cleaned wound with 0.9% sodium chloride solution. (See care plan for dressing change orders.) Pt. states, "My arm is really throbbing." Administered Darvocet-N and repositioned patient to semi-Fowler's position with left arm supported on pillow. Susan Gionet, Wound Care Specialist, notified of change and increase in drainage. ———————— Louise Davis, RN

This example refers to a practice guideline or standard of care for patients with a nursing diagnosis of impaired skin integrity. Because this protocol mandates cleaning with normal saline solution and culture and sensitivity testing for a patient with purulent wound drainage, no further orders or clarification are required.

The note also directs the reader to the patient's care plan for specific dressing change methods. The reader would also know to check the MAR for specific information about the pain medication given.

The note goes on to specify information about the other pain-relief measure implemented as well as the patient's comments about the pain's characteristics. It doesn't repeat information recorded elsewhere in the chart, so it's concise yet informative.

PATIENT TEACHING

With each patient, you'll need to implement the teaching plan you've created and evaluate its effectiveness. Of course, you'll also need to clearly and completely document your teaching sessions and the results. Doing so provides a permanent legal record of the extent and success of teaching. Thus, your documentation may serve as your defense against charges of insufficient patient care—even years later. Clear documentation also helps administrators gauge the overall worth of a specific patient-education program as well as helping you support your requests for improving patient care.

Direct benefits

Documenting exactly what you've taught the patient also saves time by preventing duplication of patient-teaching efforts by other staff members. By checking your notes, another nurse can determine precisely what has been covered and what she should teach next, without skipping essential information. This is important for patients with complicated needs who may receive care from several nurses.

Take the case of a hypertensive patient who requires instruction in several areas, including diet, medication, exercise, and self-care. Successful teaching hinges on a clear record of what has been taught by everyone involved in his care. When staff members communicate by documenting what they've taught and how well the patient has learned, the teaching plan can be evaluated and revised as needed, and the patient will get the care he needs.

You can also use your documentation to help motivate your patient. As appropriate, show him your record of his learning successes and encourage him to continue. Moreover, by recording the patient's response to your teaching and your assessment of his progress, you're gathering some of the data necessary to evaluate the effectiveness of your teaching, the patient's degree of knowledge or competency, and the appropriateness of his learning outcomes.

Documentation tools

In many facilities, you'll document patient teaching on preprinted forms that become part of the clinical record. Using these forms not only makes documentation quicker, but also ensures that it's complete. If your facility doesn't have a preprinted form, you might talk to your supervisor about developing one. In the meantime, write accurate, detailed narrative notes to document your patient teaching.

Whether you use a preprinted form or narrative notes, keep these tips in mind:
▶ Check your facility's policies and procedures regarding when, where, and how to document your teaching.
▶ Each shift, ask yourself these questions: "What part of the teaching plan did I complete?" and "What other teaching have I given this patient or his family members?" Then document your answers.
▶ Make sure that your documentation indicates that the patient's ongoing educational needs are being met.
▶ Before discharge, document the patient's remaining learning needs.

PATIENT DISCHARGE
The Joint Commission requirements specify that when preparing a patient for discharge, you must document your assessment of his continuing care needs as well as referrals for such care. To facilitate this documentation (and to save charting time), many facilities have developed forms that combine discharge summaries and patient instructions. (See *Discharge summaries.*)

This documentation tool combines all the essential information required on a discharge summary as well as the instructions given to the patient. Typically, you'll keep one copy of the form in the medical record and give one copy to the patient. The form is usually signed by the patient or authorized representative, as well as the discharging nurse and practitioner.

Of course, not all facilities use these forms; some still require a narrative discharge summary. If you must use this type of documentation, be sure to include the following information:
▶ patient's status on admission and discharge
▶ significant highlights of the hospitalization
▶ outcomes of your interventions
▶ resolved and unresolved patient problems, continuing care needs for unresolved problems, and specific referrals for continuing care
▶ instructions given to the patient or family member about treatments, activity, diet, refer-

ChartWizard

Discharge summaries

By combining the patient's discharge summary with instructions for care after discharge, you can fulfill two requirements with a single form. When using this documentation method, be sure to give one copy to the patient and keep one for the medical record.

DISCHARGE INSTRUCTIONS

1. **Summary** _Tara Nicholas is a 55-year-old woman admitted with complaints of severe headache and diagnosed with hypertensive crisis._
Treatment: Nitroprusside gtt for 24 hours
Started Lopressor for hypertension
Recommendation: Lose 10–15 lbs
Follow low-sodium, low-cholesterol diet

2. **Allergies** _penicillin_

3. **Medications (drug, dose time)** _Lopressor 25 mg at 6am and 6pm. Temazepam 15 mg at 10pm. Medication list given to patient, instructed to bring to each visit._

4. **Diet** _Low-sodium, low-cholesterol_

5. **Activity** _As tolerated_

6. **Discharged to** _Home_

7. **If questions arise, contact Dr.** _James Pritchett_   **Telephone No.** _525-1448_

8. **Special instructions**

9. **Return visit Dr.** _Pritchett_   **Location** _Health Care Clinic_
   On Date _2/19/07_   **Time** _8:45 am_

Tara Nicholas	_Joann Phillips, RN_	_JE PRITCHETT MD_
Signature of patient for receipt of instructions from practitioners	**Signature of registered nurse reviewing discharge instructions**	**Signature of practitioner giving instructions**

---

rals, and follow-up appointments as well as any other special instructions

▶ a complete list of the patient's medications. According to the most recent Joint Commission Patient Safety Goals, an accurate, updated, and complete list of medications must be given to the patient at discharge. An accurate medication list for that patient must then be communicated to the next care provider, whether that care provider is within or outside the organization.

Evaluation

The current emphasis on evaluating your interventions has changed documentation. Traditional documentation methods didn't always reflect the end results of nursing care. Today, however, your progress notes must include an assessment of your patient's progress toward the expected outcomes you established in the care plan.

This new method, called *outcomes and evaluation documentation,* focuses on the patient's response to nursing care and thus enables the nurse to provide high-quality, cost-effective care. It's now replacing narrative charting and lengthy, handwritten care plans. (See *Writing clear evaluation statements.*)

The belief that hands-on care is more important than documentation is one reason why nurses often focus more on nursing interventions than on documenting patient responses. Outcomes and evaluation documentation forces nurses to focus on patient responses. When you evaluate the results of your interventions, you help ensure that your plan is working.

Evaluation of care gives the nurse a chance to:
▶ determine if her original assessment findings still apply
▶ uncover complications
▶ analyze patterns or trends in the patient's care and his responses to it
▶ assess the patient's response to all aspects of care, including medications, changes in diet or activity, procedures, unusual incidents or problems, and teaching
▶ determine how closely care conforms to established standards
▶ measure how well the patient was cared for

▶ assess the performance of other members of the health care team
▶ identify opportunities to improve the quality of care.

When to perform evaluation

Although evaluation is an ongoing process that takes place whenever you see your patient, how often you're required to make evaluations will be influenced by several factors, including where you work. If you work in an acute care setting, your facility's policy may require you to review care plans every 24 hours. If you work in a long-term care facility, the required interval between evaluations may be up to 30 days. In either case, this doesn't mean that you shouldn't evaluate and revise the care plan more often, if warranted.

Evaluating expected outcomes

Evaluation includes gathering reassessment data, comparing findings with the outcome criteria, determining the extent of outcome achievement (outcome met, partially met, or not met), writing evaluation statements, and revising the care plan.

Revision starts with determining whether the patient has achieved the expected outcomes. If they've been fully met, and you decide that the problem is resolved, the plan can be discontinued. If the problem persists, the plan continues—with new target dates—until the desired status is achieved.

If outcomes have been partially met or unmet, you must identify interfering factors, such as misinterpreted information, and revise the plan accordingly. This may involve the following:

Smarter charting

Writing clear evaluation statements

Below, you'll find examples of clear evaluation statements describing common outcomes. Note that they include specific details of care provided and objective evidence of the patient's response to care.

RESPONSE TO P.R.N. MEDICATION WITHIN 1 HOUR OF ADMINISTRATION

▶ "Pt. states pain decreased from 8 to 4 (on a scale of 0 to 10) 10 minutes after receiving I.V. morphine sulphate."
▶ "Vomiting subsided 1 hr after given 25 mg P.O. of prochlorperazine."

RESPONSE TO PATIENT EDUCATION

▶ "Able to describe the signs and symptoms of a postoperative wound infection."'
▶ "Despite repeated attempts, pt. couldn't identify signs or symptoms of hypoglycemia."

TOLERANCE OF CHANGE OR INCREASE IN ACTIVITY

▶ "Able to walk across the room, approximately 15 feet, without dyspnea."
▶ "Became fatigued after 5 minutes of assisted ambulation."

ABILITY TO PERFORM ACTIVITIES OF DAILY LIVING, PARTICULARLY THOSE THAT MAY INFLUENCE DISCHARGE PLANNING

▶ "Unable to wash self independently because of left-sided weakness."
▶ "Requires a walker to ambulate to bathroom."

TOLERANCE OF TREATMENTS

▶ "Consumed full liquid lunch; pt. stated she was hungry and wanted solid food."
▶ "Skin became pink and less dusky 15 minutes after nasal O_2 was administered at 4 L/min."
▶ "Unable to tolerate having head of bed lowered from 90 degrees to 45 degrees; became dyspneic."

▶ clarifying or amending the database to reflect newly discovered information
▶ reexamining and correcting nursing diagnoses
▶ establishing outcome criteria that reflect new information and new or amended nursing strategies
▶ adding the revised nursing care plan to the original document
▶ recording the rationale for the revisions in the nurse's progress notes.

Documenting evaluation

Evaluation statements should indicate whether expected outcomes were achieved and should list evidence supporting this conclusion. Base these statements on outcome criteria from the care plan, and use active verbs, such as "demonstrate" or "ambulate." Include the patient's response to specific treatments (such as medication administration or physical therapy), and describe the conditions under which the response occurred or failed to occur. Document patient teaching and palliative or preventive care as well.

After evaluating the outcome, be sure to record it in the patient's chart with clear statements that demonstrate the patient's progress toward meeting the expected outcomes.

Selected references

Austin, S. "Ladies & Gentlemen of the Jury, I Present...The Nursing Documentation," *Nursing* 36(1):57-62, January 2006.

Berwick, D.M., et al. "The 100,000 Lives Campaign: Setting a Goal and a Deadline for Improving Health Care Quality," *JAMA* 295(3):324-7, January 2006.

Carpenito-Moyet, L.J. *Understanding the Nursing Process—Concept Mapping and Care Planning for Students.* Philadelphia: Lippincott Williams & Wilkins, 2007.

Charting Made Incredibly Easy, 3rd ed. Philadelphia: Lippincott Williams & Wilkins, 2005.

Chart Smart: The A-to-Z Guide to Better Nursing Documentation, 2nd ed. Philadelphia: Lippincott Williams & Wilkins, 2007.

Comprehensive Accreditation Manual for Hospitals: The Official Handbook, The Joint Commission on Accreditation of Healthcare Organizations, Oakbrook Terrace, IL, 2007.

Dochterman, J.M., and Bulechek, G.M. *Nursing Interventions Classification (NIC),* 4th ed. St. Louis: Mosby, 2004.

Doyle, M. "Promoting Standardized Nursing Language Using an Electronic Medical Record System," *AORN Journal* 83(6):1336-42, June 2006.

Figoski, M.R., and Downey, J. "Facility Charging and Nursing Intervention Classification (NIC): The New Dynamic Duo," *Nursing Economic* 24(2):102-11, 115, March-April 2005.

Gugerty, B. "Progress and Challenges in Nursing Documentation, Part I," *Journal of Healthcare Information Management* 20(2):18-20, Spring 2006.

Institute for Healthcare Improvement Web site: http://www.ihi.org.

Iyer, P., et al. *Medical Legal Aspects of Medical Records.* Tucson: Lawyers & Judges Publishing Company, Inc., 2006.

Johnson, M., et al., eds. *NANDA, NOC, and NIC Linkages,* 2nd ed. St. Louis: Mosby, 2006.

Joint Commission Web site: http://www.jointcommission.org.

Lunney, M. "Helping Nurses Use NANDA, NOC, and NIC: Novice to Expert," *Nurse Educator* 31(1):40-6, January-February 2006.

Macnee, C.L., et al. "Evaluation of NOC Standardized Outcome of 'Health Seeking Behavior' in Nurse-Managed Clinics," *Journal of Nursing Care Quality* 21(3):242-7, July-September 2006.

NANDA Nursing Diagnoses: Definitions & Classification 2007-2008. Philadelphia: NANDA International, 2007.

Pullen, Richard L. "Applying Nursing Process: A Tool for Critical Thinking," *Nurse Educator* 30(6): 238-239, November/December 2005.

Smith, L.S. "Documenting Discharge Planning," *Nursing* 36(5):18, May 2006.

DOCUMENTATION IN PRACTICE SETTINGS

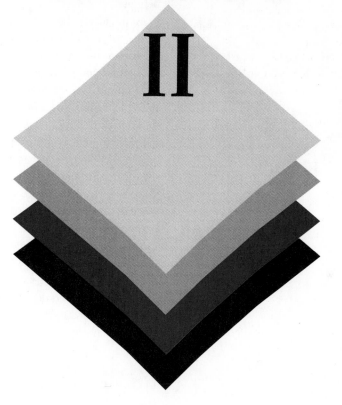

II

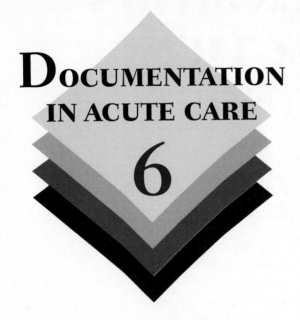

DOCUMENTATION IN ACUTE CARE

6

If you're like most nurses, you probably feel discouraged—even overwhelmed—by the number of forms you have to complete each day. Undeniably, paperwork takes time away from your chief priority—patient care. But being familiar with all the forms your health care facility requires and knowing how to use them efficiently bring major benefits.

A medical record with well-organized, completed forms will help you communicate patient information to the health care team, garner accreditation and reimbursements, and protect you and your employer legally. In the long run, taking the time initially to commit patient information to a standard, easy-to-use format will allow you to spend more time providing direct patient care.

On the following pages, you'll find the charting forms and methods commonly used in hospital settings. Among the forms and notations you'll find in the medical record of a hospitalized patient are the nursing admission assessment form, progress notes, Kardexes, graphic forms, flow sheets, clinical pathways, patient-teaching documents, discharge summary–patient instruction forms, dictated documentation, patient self-documentation, and adapted or new forms. Let's look at each of these in turn.

Nursing admission assessment form

Also known as a *nursing database,* the nursing admission assessment form contains your initial patient assessment data. You'll take this step in the nursing process when you first meet the patient. Completing the form itself involves collecting relevant information from various sources and analyzing it to assemble a complete picture of the patient. (For more information on documenting nursing assessments, see chapter 5, Documentation of the Nursing Process.)

The nursing admission assessment form may be configured in various ways. Some facilities use a form organized by patient responses, such as relating, choosing, exchanging, and communicating, while others organize the form by body systems.

The nursing admission assessment form records your nursing observations, the patient's health history, and your physical examination findings. It includes data on the patient's medications; known allergies to foods, drugs, and other substances; nursing findings related to activities of daily living (ADLs); current pain level; impressions of the patient's support systems; and documentation of the patient's advance directives, if any.

How you complete this form depends on your health care facility. You may need to fill in blanks, check off boxes, or write narrative notes. (See *Completing the nursing admission assessment,* pages 148 and 149.)

Advantages

When carefully completed, the form provides pertinent physiologic, psychosocial, spiritual, and cultural information. It contains subjective and objective data about the patient's current health status and clues about actual or potential health problems. It reveals the patient's ability to comply with treatments, his expectations for treatment, and details about lifestyle, family relationships, and cultural influences.

Using this information can guide you through the nursing process by helping you readily formulate nursing diagnoses, create patient problem lists, construct care plans, and begin discharge planning.

As you complete the form, keep in mind that The Joint Commission, quality improvement groups, and other parties use admission assessment information to continue accreditation, justify requests for reimbursement, and maintain or improve the standards of quality patient care. The recorded data also serve as a baseline for later comparison with the patient's progress.

Another advantage of this form is its usefulness in describing the patient's living arrangement, caregivers, resources, support groups, and other relevant information needed for discharge planning.

Disadvantages

Sometimes, through no fault of your own, you'll be unable to complete the nursing admission assessment form, especially if the patient is too sick to answer questions or a family member can't answer for him. Check your facility policy on documenting incomplete initial assessment data.

Documentation style

Admission assessment forms have typically followed a medical format, emphasizing initial symptoms and a comprehensive review of body systems. Although many facilities still use this format, others have opted for formats that reflect the nursing process. (See chapter 5, Documentation of the Nursing Process.) Regardless of which format you use, document admission assessments in one or a combination of three styles: open-ended, closed-ended, and narrative. (See *Writing a narrative admission assessment,* pages 150 and 151.)

STANDARD OPEN-ENDED STYLE

In standard open-ended style, the assessment form has standard fill-in-the-blank pages with preprinted headings and questions. Information

(*Text continues on page 153.*)

ChartWizard

Completing the nursing admission assessment

Most health care facilities use a combined checklist and narrative admission form such as the one below. The nursing admission assessment becomes a part of the patient's permanent medical record.

ADMISSION DOCUMENT
(To be completed on or before admission by admitting RN)

Name: *Raymond Bergstrom*
Age: *70*
Birth date: *4/15/36*
Address: *3401 Elmhurst Ave,*
Jenkintown, PA 19046
Hospital I.D. No.: *4227*
Insurer: *Aetna*
Policy No.: *60531OP*
Physician: *Joseph Milstein*
Admission date: *1/28/07*
Unit: *3N*

Preoperative teaching according to standard?
☑ Yes ☐ No
Preoperative teaching completed on *1/28/07*
If no, ☐ Surgery not planned
☐ Emergency surgery

Signature *Kate McCauley, RN*

T *101° F*   P *120*   R *24*
BP (Lying/sitting) Left: _____
Right: *120 / 68*

Height *5'7"*   Weight *160*

Pulses:
L: *P* Radial *P* DP *P* PT
R: *P* Radial *P* DP *P* PT
Apical pulse *120*
☑ Regular ☐ Irregular
P = Palpable D = Doppler O = Absent

Admitted from:
☐ Emergency room
☐ Home
☑ Practitioner's office
☐ Transfer from

Mode:
☐ Ambulatory
☑ Wheelchair
☐ Stretcher
Accompanied by: *Wife*

Pain:
⓪ 1 2 3 4 5 6 7 8 9 10
("0" indicates no pain; "10" indicates worst pain imaginable)

Signature *Kate McCauley, RN*

Medical & surgical history

Check (P) if patient or (R) if a blood relative has had any of the following. Check (H) if patient has ever been hospitalized. If it isn't appropriate to question patient because of age or sex, cross out option, e.g., ~~infertility.~~

	(H) (P) (R) Interviewer comments		(H) (P) (R) Interviewer comments		(H) (P) (R) Interviewer comments
Addictions (e.g., alcohol, drugs)	☐☐☐	Eye problems (not glasses)	☐☐☐	Memory loss	☐☐☐
Angina	☐☐☐	Fainting	☐☐☐	Mood swings	☐☐☐
Arthritis	☐☐☐	Fractures	☐☐☐	Myocardial infarction	☐☐☐
Asthma	☑☑☐ *lungs clear*	Genetic condition	☐☐☐	Prostate problems	☐☐☐
Bleeding problems	☐☐☐	Glaucoma	☐☐☐	Rheumatic fever	☐☐☐
Blood clot	☐☐☐	Gout	☐☐☐	Sexually trans. disease	☐☐☐
Cancer	☐☐☐	Headaches	☐☐☐	Thyroid problems	☐☐☐
Counseling	☐☐☐	Hepatitis	☐☐☐	TB or positive test	☐☐☐
CVA	☐☐☐	High cholesterol	☐☑☐	Other	☐☐☐
Depression	☐☐☐	Hypertension	☐☐☐		
Diabetes	☐☐☑	~~Infertility~~	☐☐☐		
Eating disorders	☐☐☐	Kidney disease/ stones	☐☐☐		
Epilepsy	☐☐☐	Leukemia	☐☐☐		

List any surgeries the patient has had:
Date   Type of surgery
_____

Has the patient ever had a blood transfusion: ☐ Y ☑ N
Reaction: ☐ Y ☐ N

Completing the nursing admission assessment *(continued)*

Unit introduction

Patient rights given to patient: ☑ Y ☐ N **Patient valuables:**   **Patient meds:**
Patient verbalizes understanding: ☑ Y ☐ N ☑ Sent home   ☑ Sent home
☑ Patient ☑ Family oriented to: ☐ Placed in safe   ☐ Placed in pharmacy
Nurse call system/unit policies: ☑ Y ☐ N   ☐ None on admission   ☐ None on admission
Smoking/visiting policy/intercom/
side rails/TV channels: ☑ Y ☐ N

Allergies or reactions

Medications/dyes ☑ Y ☐ N   *PCN*
Anesthesia drugs ☐ Y ☑ N
Foods ☐ Y ☑ N
Environmental (e.g., tape, latex, bee
stings, dust, pollen, animals, etc.) ☑ Y ☐ N   *Dust, pollen, cats*

Advance directive information

1. Does patient have health care power of attorney?   ☐ Y ☑ N
   Name:_____ Phone:_____
   If yes, request copy from patient/family and place in chart. Date done:_____ Init._____
2. Does patient have a living will?   ☑ Y ☐ N
3. Educational booklet given to patient/family?   ☑ Y ☐ N
4. Advise attending physician if there is a living will or power of attorney.   ☑ Y ☐ N

Organ & tissue donation

1. Has patient signed an organ and/or tissue donor card?   ☑ Y ☐ N
   If yes, request information and place in chart. Date done: *1/28/07*
   If no, would patient like to know more about the subject of donation?   ☐ Y ☐ N
2. Has patient discussed his wishes with family?   ☑ Y ☐ N

Medications

Complete medication reconciliation form for all medications.

Vaccines:
☐ Influenza, date:_____
☐ Pneumonia, date:_____
☐ Does not remember

Signature *Kate McCauley, RN*_____ Date *1/28/07*_____

ChartWizard

Writing a narrative admission assessment

Here's an example of a nursing admission assessment form documented in narrative style. The data begin with the patient's health history.

Patient's name:	James McGee
Address:	20 Tomlinson Road, Elgin, IL 60120
Home phone:	(555) 203-0704
Work phone:	(555) 389-2050
Sex:	Male
Age:	52
Birth date:	5/11/54
Hospital I.D. no.:	20074228
Place of birth:	Waterbury, CT
Race:	Caucasian
Nationality:	American

Culture: Irish-American
Marital status: Married, Susan, age 45
Dependents: James, age 14; Gretchen, age 12
Contact person: Wife (same address as patient) or Clare Hennigan, sister (1214 Ridge Road, De Kalb, IL 60115; phone (555) 203-1212)
Religion: Roman Catholic
Education: M.S. Degree
Occupation: Chemistry teacher, Park Ridge High School

Chief health complaint

Pt. states, "I've had several episodes of gnawing pain in my stomach, and I feel very tired. My doctor examined me and told me I should have some tests to find out what's wrong."

Health history

Pt. has been feeling unusually tired for about one month. States he lost 12 lb last month and about 5 lb before that without trying. States that he's busier at work than usual. He thinks his fatigue may be caused more by his schedule than by physical problems.

Past health: Had measles, mumps, chickenpox as child. Hospitalized at age 6 for tonsillectomy and adenoidectomy. Had a concussion and a fractured left leg at age 17 from a football accident. Has had no complications from that. Immunizations are up-to-date. Last tetanus shot 5 years ago; received hepatitis B vaccine 1 year ago.

Functional health: Describes himself as having a good sense of humor. Feels good about himself; feels he gets along fairly well with people and has many friends.

Cultural and religious influences: Pt. says he has strong religious background, goes to church regularly — important part of his life.

Family relationships: Because he's enrolled in a doctorate program at night, pt. regrets he doesn't get to spend much time with wife and children.

Jimmy and Gretchen get along well together, but sometimes compete for time with him.

Pt. says he's usually easygoing but lately blows up at the kids when stress and deadlines from school have him tied in knots.

Describes relationship with wife, father, and sister as good (mother deceased).

Sexuality: Says he and wife had a "decent [adequate] sex life" before he started work toward PhD. Now he's too tired.

Social support: Has many close friends who live in his neighborhood. Would like to socialize more with friends but schoolwork claims most of his time.

Other:

(continued)

Writing a narrative admission assessment *(continued)*

Personal health perception and behaviors: *Smokes cigarettes—between 1 and 2 packs per day. Never used recreational drugs. Takes vitamin and mineral supplements and occasional nonprescription cold medicines. Diet is eat and run—usually goes to fast-food place for dinner before night class. Drinks 1 or 2 glasses of beer a week when he has time for dinner at home. Drinks 6 to 8 cups black coffee daily.*

Rest and sleep: *Describes himself as a morning person. Gets up at 6:30 a.m., goes to bed between 11:30 p.m. and midnight. Likes to get about 8 hours of sleep, but rarely does. Needs to study at night after kids are asleep.*

Exercise and activity: *Says he'd like to be more active but can't find the time. Occasionally takes a walk in the evening but has no regular exercise regimen.*

Nutrition: *24-hour recall indicates deficiency in iron, protein, and calcium. Takes vitamin and mineral supplements. Skips lunch often. States he's been losing weight without trying.*

Recreation: *Likes swimming, hiking, and camping. Tries to take family camping at least once each summer. Wishes he had more time for recreation.*

Coping: *Describes his way of coping as avoiding problems until they get too big. Feels he copes with day-to-day stresses O.K. Says job is busy and stressful most days. Says he's feeling a lot of pressure trying to juggle family, career, and educational responsibilities.*

Socioeconomic: *Employed full time. Has health insurance and retirement benefits through job. Wife Susan is a secretary.*

Environmental: *No known environmental hazards. Lives in 3-bedroom house in town.*

Occupational: *Works 7 hours a day with 1/2 hr for lunch. Gets along well with coworkers. Feels pressure to attain doctorate to advance his career into educational administration. Has had present position for 12 years.*

Family health history

Maternal and paternal grandfathers are deceased. Both grandmothers are alive and well at ages 94 and 96. Father is alive and well at age 75; mother is deceased (at age 59, of breast cancer). Younger sister is alive and well.

Physical status

General health: *Complains of recent stomach pain and fatigue. Had two head colds last winter. No other illnesses or complaints.*

Skin, hair, and nails: *Pallor, no skin lesions. Hair receding, pale nails*

Head and neck: *Headaches occasionally, relieved by aspirin. No history of seizures. Reports no pain or limited movement*

Nose and sinuses: *No rhinorrhea, has occasional sinus infections, no history of nosebleeds*

Mouth and throat: *Last dental exam and cleaning 6 months ago*

Eyes: *Last eye exam 1 year ago. Reports 20/20 vision.*

Ears: *Reports no hearing problems. No history of ear infections. Last hearing evaluation 2 years ago.*

Respiratory system: *No history of pneumonia, bronchitis, asthma, or dyspnea.*

Cardiovascular system: *No history of murmurs or palpitations. No history of heart disease or hypertension.*

Breasts: *Flat*

GI system: *Frequent episodes of indigestion, sometimes relieved by several doses of an antacid (usually Mylanta). Currently complains of gnawing stomach pain. Rates pain as 5 on a scale of 0 (no pain) to 10 (worst pain imaginable). Regular bowel movements but recently noticed dark, tarry stools.*

Urinary system: *No history of kidney stones or urinary tract infections. Voids clear yellow urine several times a day without difficulty. Denies nocturia.*

Reproductive system: *No history of sexually transmitted disease. Is currently sexually active in monogamous relationship. States that sexual relationship with marriage partner is "fine."*

Nervous system: *Reports no numbness, tingling, or burning in extremities*

Musculoskeletal: *Reports no muscle or joint pains or stiffness*

Immune and hematologic systems: *Pt. says doctor told him his hemoglobin was low. Reports no lymph gland swelling.*

Endocrine system: *No history of thyroid disease*

ChartWizard

Medication reconciliation

Below is an example of a completed medical reconciliation form.

Name: Benjamin Henry   **Medical record #:** 13011976   **Admission date:** 1/19/07

Information Source:
- ☑ Patient
- ☐ Family
- ☐ Caregiver
- ☐ Medication bottle
- ☐ Other: _____

Allergies:
NKDA

☐ Unable to obtain Medication History – Reason:

Reconciliation
(Check yes if drug is ordered, no if drug is not ordered or the dose/frequency/route has been changed. Complete the comment section using the comment codes provided)

| Medications on Admission | | | | | | | Admission Reconciliation (must be completed within 24 hours) | | | |
Medication	Dose	Route	Frequency	Date/time of last dose	Date & initials	Reason for medication	Yes	No	Comment*	Date & initials
Zetia	10 mg	P.O.	daily	1/18/07 2100	1/19/07 MG	high cholesterol	✔			1/19/07 MG
lisinopril	5 mg	P.O.	daily	1/18/07 2100	1/19/07 MG	hypertension	✔			1/19/07 MG
aspirin	81 mg	P.O.	daily	1/18/07 2100	1/19/07 MG	prophylactic	✔			1/19/07 MG

Signature & initials: Millie Gondek, RN   MG   Signature & initials: _____

Signature & initials: _____   Signature & initials: _____

NOTE:
- ► Place form on top of the current practitioner order sheet until admission reconciliation is complete.
- ► Place form with discharge instructions once admission reconciliation is completed.

*Comment Codes:
DFR: Dose/frequency/route changes (see practitioner order)
N/A: Not applicable based on diagnosis
NPO: Patient status is NPO and an alternate route is not indicated

TS: Therapeutic substitution
PA: Practitioner aware
Other: Note reason and continue on flowsheet or progress note as needed

THIS IS NOT A PRACTITIONER ORDER SHEET

is organized into specific categories, so you can easily record and retrieve it. Use phrases and approved abbreviations to complete this form.

STANDARD CLOSED-ENDED STYLE

Arranged categorically with preprinted headings, checklists, and questions, a closed-ended admission assessment form requires you simply to check off the appropriate responses. This eliminates the problem of illegible handwriting and makes reviewing documented information easy. The form also clearly establishes the type and amount of information required by the health care facility.

NARRATIVE NOTES

Handwritten or computer-generated, narrative notes summarize information obtained by general observation, the health history interview, and a physical examination. They allow you to list your findings in order of importance. They can be quite time-consuming to write and to read because they require you to remember and record all significant information in a detailed, logical sequence.

The current trend in hospitals and home care agencies is to avoid writing long narrative note entries. Nursing documentation is no longer judged by quantity but by quality. The narrative note content should be concise, pertinent, and evaluatory. If it's too lengthy, it will interfere with efficient data retrieval.

Documentation guidelines

Acute illness, short hospital stays, and staff shortages sometimes make conducting a thorough and accurate initial interview difficult. In certain circumstances, you can ask the patient to complete a questionnaire about his past and present health status and use this to document his health history. If he's too ill to be interviewed

and family members aren't available, base your initial assessment on your observations and physical examination. Just be sure to document on the admission form why you couldn't obtain complete data.

Conduct an interview and record the complete information on the admission form or progress notes as soon as possible, noting the date and time of the entry. Remember that new information may require you to revise the care plan accordingly. Another form that should be completed during your initial patient assessment is the medication reconciliation form (see *Medication reconciliation*). The purpose of this form is to prevent drug omissions, duplications, or transcription errors by comparing a patient-provided list of medications with prescribed medications. Practitioners should convey this list to the next health care provider when the patient is discharged or transferred.

Before completing the admission assessment form, consider the patient's ability and readiness to participate. For example, if he's sedated, confused, hostile, angry, having difficulty breathing, or in pain, ask only the most essential questions. You can perform an in-depth interview later when his condition improves. In the meantime, try to find secondary sources (relatives, for example) to provide needed information. Be sure to document your source.

During your interview, try to alleviate as much of the patient's discomfort and anxiety as possible. Also try to create a quiet, private environment for the interview.

Progress notes

After you've completed your nursing assessment and devised an initial care plan, use progress notes to record the patient's status and track changes in his condition. Progress notes de-

ChartWizard

Keeping standard progress notes

Use the following example as a guide for completing your progress notes.

PROGRESS NOTES

Date	Time	Comments
2/20/07	0900	Notified Dr. Watts re Ⓛ lower lobe crackles and ineffective cough. R 40 and shallow. Skin pale. Nebulizer treatment ordered. —————————— Ruth Bullock, RN
2/20/07	1030	Skin slightly pink after nebulizer treatment. Lungs clear. R 24. Showed pt. how to do pursed-lip and abdominal breathing. —————————— Ruth Bullock, RN
2/20/07	1400	Ⓛ leg wound 3 cm x 1 cm wide x 1 cm deep. 1 cm diameter spot of pink-yellow, non-odorous drainage noted on dressing. Surrounding skin reddened and tender. Wound irrigated and dressed as ordered. —————————— Ruth Bullock, RN
2/20/07	1930	Pt. instructed about upper GI test. Pt. related correct understanding of test purpose and procedure. —————————— Ann Barrow, RN

scribe, in chronological order, patient problems and needs, pertinent nursing observations, nursing reassessments and interventions, patient responses to interventions, and progress toward meeting expected outcomes.

These notes promote effective communication among all members of the health care team and continuity of care. Standard progress notes have a column for the date and time and a column for detailed comments. (See *Keeping standard progress notes.*)

Advantages

Because progress notes are written chronologically and usually reflect the patient's problems (the nursing diagnoses), retrieving information can be easy. Also, progress notes contain information that doesn't fit into the space or format of other forms.

Disadvantages

If the notes aren't well organized, you may have to read through the entire form to find what you're looking for. Nurses may also waste time recording information on progress notes that they've already recorded on other forms. In addition, the notes may contain insignificant information because the documenter feels compelled to fill in space with a lengthy note.

Documentation guidelines

When writing a progress note, include the date and time of the care given or your observations, what prompts the entry, changes in the patient's condition, and other pertinent data.

Some progress notes are designed to focus on the nursing diagnoses. If your facility uses this type of progress note, be sure to record each nursing diagnosis, problem, goal, or expected outcome that relates to your entry. For example, the nursing diagnosis *Acute pain* and related problems, such as pain relief and the effective-

ChartWizard

Using nursing diagnoses
to write progress notes

Progress notes can be written using a nursing diagnosis, as the example below shows.

Patient identification information   Generic Hospital, Van Nuys, CA
John Adams
DOB: 6/14/49
Admit date: 1/3/07
MR#: 20070139

PROGRESS NOTES

Date and time	Nursing diagnosis and related problems	Notes
1/9/07 —2300	Acute pain related to pressure ulcer on Ⓛ elbow.	Pt. rates pain an 8 on a scale of 0 to 10, with 0 being no pain and 10 being the worst pain ever experienced. Pt. frowning when pointing to wound. BP 130/84; P 96. Pain aggravated by dressing change @ 2200. Percocet ⊤ given P.O. and pt. repositioned on Ⓡ side. ———— *Anne Curry, RN*
1/9/07 —2330	Acute pain related to pressure ulcer on Ⓛ elbow.	Pt. states that pain is relieved (0/10 on pain scale). Will give Percocet ½ hour before next dressing change and before future dressing changes. ———— *Anne Curry, RN*

ness of analgesics, may be the focus of a nursing progress note. (See *Using nursing diagnoses to write progress notes.*)

CHART TIMES

Make sure that every progress note has the specific date and time of the care given or the observation noted. Don't record entries in blocks of time ("1500 to 2330 hours," for example). In the past, when nurses were required to write progress notes every 2 hours, charting blocks of time was common. Today most nurses use a flow sheet to chart how often they check on a patient. Together, flow sheets and progress notes usually provide adequate evidence of nursing care.

CHART CHANGES IN CONDITION

Be sure to document new patient problems ("onset of seizures," for example); resolution of old

problems (such as "no complaint of pain in 24 hours"); or deteriorations in the patient's condition (for example, "Pt. has increasing dyspnea, causing him to remain on bed rest. ABG values show PaO_2 of 52. O_2 provided by rebreather mask as ordered.").

RECORD OBSERVATIONS

Document your observations of the patient's response to the care plan. If the patient's behaviors are similar to agreed-upon objectives, document that the goals are being met. If the reverse is true, document that the goals aren't being met. For example, you might record:

2/9/07	1600	Dyspnea resolving. Pt. can perform ADLs and ambulate 20 feet 5̄ SOB. ———— *Lois Cahn, RN*

Or you might write:

2/9/07	2000	Dyspnea unrelieved. Pt. con-
		tinues to have tachypnea
		and tachycardia 1 hr after
		receiving O₂ by rebreather
		mask. Blood drawn for ABG
		analysis shows PO₂ 70; PCO₂
		32; pH, 7.40 —— Carol Davis, RN

DON'T REPEAT YOURSELF

Generally, avoid including information that's already on the flow sheet. The exception: a sudden change in the patient's condition, such as a decreased level of consciousness, a change in skin condition, or swelling at an I.V. site.

BE SPECIFIC

Avoid vague wording when you write a progress note. For example, using a phrase such as "appears to be" indicates that you aren't sure about what you're charting. Phrases such as "no problems" and "had a good day" are also ambiguous and subject to interpretation. Instead, chart specifics, such as the details found in the following example:

1/06/07	1000	Pt. ate 80% of breakfast
		and 75% of lunch; OOB to
		bathroom and walked in
		hallway 3 times for a
		distance of 10 feet with no
		shortness of breath.————
		————K. Comerford, RN

RESPOND TO NEEDS OR COMPLAINTS

Sometimes nurses document a problem but fail to describe what they did about it. Outline your interventions clearly—how and when you notified the practitioner, what his orders were, when you followed through, and how and when you

followed through on a request for nursing orders, information, or services. Here's an example:

1/10/07	1400	Pt. wants to know when he'll
		be getting chemotherapy.
		Dr. Milstein notified. Pt.
		informed that Dr. Milstein
		ordered chemotherapy to
		start this afternoon.———
		———— Esther Blake, RN

Kardex

In use for decades, the patient care Kardex (sometimes called the *nursing Kardex*) gives a quick overview of basic patient care information. A Kardex typically contains boxes for you to check off what applies to each patient as well as current orders for medications, patient care activities, treatments, and tests. You'll refer to the Kardex during change-of-shift reports and throughout the day. A Kardex can come in various shapes, sizes, and types. It may also be computer-generated.

A Kardex may include the following data:
▶ the patient's name, age, marital status, and religion (usually on the address stamp)
▶ allergies
▶ medical diagnoses, listed by priority
▶ nursing diagnoses, listed by priority
▶ current practitioners' orders for medication, treatments, diet, I.V. therapy, diagnostic tests, procedures, and other measures
▶ do-not-resuscitate status
▶ consultations
▶ results of diagnostic tests and procedures
▶ permitted activities, functional limitations, assistance needed, and safety precautions
▶ emergency contact numbers.

A Kardex can be made more effective by tailoring the information to the needs of a particular setting. For instance, a home health care Kardex should have information on family contacts, practitioners, other services, and emergency referrals. Some facilities have eliminated the Kardex and incorporated the information into the patient's care plan.

Some health care facilities use a Kardex specifically to document medication information or other data, such as test results or nonnursing information, which avoids duplicating what's already written in the nursing care plan.

Medication Kardex

If your health care facility uses a separate medication Kardex on acute care units, you'll find this document on a medication cart or in a locked cabinet at the patient's bedside that also contains his medications. The medication Kardex contains a permanent record of the patient's medications. (For a sample of a completed medication Kardex, see chapter 10, Documentation of Everyday Events.) Many facilities have made the transition to computerized practitioner ordering and computerized medication documentation systems.

Computer-generated Kardex

Typically used to record laboratory or diagnostic test results and X-ray findings, a computerized Kardex usually includes information regarding medical orders, medication orders and administration times, referrals, consultations, specimens (for example, for culture and sensitivity tests or for blood glucose analysis), vital signs, diet, activity restrictions, and so forth. (See *Characteristics of a computer-generated Kardex,* pages 158 and 159.)

ADVANTAGES

A patient care Kardex provides quick access to data about task-oriented interventions, such as medication administration and I.V. therapy. Although it duplicates information, the care plan may be added to the Kardex to provide all the necessary data for patient care.

DISADVANTAGES

Kardexes are only as useful as nurses make them. A Kardex won't be effective if it doesn't have enough space for appropriate data, if it isn't updated frequently, if it isn't completed, or if the nurse doesn't read it before giving patient care.

Make sure the Kardex doesn't become the working care plan. Whenever the Kardex is updated, the care plan should also be updated. At many facilities, a Kardex isn't part of the permanent record and is discarded after the patient is discharged.

DOCUMENTATION GUIDELINES

The most effective types of Kardex are designed for specific units and reflect the needs of the patients on those units. Keep in mind that you should record information that helps nurses plan daily interventions (for example, the time a particular patient prefers to bathe, his food preferences before and during chemotherapy, and which analgesics or positions are usually required to ease pain).

If you're documenting on a medication Kardex, here are some tips:
▶ Be sure to include the date; the administration time; the medication dose, route, and frequency; and your initials.
▶ Indicate when you administer a stat dose and, if appropriate, the specific number of doses, as ordered, or the stop date.
▶ Write legibly, using only standard abbreviations accepted or approved by your facility.

(*Text continues on page 160.*)

ChartWizard

Characteristics of a computer-generated Kardex

In the computer-generated Kardex shown below, you'll find a detailed list of medical orders and other patient care data.

```
2/10/07      539                                          Page 001
= = = = = = = = = = = = = = = = = = = = = = = = = = = = = = = = =
Stevens, James                          M 65
MR#: 000310593                 Acct#: 9400037290
DR: J. Carrio                          2/W 204-01
DX: Unstable angina            Date: 2/10/07
= = = = = = = = = = = = = = = = = = = = = = = = = = = = = = = = =
SUMMARY: 2/10      0701 to 1501

PATIENT INFORMATION
    2/10      ADVANCE DIRECTIVE: No.
              Advance directive does not exist
    2/10      ORGAN DONOR: Yes
    2/10      ADMIT DX: Unstable angina
    2/10      MED ALLERGY: None known
    2/10      ISOLATION: Standard precautions

MISC. PATIENT DATA

NURSING CARE PLAN PROBLEMS
2/10    Acute pain R/T: anginal pain

ALL CURRENT MEDICAL ORDERS

NURSING ORDERS:
    2/10      Activity, OOB, up as tol.
    2/10      Routine vital signs q 8 h
    2/10      Telemetry
    2/10      If 1800 PTT less than 50, increase heparin drip to 1,200 units
              per hr. If 50 to 100, maintain 1,000 units per hr. If greater
              than 100, reduce to 900 units per hr.
    2/10      Please contact M. Sweeney to see pt. regarding diabetic man-
              agement and insulin treatment.
DIET:
    2/10      Diabetic: 1,600 cal., start with lunch today
I.V.s.:
    2/10      Peripheral line #1. . . . Start D₅W 250 ml with heparin 25,000
              units: rate, 1,000 units per hr.
```

Characteristics of a computer-generated Kardex *(continued)*

```
2/10/07     539                                    Page 002
= = = = = = = = = = = = = = = = = = = = = = = = = = = = = = = = = =
Stevens, James                         M 65
MR#: 000310593             Acct#: 9400037290
DR: J. Carrio                          2/W 204-01
DX: Unstable angina        Date:  2/10/07
= = = = = = = = = = = = = = = = = = = = = = = = = = = = = = = = = =
SUMMARY: 2/10      0701 to 1501

SCHEDULED MEDICATIONS:
    2/10     Nitroglycerin oint 2%, 1-1/2 inches, apply to chest wall
             q 8 h, starting on 3/10, 1800 hrs.
    2/10     Diltiazem tab 90 mg, #1, P.O., q 6 h 0800, 1400, 2000,
             0200
    2/10     Furosemide tab 40 mg, #1, P.O., daily 0900
    2/10     Potassium chloride tab 10 mEq, #1, P.O. daily 0900
    2/10     Labetalol tab 100 mg, #1 or 2 P.O. bid 0900, 1800

STAT/NOW MEDICATIONS:
    2/10     Furosemide tab 40 mg, #1, P.O., now
    2/10     Potassium chloride tab 10 mEq, #1, P.O., now

PRN MEDICATIONS:
    2/10     Procardia nifedipine cap 10 mg, #1, subling. q 6 h, prn
             SBP greater than 170 or DSBP greater than 105
    2/10     Acetaminophen tab 325 mg, #2, P.O., q 4 h, prn for pain
    2/10     Temazepam cap 15 mg, #1, P.O., at bedtime, prn
    2/10     Alprazolam tab 0.25 mg, #1/2, P.O., q 8 h, prn

LABORATORY:
    2/10     CK & MB 1800 today
    2/10     CK & MB 0200 tomorrow
    2/10     Urinalysis floor to collect
    2/10     PTT 1800 today

ANCILLARY:
    2/10     Stress test persantine, prep H1, Patient handling:
             wheelchair, Schedule: tomorrow

                        Last page
```

When in doubt about how to abbreviate a term, spell it out.

▶ After giving the first dose of a medication, sign your full name, your licensure status, and your initials in the appropriate space.

▶ After withholding a medication dose, document which dose wasn't given (usually by circling the time it was scheduled or by drawing an asterisk) and the reason it was omitted (for example, withholding oral medications from a patient the morning of scheduled surgery).

If you give all medications according to the care plan, you don't need further documentation. However, if your medication administration record (MAR) doesn't have space for information, such as the parenteral administration site, the patient's response to medications given as needed, or deviations from the medication order, you'll need to record this information in the progress notes. Here's an example:

1/12/07	0800	Withheld Procardia per or-
		der of Dr. Patel because pt.'s
		BP: 98/58. —— Dave Bevins, RN

Graphic forms

Used for 24-hour assessments, graphic forms usually have a column of data printed on the left side of the page, times and dates printed across the top, and open blocks within the side and top borders. You'll use graphic forms to plot various changes—in the patient's vital signs, weight, intake and output (stools, urine, and vomitus), appetite, and activity level, for instance.

Advantages

Graphic forms present information at a glance, allowing you to trend data and identify patterns.

For example, blood pressure that rises, falls, or fluctuates over time can be detected much more readily on a graph than in a narrative accounting of raw numbers. Also, health care personnel such as licensed practical nurses are typically permitted to document measurements on a graphic form, thereby saving registered nurses valuable time.

Disadvantages

Data placed on the graph must be accurate, legible, and complete. Every vital sign you take should be transcribed onto this form. If these guidelines aren't followed, the form loses its value. For accuracy, double-check the graph after transcribing any information onto it.

Avoid using the information on a graph alone; instead, combine it with narrative documentation to present a complete picture of the patient's clinical condition.

Documentation guidelines

For greater accuracy, try to chart on graphic forms at the same time each day. Document the patient's vital signs on both the graphic form and the progress notes when you give an analgesic, antihypertensive, or antipyretic drug, for example. This provides a record of the patient's response to a drug that may produce a change in a particular vital sign.

Also document vital signs on both forms for such events as chest pain, chemotherapy, a seizure, or a diagnostic test to indicate the patient's condition at that time.

Be sure to chart legibly, to put data in the appropriate time line, and to make the dots on the graph large enough to be seen easily. Connect the dots if your facility requires you to do so. (See *Using a graphic form.*)

ChartWizard

Using a graphic form

Plotting information on a graphic form, such as the sample shown below, helps you visualize changes in your patient's temperature, blood pressure, heart rate, weight, and intake and output.

GRAPHIC FORM

Instructions: Indicate temperature in "O" and pulse in "X"

DATE		2/5/07			2/6/07																					
POSTOP. DAY			2			3																					
		4	8	12	4	8	12	4	8	12	4	8	12	4	8	12	4	8	12	4	8	12	4	8	12	4	8

PULSE	TEMP.
150	106°
140	105°
130	104°
120	103°
110	102°
100	101°
90	100°
80	99°
	98.6°
70	98°
60	97°
50	96°
	95°

RESPIRATION	18		22	20	18

BLOOD PRESSURE	120/80		138/80	140/90	132/74

INTAKE	7-3	3-11	11-7	7-3	3-11	11-7	7-3	3-11	11-7	7-3	3-11	11-7	7-3	3-11	11-7	7-3	3-11	11-7	7-3	3-11	11-7
P.O.	480	800	600	300	250																
I.V.		100	100	50	100																
Blood/Colloid	250	900	0	0	0																
8-hour	730	1800	700	350	350																
24-hour		3230																			
OUTPUT	7-3	3-11	11-7	7-3	3-11	11-7	7-3	3-11	11-7	7-3	3-11	11-7	7-3	3-11	11-7	7-3	3-11	11-7	7-3	3-11	11-7
Urine	800	550	500	450	225																
NG/Emesis	0	50	0	0	0																
Other	0	0	0	0	0																
8-hour	800	600	500	450	225																
24-hour		1900																			
WEIGHT		150 lb																			
STOOL	0	0	†	0	†																

Flow sheets

Also called *abbreviated progress notes*, flow sheets have vertical or horizontal columns for recording dates, times, and interventions. You can insert nursing data quickly and concisely, preferably at the time you give care or observe a change in the patient's condition. Because flow sheets provide an easy-to-read record of changes in the patient's condition over time, they allow all members of the health care team to compare data and assess the patient's progress.

Using flow sheets doesn't exempt you from narrative charting to describe your observations, patient teaching, patient responses, detailed interventions, and unusual circumstances. However, flow sheets are handy for charting data related to a patient's ADLs, fluid balance, nutrition, pain management, and skin integrity. They're also useful for recording nursing interventions.

In response to a request by The Joint Commission, nurses use these forms to document basic assessment findings and wound care, hygiene, and routine care interventions. In addition, many facilities document I.V. therapy and patient education on flow sheets. The style and format of flow sheets vary to fit the needs of patients on particular units. (See *Using a flow sheet to record routine care.*)

Advantages

Because of their concise format, flow sheets let you evaluate patient trends at a glance, especially if you keep the forms conveniently near the patient's bedside in a secure location that maintains patient confidentiality. The format of flow sheets also reinforces nursing standards of care and allows precise nursing documentation.

Disadvantages

Because flow sheets have little space, they aren't well suited for recording unusual events. Also, overuse of these forms can lead to incomplete or fragmented documentation that obscures the patient's clinical picture. In addition, flow sheets may cause legal problems if they aren't consistent with the progress notes, which may happen if the nurse hurriedly checks off whatever the nurse on the previous shift checked off and then charts the actual care in the progress notes.

In some cases, the flow sheet format fails to reflect the needs of the patients and the documentation needs of the nurses on each unit. If the flow sheet doesn't take these needs into account or isn't revised as needs change, it becomes more of a liability than an asset.

In addition, flow sheets add bulk to the medical record, causing handling and storage problems and duplication of documentation.

Documentation guidelines

Ideally, you'll use flow sheets to document all routine assessment data and nursing interventions, such as repositioning or turning the patient, range-of-motion exercises, patient education, wound care, and medication administration. Then your progress notes need only include the patient's progress toward achieving desired outcomes and any unplanned assessments.

Make sure data on the flow sheet are consistent with data in your progress notes. Of course, all entries should accurately reflect the care given. Discrepancies can damage your credibility and increase your chance of liability.

Sometimes recording only the information requested isn't sufficient to give a complete picture of the patient's status. In such cases, record additional information in the space provided on

(*Text continues on page 166.*)

ChartWizard

Using a flow sheet to record routine care

As this sample shows, a patient care flow sheet lets you quickly document your routine interventions.

PATIENT CARE FLOW SHEET

Date 1/22/07	2300–0700	0700–1500	1500–2300
Respiratory			
Breath sounds	Clear 2330	Crackles @LL 0800	Clear 1600
Treatments/results	———	Nebulizer 0830	———
Cough/results	———	Mod. amt. tenacious yellow mucus, 0900	———
O₂ therapy	Nasal cannula at 2 L per min	Nasal cannula at 2 L per min	Nasal cannula at 2 L per min
Cardiac			
Chest pain	None	None	None
Heart sounds	Normal S_1 and S_2	Normal S_1 and S_2	Normal S_1 and S_2
Telemetry	N/A	N/A	N/A
Pain			
Type and location	© flank 0400	© flank 1000	© flank 1600
Intervention	Morphine 0415	Repositioned and morphine 1010	Morphine 1615
Pt. response	Improved from #9 to #3 in ½ hr	Improved from #8 to #2 in 45 min.	Complete relief in 1 hr
Nutrition			
Type	———	Regular	Regular
Toleration %	———	90%	80%
Supplement	———	1 can Ensure	———
Elimination			
Stool appearance	N/A	N/A	✝ soft dark brown
Enema	N/A	N/A	N/A
Results	———	———	———
Bowel sounds	Present all quadrants 2330	Present all quadrants 0800	Hyperactive all quadrants 1600
Urine appearance	Clear, amber 0400	Clear, amber 1000	Dark yellow 1500
Indwelling urinary catheter	N/A	N/A	N/A
Catheter irrigations	———	———	———
Signature/Title	Pam Watts, RN	Susan Reynolds, RN	Mary La Farge, RN

(continued)

Using a flow sheet to record routine care *(continued)*

PATIENT CARE FLOW SHEET

Date 1/22/07	2300–0700	0700–1500	1500–2300
I.V. therapy			
Tubing change	————	1100	————
Dressing change	————	1100	————
Site appearance	No edema, no redness 2330	No redness, no edema, no drainage 0800	No redness, no edema 1600
Wound			
Type	Ⓛ flank incision 2330	Ⓛ flank incision 1200	Ⓛ flank incision 2000
Dressing change	Dressing dry and intact 2330	1200	2000
Appearance	Wound not observed	See progress note.	See progress note.
Tubes			
Type	N/A	N/A	N/A
Irrigation	————	————	————
Drainage appearance	————	————	————
Hygiene			
Self/partial/complete	————	Partial 1000	Partial 2100
Oral care	————	1000	2100
Back care	0400	1000	2100
Foot care	————	1000	————
Remove/reapply elastic stockings	0400	1000	2100
Activity			
Type	Bed rest	OOB to chair X 20 min. 1000	OOB to chair X 20 min. 1800
Toleration	Turns self	Tol. well	Tol. well
Repositioned	2330 Supine 0400 Ⓛ side	Ⓛ side 0800 Ⓡ side 1400	Self
ROM	————	1000 (active) 1400 (active)	1800 (active) 2200 (active)
Signature/Title	Pam Watts, RN	Susan Reynolds, RN	Mary La Farge, RN

Using a flow sheet to record routine care *(continued)*

PATIENT CARE FLOW SHEET

Date 1/22/07	2300–0700	0700–1500	1500–2300
Sleep			
Sleeps well	0400 0600	N/A	N/A
Awake at intervals	2330 0400	————	————
Awake most of the time	————	————	————
Safety			
ID bracelet on	2330 0200 0400	0800 1200 1500	1600 2200
Side rails up	2330 0200 0400	0800 1200 1500	1600 2200
Call button in reach	2330 0200 0400	0800 1200 1500	1600 2200
Equipment			
Type IVAC pump	Continuous 2300	Continuous 0800	Continuous 1600
Teaching			
Wound splinting	0400	1000	————
Incentive Spirometry	0400	1000	1600
Signature/Title	Pam Watts, RN	Susan Reynolds, RN	Mary La Farge, RN

PROGRESS SHEET

Date	Time	Comments
1/22/07	1200	Ⓛ flank dressing saturated with serosang. drng. Dressing removed. Wound edges well-approximated except for 2–cm opening noted at lower edge of incision. Small amount serosang. drng noted oozing from this area. No redness noted along incision line. Sutures intact. Five 4" x 4" gauze pads applied and taped in place. Dr. Wong notified of increased amt. of drng.
		———————————————— Susan Reynolds, RN
1/22/07	2000	Dr. Wong to see pt. Ⓛ flank drsg. removed. 2 cm opening noted at lower edges of incision. Otherwise, wound edges well-approximated. Dr. Wong sutured opening with one 3–0 silk suture. No redness or drng. noted along incision line. Applied two 4" x 4" gauze pads. Taped drsg. in place.
		———————————————— Mary La Farge, RN.

the flow sheet. If additional information isn't necessary, draw a line through this space to indicate that further information isn't required. If your flow sheet doesn't have additional space, and you need to record more information, use the progress notes.

Fill out flow sheets completely, using the key symbols provided, such as a check mark, an "X," initials, circles, or the time to indicate that a parameter was observed or an intervention was carried out. When necessary, use the abbreviation "N/A" (not applicable) or another abbreviation recognized by your facility.

Don't leave blank spaces—they imply that an intervention wasn't completed, wasn't attempted, or wasn't recognized. If you have to omit something, document the reason.

Clinical pathways

A clinical pathway (also known as a *critical pathway*) integrates the principles of case management into nursing documentation. It outlines the standard of care for a specific diagnosis-related group (DRG). It incorporates multidisciplinary diagnoses and interventions, such as nursing-related problems, combined nursing and medical interventions, and key events that must occur for the patient to be discharged by a target date.

These events include consultations, diagnostic tests, treatments, medications, procedures, activities, diet, patient teaching, discharge planning, and anticipated outcomes. Other events or interventions may be added, and the pathway's categories may be presented in various formats and combinations.

Within the managed care system, clinical pathways set the standard for patient progress and track it as well. They provide the nursing staff with necessary written criteria to guide and monitor patient care. In some health care facilities, the nursing diagnosis forms the clinical pathway's basis for patient care, although critics believe that structuring the pathway in this way interferes with communication and coordination of care among nonnursing members of the health care team.

A clinical pathway is usually organized by categories according to the patient's diagnosis, which dictates his expected length of stay, daily care guidelines, and expected outcomes. The care guidelines specified for each day may be organized into such categories as activity, diet or nutrition, treatments, medications, patient teaching, discharge planning, and so forth.

The structure and categories may vary from one facility to the next and depend on which are appropriate for the specific DRG. (For an example of a completed clinical pathway, see "Take the clinical pathway," in chapter 5, pages 130 and 131.)

Advantages

Using a clinical pathway form as a permanent documentation tool can eliminate duplicate charting. Narrative notes need only be written when a standard on the pathway remains unmet or when the patient's condition warrants a deviation in care as planned on the pathway. Like the traditional care plan, the clinical pathway becomes part of the patient's permanent record.

As long as standardized orders or standing protocols have been determined and accepted, nurses can advance the patient's activity level, diet, and treatment regimens without waiting for a practitioner's order. Also, practitioners receive fewer phone calls because nurses have the freedom to make nursing decisions.

Clinical pathways improve communication among all members of the health care team because everyone works from the same plan. Proponents of clinical pathways believe that shared accountability for patient outcomes also improves the overall quality of care.

Some health care facilities adapt certain clinical pathways for distribution to patients, finding that many patients feel less anxiety and cooperate more with therapy because they know what to expect. Furthermore, some patients seem to recover more quickly and go home sooner than anticipated. A secondary benefit of clinical pathways seems to be improved patient teaching and discharge planning.

Disadvantages

Clinical pathways prove most effective for a patient who has only one diagnosis; they're less effective for a patient with several diagnoses or one who experiences complications (because of the difficulty establishing a time line for such a patient). For example, treatment progress is usually predictable for a patient who undergoes a cholecystectomy and is otherwise healthy. However, if the same patient has diabetes and coronary artery disease, the expected treatment course is fairly unpredictable. Furthermore, the care plan is likely to change, which results in lengthy and fragmented documentation.

Documentation guidelines

When developing a clinical pathway to distribute to patients, use simple vocabulary and keep your instructions short. Avoid unapproved abbreviations and complex medical terminology. Ideally, this version of the pathway should explain the diagnosis, review any tests and care the patient can expect, and inform him about activity restrictions, diet, medications, and home health care services.

When writing a clinical pathway, you'll need to collaborate with the practitioner and other members of the health care team. Keep in mind that the standardized orders for the clinical pathway require the practitioner's signature on admission of the patient.

To ensure consistent documentation from shift to shift, review the clinical pathway during the change-of-shift report with the nurse who is taking over. Point out any critical events, note any changes in the patient's expected length of stay, and discuss any variances that may have occurred during your shift.

If an objective for a particular day remains unmet, document this fact on the appropriate form. Variances from the plan may result for several reasons: the plan itself, patient complications, or unforeseeable events.

Document variances as justifiable or unjustifiable. For instance, you may have a patient who doesn't walk in the hall as scheduled. If he has a secondary infection that prevents him from walking, the variance is justifiable. If he prefers to stay in bed to read or watch TV, the variance is unjustifiable. You'll need to take steps to correct the problem and then document your interventions.

Patient-teaching documents

A preprinted patient-teaching form lets you clearly and completely document the dates, times, and results of your patient-teaching sessions. The form provides evidence that you implemented a teaching plan and that you're evaluating its effectiveness. Completed, the form also documents the patient's progress toward an acceptable level of self-care or assisted care.

Of course, you'll need to construct a patient-teaching plan before you can perform patient-teaching services, complete patient-teaching forms, or distribute educational materials.

Patient-teaching plans

Because standard-setting and reimbursing agencies require the health care facility to instruct patients about their condition and treatment regimen, you'll need to develop teaching plans to meet your patient's particular needs.

Beginning with your assessment findings—including what the patient already knows about the topic, the patient's cognitive level, and any barriers to learning (such as language, hearing loss, illiteracy, or others)—compile a list of topics and strategies that the patient needs to know or perform to attain his maximum level of health and self-care. These are called *learning outcomes* or *objectives*. Next, devise teaching activities, methods, and tools (such as brochures, one-on-one discussions, and videotapes) to convey and reinforce the information. Then design a way to evaluate your teaching effectiveness, such as a return demonstration or an oral question-and-answer session. (See *Filing a teaching plan,* pages 170 and 171.)

Identifying what needs to be learned and how you'll teach it constitutes the patient-teaching plan. Translated into reality, the instructive elements and activities should:

▶ define the patient's condition. If the patient has hypertension, the plan will probably begin with a working definition of normal blood pressure—both systolic and diastolic—and the roles played by the heart and blood vessels. The lesson will continue with an explanation of what happens in abnormal blood pressure.

▶ identify risk factors associated with the patient's condition. General risk factors usually have something to do with family history, age, race, diet, activity patterns, personal habits (such as smoking cigarettes or drinking alcohol), and so forth.

▶ explain what causes the patient's condition. For example, a patient-teaching plan for hypertension would include a simplified lesson on the dynamics of cardiac output and peripheral vascular resistance. (The teacher might use a model blood vessel for illustration.) If appropriate, the teaching plan should include an explanation of variations of the patient's condition (such as essential or secondary hypertension).

▶ point out the importance of therapy, emphasizing, if necessary, the consequences of untreated disease. (In untreated hypertension, for example, consequences include cardiovascular disease, stroke, and kidney damage.)

▶ explain the goals of treatment and identify the components of the treatment plan. In hypertension, for example, the goal of treatment would be stable, normal blood pressure; the components of the treatment plan might include dietary modifications, weight reduction, medications, exercise, stress management, self-monitoring, and regular health care follow-up.

▶ define the patient's anticipated learning outcomes and provide a time frame. Again using hypertension as an example, some timed learning outcomes might include:
– By discharge, the patient will be able to plan three well-balanced, low-sodium meals from the food list supplied by the nutritionist.
– Within 48 hours, the patient will be able to name his medications, explain their purposes, state how and when to take them, and list related adverse reactions that he should report to the practitioner or nurse.
– By discharge, the patient will develop a practitioner-approved exercise program.

ADVANTAGES

Though the patient teaching plan doesn't stand alone as a document in the medical record, it's part of the patient's care plan, which is part of the medical record. The teaching plan tells health care team members at a glance what the patient learned and what he still needs to learn and do about his health condition. It also shows quality-improvement measures in progress and meets professional and accrediting requirements as well.

DISADVANTAGES

Constructing individual teaching plans requires time and thought. Fortunately, some health care facilities have patient-education departments that focus on developing and implementing standard teaching plans for many common disorders.

DOCUMENTATION GUIDELINES

Check your facility's policies and procedures to learn where you're expected to file the patient-teaching plan—for example, within the care plan, on charts, in progress notes, in the patient-education office, or elsewhere.

When writing the teaching plan, be sure to follow the nursing process. Assess the patient's learning needs first, formulate a list of learning diagnoses (or learning outcomes), plan ways to meet the patient's learning needs, implement the plan, and periodically evaluate the results of your teaching by assessing your patient's responses.

Be sure to keep the plan succinct and precise. Most important, be sure to talk with the patient about the patient-teaching plan and agree on realistic learning outcomes.

Encourage and expect the patient's participation in the plan. Doing so usually increases his cooperation and your effectiveness.

Patient-teaching forms

Despite their similar content, patient-teaching forms vary according to the health care facility. For the most part, they contain general information about the patient's learning abilities, goals to be met, and skills to be acquired by the time of discharge. They may also focus on teaching aspects as they relate to a patient's particular disease. You can document information by filling in blanks, checking boxes, or writing brief narrative notes. (See *Documenting your teaching,* pages 172 to 175.)

ADVANTAGES

Patient-teaching forms make documenting your patient education quicker and easier by creating

(Text continues on page 175.)

ChartWizard

Filing a teaching plan

Your teaching plan should include your assessment findings; projected learning outcomes, along with the activities, methods, and tools needed to accomplish the outcomes; and the techniques you'll use to evaluate the effectiveness of teaching.

The teaching plan below was structured for Harold Harmon, a patient who has heart failure.

Assessment findings	Learning outcomes	Activities
Mr. Harmon needs to understand the action of his medication.	Mr. Harmon will: —explain the action of digoxin. —state when to take the drug.	—Present written brochures. —Discuss content. —Assess Mr. Harmon's knowledge.
Mr. Harmon needs to learn how to take his pulse.	Mr. Harmon will take his pulse and come within two beats of his practitioner's or nurse's results.	—Show Mr. Harmon a videotape that includes instruction on how to take a pulse. —Instruct him to study printed materials. —Demonstrate the procedure. —Provide feedback and practice time. —Ask Mr. Harmon to demonstrate the procedure.
Mr. Harmon reports feeling increased anxiety. He needs to learn how to cope with this anxiety and to control stress in his life.	Mr. Harmon will explain two techniques that he'll use to help him reduce his anxiety.	—Invite Mr. Harmon to watch a videotape on how to control stress. —Encourage him to read printed materials (booklets, pamphlets) on techniques to reduce stress. —Demonstrate deep-breathing and progressive muscle relaxation techniques. —Role-play a guided imagery scene. —Present a case study on how other people have successfully coped with stress.

Teaching methods	Teaching tools	Evaluation methods
—One-on-one discussion	—Printed materials describing digoxin's action	—Question and answer
	—Patient-teaching aid on digoxin	
	—Illustration of a medication clock	
—Demonstration	—Videotape	—Question and answer
—Supervised practice sessions	—Printed materials	—Return demonstration
—One-on-one discussion	—Photographs or illustrations of key steps in the procedure	
—One-on-one discussion	—Printed materials	—Question and answer
—Group discussion (with family)	—Videotape	—Interview
—Role-playing		—Observation
—Case study		—Return demonstration of relaxation techniques
—Self-monitoring		

ChartWizard

Documenting your teaching

Use the model patient-teaching form below—for a patient with diabetes mellitus—as a guideline for documenting your teaching sessions clearly and completely.

PATIENT TEACHING
Instructions for Diabetic Patients

County Hospital, Waltham, MA

Patient name: _Justin Bridge_
Medical record number: _198125_
Admission date: _1/3/07_   **Anticipated discharge:** _1/8/07_   **Diagnosis:** _TIA/type 2 diabetes_

Educational assessment

Comprehension level
Ability to grasp concepts
- ☑ High
- ☐ Average
- ☐ Needs improvement
Comments: _____

Motivational level
- ☑ Asks questions
- ☐ Eager to learn
- ☐ Anxious
- ☐ Uncooperative
- ☐ Disinterested
- ☐ Denies need to learn
Comments: _____

Knowledge and skill levels
Understanding of health condition and how to manage it
- ☐ High (greater than 75% working knowledge)
- ☐ Adequate (50% to 75% working knowledge)
- ☑ Needs improvement (25% to 50% working knowledge)
- ☐ Low (less than 25% working knowledge)
Comments: _____
_____

Learning barriers
- ☐ Language (specify: foreign, impairment, laryngectomy, other): _____
- ☐ Vision (specify: blind, legally blind, other): _____
- ☐ Hearing (impaired, deaf)
- ☐ Memory
  - ☐ Change in long-term memory (specify):
  - ☐ Change in short-term memory (specify):
- ☐ Other (specify): _____
Instructor's initials: _CW_

Anticipated outcomes
Patient will be prepared to perform self-care at the following level:

- ☑ High (total self-care)
- ☐ Moderate (self-care with minor assistance)
- ☐ Minimal (self-care with more than 50% assistance)

Documenting your teaching *(continued)*

Key
P	=	patient taught	N/A	=	not applicable	C	=	expressed denial, resistance
F	=	caregiver or family taught	A	=	asked questions	D	=	verbalized recall
R	=	reinforced	B	=	nonattentive, poor concentration	E	=	demonstrated ability

	1/4/07	1/5/07	1/5/07	1/5/07	1/6/07	1/7/07	1/7/07	1/8/07	
Date									
Time	1900	0800	1330	1830	1000	0800	1830	0800	
Assessed educational needs Assessment of patient's (or caregiver's) current knowledge of disease (include medical, family, and social histories)	A								
Assessment of learner's reaction to diagnosis (verbal and nonverbal responses)	A								
General diabetic education goals The patient (or caregiver) will:									
▪ define diabetes mellitus.	P/A	R	D					D	
▪ state hormone produced in the pancreas.	P/A	R	D					D	
▪ identify three signs and symptoms of diabetes.	P	R	D					D	
▪ discuss risk factors associated with the disease.	P	R	D					D	
▪ differentiate between type 1 and type 2 diabetes.	P/A	R	D					D	
Survival skill goals The patient (or caregiver) will:									
▪ identify the name, purpose, dose, and time of administration of medication ordered.		P	R	D				D	
▪ properly administer insulin.	N/A								
– draw up insulin properly.	N/A								
– discuss and demonstrate site selection and rotation.	N/A								
– demonstrate proper injection technique with needle angled appropriately.	N/A								
– explain correct way to store insulin.	N/A								
– demonstrate correct disposal of syringes.	N/A								
▪ distinguish among types of insulin.	N/A								
– regular	N/A								
– NPH (longer acting)	N/A								
▪ Properly administer mixed insulins.	N/A								
– demonstrate injecting air into vials.	N/A								
RN initials	CW	EG	ME	LT	EG	EG	LT	EG	

(continued)

Documenting your teaching *(continued)*

Date	1/4/07	1/5/07	1/5/07	1/5/07	1/6/07	1/7/07	1/7/07	1/8/07	
Time	1900	0800	1330	1830	1000	0800	1830	0800	
– draw up mixed insulin properly (regular before NPH).	N/A								
■ demonstrate knowledge of oral antidiabetic agents.									
– identify name of medication, dose, and time of administration.		P	A		D	F	R	D	
– identify purpose of medication.		P	A		D	F	R	D	
– state possible adverse effects.		P	A		D	F	R	D	
■ list signs and symptoms, causes, implications, and treatments of hyperglycemia and hypoglycemia.		P	A			F		D	
■ monitor blood glucose levels satisfactorily.									
– demonstrate proper use of blood glucose monitoring device.				P	E	E	R	E	
– perform fingerstick.				P	E	E	R	E	
– obtain accurate blood glucose reading.				P	E	E	R	E	
Healthful living goals The patient (or caregiver) will:									
■ consult with the nutritionist about meal planning.			P	R	A			D	
■ follow the diet recommended by the American Diabetes Association.			P	R	A			D	
■ state importance of adhering to diet.			P	R	A			D	
■ give verbal feedback on 1-day meal plan.			P	D	A			D	
■ state the effects of stress, illness, and exercise on blood glucose levels.			P	D	A			D	
■ state when to test urine for ketones and how to address results.			P	D	A			D	
■ identify self-care measures for periods when illness occurs.			P	D	A			D	
■ list precautions to take while exercising.			P	D	A			D	
■ explain what steps to take when patient doesn't want to eat or drink on proper schedule.			P	D	A			D	
■ agree to wear medical identification (for example, a Medic Alert bracelet).			P	A				D	
RN initials	CW	EG	ME	LT	EG	EG	LT	EG	

Documenting your teaching (continued)

Date	1/4/07	1/5/07	1/5/07	1/5/07	1/6/07	1/7/07	1/7/07	1/8/07	
Time	1900	0800	1330	1830	1000	0800	1830	0800	
Safety goals The patient (or caregiver) will:									
■ state the possible complications of diabetes.	P	R		D		F		D	
■ explain the importance of careful, regular skin care.	P	R		D		F		D	
■ demonstrate healthful foot care.	P	R		D		F		D	
■ discuss the importance of regular eye care and examinations.	P	R		D					
■ state the importance of oral hygiene	P	R		D					
RN initials	CW	EG	ME	LT	EG	EG	LT	EG	
Individual goals									

Initial	Signature								
CW	Carol Witt, RN, BSN								
EG	Ellie Grimes, RN, MSN								
ME	Marianne Evans, RN								
LT	Lynn Tata, RN, BSN								

a record of a patient's outcomes, responses, and level of learning. Correct use of these forms may be your legal defense for many years against charges of inadequate patient care. These forms also prevent duplication of patient-teaching efforts by other staff members. There are no disadvantages of using patient-teaching forms.

DOCUMENTATION GUIDELINES

Aim to have your completed patient-teaching forms include the patient's learning ability, his response to teaching, and the outcomes. If your facility doesn't have a preprinted form, talk to your supervisor about developing one. In the meantime, document your patient teaching in accurate, detailed progress notes. (See chapter 5, Documentation of the Nursing Process, for more information on patient-teaching forms.)

Whether you chart on a preprinted form or on progress notes, remember these tips:
▶ Check your facility's policies and procedures regarding when, where, and how to document your teaching.
▶ Each shift, ask yourself these questions: What part of the teaching plan did I complete? What other instruction did I give the patient or his family? Document your answers.
▶ Be sure to document that the patient's ongoing educational needs are being met.
▶ Before discharge, document the patient's remaining learning needs and note whether you provided him with printed or other patient-teaching aids.
▶ Be sure to evaluate your teaching. One way is by using a checklist. (See *Evaluating your teaching: The checklist method,* page 176.)

Evaluating your teaching: The checklist method

A checklist is a simple, quick way of obtaining information, evaluating your teaching, and gauging your patient's progress at various learning stages. It clearly shows you and the patient which goals he has achieved and which goals remain. To devise a useful checklist, follow these tips:
► Make sure the list is concise but wide-ranging enough to cover all aspects of the skill or activity being evaluated.
► Limit the items on the checklist to a group of related activities, such as the steps in tracheostomy care or the segments of a cardiac rehabilitation plan.
► Arrange items in a logical order—sequentially, chronologically, or in order of importance.
► Identify the essential steps of the activities or behavior you're evaluating.
► Relate items on the list to the patient's learning goals and to your teaching methods.
► Use only one idea or concept for each item.
► Phrase each item succinctly and accurately.
► Test your checklist on at least two patients before adopting it permanently.
► Use the checklist along with other evaluation tools to promote balance and avoid giving it undue importance.

The sample checklist below might be used for evaluating how well a diabetic patient has learned to draw up insulin.

DRAWING UP INSULIN

Yes	No	
☐	☐	Disinfects top of vial thoroughly
☐	☐	Inserts needle into vial without contamination
☐	☐	Withdraws proper amount of insulin
☐	☐	Expels air from syringe
☐	☐	Retains exact dose of insulin in syringe
☐	☐	Replaces cap on needle without contamination

Discharge summary–patient instruction forms

To comply with The Joint Commission requirements related to discharge planning, you must document your assessment of a patient's continuing care needs as well as any referrals for such care. To facilitate this kind of documentation, many health care facilities combine discharge summaries and patient instructions in one form. This form contains sections for recording discharge documentation, patient assessment, patient education, and detailed special instructions. On such forms, a narrative style coexists with open- and closed-ended styles.

Another form summarizes the discharge plans made by the different services on one page, emphasizing and documenting a team approach to discharge planning. This form is started at admission, updated during the hospital stay, and completed as discharge arrangements are finalized. (See *Using a multidisciplinary discharge document.*)

ChartWizard

Using a multidisciplinary discharge document

Many health care facilities use a multidisciplinary discharge form. The sample form below has spaces that can be filled in by the nurse, practitioner, and other health care providers.

ADMISSION/DISCHARGE DOCUMENT

Patient name: _Mary Mayer_   Patient no.: _347/9284_
Address: _312 Woodlake Drive_   HMO no.: _43217575_
Philadelphia, PA 19111   Physician: _Dr. Michael Bloom_
Birth date: _4/12/41_   Discharge date: _2/9/07_   Unit: _SN_
Date of admission: _2/1/07_

Discharged to:	Discharged by:	Accompanied by:		
☑ Home	☐ Ambulatory	_husband_	Valuables w/patient	☑ Y ☐ N
☐ Transfer to: _____	☑ Wheelchair		Meds w/patient	☑ Y ☐ N
	☐ Stretcher		I.V. access DC'd	☑ Y ☐ N

Discharge planning   Family/Friend contacts

1. Name _Frank Mayer_	Relationship _Husband_	Phone (H) _492-7342_ (W)
2. Name _Rose Hayes_	Relationship _Sister_	Phone (H) _492-1965_ (W)
3. Name	Relationship	Phone (H) (W)
4. Name	Relationship	Phone (H) (W)
5. Name	Relationship	Phone (H) (W)

Medications

Medication name	Dosage	Frequency
Lasix	_40 mg by mouth_	_twice daily_
Aspirin	_81 mg by mouth_	_once daily_
Prinivil	_10 mg by mouth_	_once daily_

Health team referrals

Date	Discipline contacted	Reason	Signature
_2/1/07_	_Nutritional services_	_Dietary compliance_	_C. Weir, RD_
_2/5/07_	_Respiratory therapy_	_Treatments_	_P. Cummins, RT_
_2/7/07_	_Physical therapy_	_Weight bearing_	_L. Doyle, PT_

Supplies/Equipment needed at home

Date	Item	Provider	Signature
_2/8/07_	_Walker_	_DME R US_	_B. Frank, MSW_
_2/8/07_	_O2 supplies_	_DME R US_	_B. Frank, MSW_

Community resources — Resource information provided (list resources)

Date		Signature	Date		Signature
_2/9/07_	1. _Meals On Wheels_	_B. Frank, MSW_		3.	
	2.			4.	

(continued)

Using a multidisciplinary discharge document *(continued)*

Education needs — Teaching topic completed (refer from 24-hour document)

Date		Signature	Date		Signature
2/1/07	1. Cardiac medications	C. Weir, RN		6.	
2/2/07	2. Low-salt diet restrictions	P. Brown, RD		7.	
	3.			8.	
	4.			9.	
	5.			10.	

Learning ability — Knowledge assessment of discharge needs

Date		Patient	Caregiver (Indicate relationship)	Signature
2/9/07	States diagnosis/disease	☑ Y ☐ N	☑ Y ☐ N husband	C. Weir, RN
2/9/07	States prognosis	☑ Y ☐ N	☑ Y ☐ N	C. Weir, RN
2/9/07	States medication regimen	☑ Y ☐ N	☑ Y ☐ N	C. Weir, RN
2/9/07	States complications	☑ Y ☐ N	☑ Y ☐ N	C. Weir, RN
2/9/07	Asks pertinent questions	☑ Y ☐ N	☑ Y ☐ N	C. Weir, RN
	Other	☐ Y ☑ N	☐ Y ☑ N	C. Weir, RN

Advantages

The combination discharge summary–patient instruction form provides useful information about additional teaching needs and points out whether the patient has the information he needs to care for himself or get further help. It establishes compliance with The Joint Commission requirements and helps to safeguard you from malpractice accusations.

A multidisciplinary discharge document allows all members of the health care team to reinforce information that may be discipline-specific. For example, the nutritionist may reinforce a special diet or a social worker may provide information regarding assistance in the home. This type of form eliminates second-guessing. There are no disadvantages of using a discharge summary–patient instruction form or a multidisciplinary discharge document.

Documentation guidelines

Upon discharge, give your patient a copy of his discharge instructions, including a complete list of his medications. Document a final physical assessment, including vital signs. Enter a final note in the narrative section or another predetermined location summarizing the patient's condition from admission to discharge with interventions. This summary should include the date, time, location, and mode of discharge.

Make sure that your discharge summary outlines the patient's care, provides useful information for further teaching and evaluation, and documents that the patient has the information he needs to care for himself or to get further help.

Dictated documentation

In some situations, nurses dictate from a nursing unit or clinical setting, and clerical personnel transcribe the information for the written clinical record. This occurs commonly among visiting nurses who may dictate into a recorder or a car phone between patient visits.

Advantages

Convenient and fast, dictated documentation can be performed without the distractions and interruptions encountered in a clinical setting. Using this documentation technique allows the nurse more time for patient care. Dictation can be done at any time of day or night, and studies show that this kind of documentation is highly accurate. Furthermore, it complies with The Joint Commission standards and may actually improve the quality of documentation.

Disadvantages

Delays in transcription time can prevent necessary documentation from being made readily available to practitioners and other health care team members. Also, supplies for recorded documentation may be more costly than for handwritten charting. In addition, the nurse

may need time to adjust to this type of documentation.

Documentation guidelines

Before dictating a report, familiarize yourself with the recording equipment. Then review the existing records and the notations you made during contact with your patient. Here are some tips for more effective dictation:

▶ Refer to your health care facility's policy and procedures manual for dictation guidelines, and consult the transcriptionist if you have related questions.

▶ Prepare a brief outline of your report so that it illustrates the nursing process.

▶ At the beginning of your dictation, name the patient and his identification number, if necessary.

▶ Tell the transcriptionist when the report begins and ends. Be sure to provide the date of the report and the date and time of the visit with the patient. Instruct the transcriptionist to provide the date of transcription. At the end of the report, include a summary, evaluation, and recommendations. Discuss your plans for the next time you'll see the patient.

▶ Use a checklist as you dictate to make sure that you include all the necessary information. For example, state the purpose of your time with the patient, list assessments performed and findings, discuss any new or changing patient problems, list interventions and patient responses, identify future care needs, explain patient teaching provided, and describe the patient's response.

▶ Try to dictate the information as near to the time that you provided care as possible so that your activities and observations are fresh in your mind.

▶ Speak clearly and slowly, avoiding unnecessary medical terminology and uncommon or unacceptable abbreviations.

▶ If you need to add information or change something you've said, give clear and specific directions to the transcriptionist.

Patient self-documentation

Although self-documentation obviously isn't feasible or desirable for every patient, it can be effective for patients who must perform considerable self-care (diabetic patients, for example) or for patients trying to discover what precipitates a problem (such as those with chronic headaches).

In using self-documentation, a patient with diabetes may record information on his diet, insulin dose, self-tested blood glucose levels, and activity level. The accumulated information can help him avoid insulin reactions and delay, prevent, or even reverse complications from hyperglycemia or hypoglycemia. Self-documentation may also provide valuable information for the practitioner as well.

A patient with chronic headaches may be asked to chart, among other things, when a headache occurred, what warning signs he noticed, and what pain-relief measures he tried. Analyzing this information may help ward off future headaches. (See *Teaching self-documentation skills.*)

The patient can document entries on preprinted forms or in journal style. Such records can be used in both inpatient and outpatient care settings. Depending on health care facility policies, they may become a permanent part of the medical record. (See *Keeping a record of monitored activity,* page 182.)

Advantages

Having the patient document data and events related to his own condition teaches him about his problem and its causes, symptoms, and treatment. It may also provide clues needed to reveal the problem's precipitators and suggest solutions to the problem.

Data recorded by the patient may actually be more accurate than data interpreted by someone else. For example, a nurse or practitioner may better understand the character of a patient's problem if the patient describes it in his own words.

Self-documentation also improves therapeutic compliance by making the patient an active participant in his treatment and providing him with some control.

Disadvantages

Self-documentation isn't difficult, but it takes time, patience, planning, motivation, and perseverance—on the part of both the nurse and the patient. The patient needs to understand how to keep careful records, what's important to document, and when to document. Otherwise, the records won't be useful and may even adversely affect his treatment and recovery.

Documentation guidelines

The patient must fully understand what needs to be documented and why it's important. If he will use preprinted forms, review each aspect of a form with him. If he will use a chart or a graph, show him how to use the form. If possible, complete a sample self-documentation form together for practice.

Identify whom the patient can contact if he has questions.

ChartWizard

Teaching self-documentation skills

For some patients, self-documentation has wide-ranging benefits. By learning to keep a log or a journal, for example, a patient may find out what triggers certain health problems (such as headaches, asthma attacks, or hypoglycemic episodes). Once the trigger emerges, the patient and caregiver can implement preventive strategies.

To help a patient learn self-documentation skills, some health care facilities use individual self-documentation forms such as the sample headache log shown at right.

REVIEWING INSTRUCTIONS

Give the patient instructions and review them with him. Tell him to complete the headache log daily. Inform him that doing so may help him to identify what triggers his headaches (for example, environmental factors, foods, or stress). Explain that information collected in the log may also help him discover effective ways to relieve a headache once it starts.

Instruct the patient to describe the details of each headache in a diary, log, or small notebook.

CHECKING THE BOXES

Review these steps with the patient:

▶ Using the log page at right as a guide, note the date and time of the headache and any warning signs.

▶ Put a check mark in the appropriate box to indicate the headache's intensity.

▶ Next, check the box to mark how long you've had the headache.

▶ Check the appropriate box for any other signs or symptoms that accompany your headache, such as nausea, vomiting, or sensitivity to light.

▶ Continue by checking the steps you took to relieve the headache (for example, medication, biofeedback, rest) as well as the effectiveness of these measures.

COMPLETING THE LOG

Urge the patient to think carefully about the events that occurred before the headache. For instance, was his headache triggered by emotional stress, by drinking a cup of coffee, or by something else? Tell him to write down the details of such potential triggers in his log.

HEADACHE LOG

Date and time headache began
2/25/07 – 5:00 p.m.

Warning signs
☑ Flashing lights   ☐ Zigzag patterns
☐ Blind spots   ☐ None
☐ Colors   ☐ Other

Intensity
☐ Mild   ☐ Severe
☑ Moderate   ☐ Disabling

Duration
☑ Less than 4 hours   ☐ 12 to 24 hours
☐ 4 to 7.5 hours   ☐ More than 1 day
☐ 8 to 11.5 hours   ☐ More than 2 days

Associated signs and symptoms
☐ Upset stomach   ☐ Sensory, motor, or
☑ Nausea or vomiting   speech disturbances
☐ Dizziness   ☐ Other
☑ Sensitivity to light

Measures for relief
☑ Medication   ☐ Biofeedback
☐ Rest   ☐ Ice pack
☑ Sleep   ☐ Relaxation exercises

Extent of relief
☐ None   ☐ Marked
☑ Mild   ☐ Complete
☐ Moderate

Possible triggers
Caffeine and sugar

ChartWizard

Keeping a record of monitored activity

In many situations, your patient can provide more information more accurately than a member of the health care team can. A case in point: a patient who wears a Holter monitor to evaluate the effect of medication on his heart and his daily activities.

Keeping this in mind, some health care facilities prepare patient instructional materials in conjunction with a diary-like chart (such as the example below), which the patient refers to and completes for the medical record.

Date	Time	Activity	Feelings
1/15/07	10:30 a.m.	Rode home from hospital in cab	Legs tired, felt short of breath
	11:30 a.m.	Watched TV in living room	Comfortable
	12:15 p.m.	Ate lunch, took propranolol	Indigestion
	1:30 p.m.	Walked next door to see neighbor	Felt short of breath
	2:45 p.m.	Walked home	Very tired, legs hurt
	3:00 to 4:00 p.m.	Urinated, took nap	Comfortable
	5:30 p.m.	Ate dinner slowly	Comfortable
	7:20 p.m.	Had bowel movement	Felt short of breath
	9:00 p.m.	Watched TV, drank one beer	Heart beating fast for about 1 minute, no pain
	11:00 p.m.	Took propranolol, urinated, and went to bed	Tired
1/16/07	8:15 a.m.	Woke up, urinated, washed face and arms	Very tired, rapid heartbeat for about 30 seconds
	10:30 a.m.	Returned to hospital	Felt better

Emphasize the benefits to the patient of self-documentation (increased knowledge about his condition and increased control of his treatment, for example). By doing so, you may help boost his interest in keeping his records updated.

Finally, show him the results of his self-documentation, pointing out how or what the data contribute to his treatment.

Adapted or new forms

You may find that one or several documentation forms you've been using no longer suit your needs. This may occur because of changes in therapies, patient populations, or reimbursement criteria. Duplicated and fragmented documentation data are among the first signs that the forms aren't filling current needs.

When developing a new form or adapting an old one, remember to ask yourself these questions:

▶ What problems exist with the old forms?

▶ What information is really needed?

▶ What changes would correct these problems?

▶ Which parts of the old forms remain valuable and need to be retained?

Even if your health care facility uses a computerized documentation system, ask staff members to help design the new form or reprogram the system. To develop an effective form, follow these guidelines:

▶ If your facility uses a specific nursing theory or framework for delivering nursing care, make sure that the nursing assessment form reflects it.

▶ If the old nursing assessment form reflects a medical format, change it to highlight the nursing process. For example, reorganize the form according to human response patterns or functional health care designs.

▶ Ask staff members who will be using the form to evaluate possible formats and indicate which they prefer. Ask for their ideas about how best to organize and document their data.

▶ List all information the form must include. Be sure to document this information to comply with professional practice standards published by such organizations as the American Nurses Association and The Joint Commission.

▶ Consider combining documentation styles in one form. Decide which style is most appropriate for each type of information included in the form. For instance, a narrative note may best suit one part of the form, whereas an open-ended style may best convey information on another part.

▶ After developing the form, write procedural guidelines for its use. Provide clear explanations and completed examples for each section.

▶ Ask staff members not involved in developing the form to analyze both the form and the guidelines. This helps identify potentially confusing sections that require more detailed explanation or revision.

▶ Before adopting the form, have staff members test it to make sure they can use it easily for entering information and retrieving it as well.

▶ If you expect the form will become a permanent part of the medical record, check the section devoted to form adoptions in your policy and procedures manual. Some health care facilities require a form to be approved by the medical records committee or certain departments before official use.

Selected references

Doran, D.M., et al. "Nursing-Sensitive Outcomes Data Collection in Acute Care and Long-Term Care Settings," *Nursing Research* 55(2 Suppl): S75-81, March-April 2006.

Hanley, E., and Higgins, A. "Assessment of Clinical Practice in Intensive Care: A Review of the Literature," *Intensive & Critical Care Nursing* 21(5): 268-75, October 2005.

Joint Commission on Accreditation of Healthcare Organizations: *Comprehensive Accreditation Manual for Hospitals: The Official Handbook,* 2007.

Joint Commission Web site: http://www.jointcommission.org.

Kirby, J., et al. "A Prospective Case Control Study of the Benefits of Electronic Discharge Summaries," *Journal of Telemedicine and Telecare* 12 (Suppl 1):20-21, 2006.

Maklebust, J., et al. "Computer-Based Testing of the Braden Scale for Predicting Pressure Sore Risk," *Ostomy/Wound Management* 51(4):40-2, 44, 46, April 2005.

Nurse's Legal Handbook, 5th ed. Philadelphia: Lippincott Williams & Wilkins, 2004.

Roberts, P., et al. "Use and Development of Clinical Pathways by Registered Nurses in an Acute Paediatric Setting," *Collegian* 12(4):22-8, October 2005.

Saufl, N.M. "Reconciliation of Medications," *Journal of Perianesthesia Nursing* 21(2):126-7, April 2006.

Smith, L.S. "Documenting Discharge Planning," *Nursing* 36(5):18, May 2006.

Watts, R., et al. "Critical Care Nurses' Beliefs about the Discharge Planning Process: A Questionnaire Survey," *International Journal of Nursing Studies* 43(3):269-79, March 2006.

Watts, R., et al. "Factors That Enhance or Impede Critical Care Nurses' Discharge Planning Practices," *Intensive & Critical Care Nursing* 21(5):302-13, October 2005.

DOCUMENTATION IN LONG-TERM CARE

7

Long-term care facilities provide continuing care for chronically ill or disabled patients. (Patients who reside in nursing homes are referred to as "residents.") Their focus of care is to attain or maintain the highest level of functioning possible; however, their role is slowly changing. Today, many long-term care facilities find that they're admitting more patients who require short-term skilled nursing services and who may eventually be discharged back into the community.

Maintaining accurate, complete documentation in long-term care is vital for the following reasons:

▶ Documentation of assessment findings, therapeutic interventions, and patient outcomes helps maintain communication among the many disciplines involved in caring for patients in a long-term care facility.

▶ State and federal agencies compile data gathered from medical record documentation into databases, where the data is compared with similar data from other long-term care facilities. Media outlets then publish the results of these comparisons for consumer information.

▶ State and federal agencies strictly regulate long-term care facilities, necessitating high standards of accurate and complete documentation. These agencies utilize documentation entered on the Minimum Data Set (MDS) form to focus the survey process on specific patients and to pinpoint reviews that statistically indicate areas of concern.

▶ The health care facility may use documentation to defend itself and its personnel in court.

▶ Documentation is now directly related to reimbursement, and good documentation ensures certification, licensure, and accreditation. Without accurate and complete charting, such programs as Medicare and Medicaid may deny payment and put the facility and practitioner under fraud and abuse scrutiny.

Your ability to document the status, care, and events affecting patients in a long-term care facility is every bit as important as it is in acute care and home health care settings. (See chapter 6, Documentation in Acute Care, and chapter 8, Documentation in Home Health Care.) Although some forms and requirements of documentation in these settings share many similarities, long-term care documentation differs in two important ways:

▶ The MDS form has become a central focus for documentation concerns in long-term care facilities. (See "Minimum data set," page 188.)
▶ Charting on intermediate care patients who stay for weeks or months in a long-term care facility may not be required as often as in the acute care setting, but specific parameters must be followed.

Levels of care

Long-term care facilities usually offer two levels of care, skilled and intermediate, but they can specialize in one or the other.

In a skilled care facility or nursing unit, patient care involves specialized nursing or other professional skills, such as I.V. therapy, parenteral nutrition, respiratory care, wound management, mechanical ventilation, and physical, occupational, or speech therapy.

An intermediate care facility or nursing unit deals with patients who have chronic illnesses and need less complex care. For example, they may simply need assistance with activities of daily living (ADLs), such as bathing, dressing, and toileting.

Patients at both levels may need short- or long-term care and may move from one level to another according to their progress or decline. Living arrangements, geography, networks, and other factors help determine the patient's length of stay. You should consider level of care and skilled needs a primary factor when documenting patient information.

Regulations and regulatory agencies

Many government programs, laws, and agencies regulate documentation in long-term care facilities, including:

▶ programs, such as Medicare and Medicaid
▶ laws such as the Omnibus Budget Reconciliation Act (OBRA) of 1987
▶ government agencies such as the Centers for Medicare and Medicaid Services (CMS) (formerly the Health Care Financing Administration)
▶ accrediting agencies such as The Joint Commission, formerly known as the Joint Commission on Accreditation of Healthcare Organizations.

Some managed care entities also have specific documentation requirements.

Medicare

Medicare is a federal health insurance program for people age 65 and older, some people with disabilities under age 65, and people with end-stage renal disease (permanent kidney failure requiring dialysis or a transplant).

The program has three parts: Part A, Part B, and Part D. Part A covers care provided as a hospital inpatient, hospice care, home health care, and care received in skilled nursing facilities. Part B helps pay for physicians' services, outpatient hospital care, and some other medically necessary services that Part A doesn't cover, such as the services of physical and occupational therapists.

Part D was enacted as part of the Medicare Prescription Drug, Improvement, and Modernization Act of 2003 and covers pharmaceutical drug insurance. This controversial drug plan became available on January 1, 2006, and is offered through private insurance plans that are then reimbursed by the CMS.

Two things must happen for a patient to receive Part A services in a skilled nursing facility: Specific criteria that are determined prior to admission must be met, and skilled services must be provided, assessed, and documented daily. Registered nurse assessment coordinators (RNACs) commonly handle this responsibility. They oversee the progress of patients receiving Part A services and ensure the timely completion of MDS assessments and related documentation requirements.

Medicaid

Medicaid is a jointly funded federal and state health insurance program for low-income people and people in need. It covers about 36 million people, including children, people who are eligible to receive federally assisted income maintenance payments, and elderly, blind, or disabled persons.

Most patients who receive care in a long-term care facility are enrolled in the state Medicaid program and receive either skilled or intermediate care. For skilled care, Medicaid requires daily documentation of all aspects of patient care. For intermediate care, Medicaid requires daily documentation of medications and treatments and restorative nursing functions.

CMS

The role of CMS, a branch of the Department of Health and Human Services, is to ensure compliance by health care facilities with federal Medicare and Medicaid standards. As part of the Nursing Home Initiative to promote quality care in nursing homes, the CMS publicizes statistical information gleaned from the MDS. Quality measures compare a nursing home against other nursing homes in such categories as pressure ulcers, pain, and ADL assistance. Nursing homes that perform poorly may be denied Medicare and Medicaid reimbursement. Therefore, you must make sure that information recorded on the MDS is accurate and complete.

OBRA

In 1987, Congress enacted OBRA, which imposed dozens of new requirements on long-term care facilities and home health care agencies to protect the rights of patients receiving long-term care. This law requires that a comprehensive assessment, or a *Resident Assessment Instrument* (RAI), be performed within 14 days of a patient's admission to a long-term care facility. This assessment helps the facility's staff gather definitive information on the patient's strengths and needs and consists of the following:

▶ *MDS*: provides key information required for patient assessment
▶ *Triggers*: conditions recorded on the MDS that indicate patients who may be at risk for

developing specific functional problems and require further evaluation using Resident Assessment Protocols (RAPs)

▶ *RAPs:* provide a problem-oriented approach for analyzing conditions triggered on the MDS.

The information from the MDS and RAPs then form the basis for developing an individualized care plan, which, under OBRA, must be developed within 7 days of completion of the RAI.

The Joint Commission

The Joint Commission accredits long-term care facilities using standards developed in conjunction with health care experts. Accreditation by The Joint Commission is voluntary but may ensure payment for services provided. Standard performance is documented in assessments, progress notes, care plans, and discharge plans. The ORYX initiative, begun in 1997, is another part of the accreditation process. It focuses on outcomes and other performance measurement data to support quality improvements in all health care organizations.

▶ Standard and required documents

Some forms are commonly used in multiple health care settings; others are specific to long-term care. Forms discussed in this section include the MDS, RAPs, care plans, the Pre-admission Screening and Annual Resident Review (PASARR), the initial nursing assessment form, other assessment forms, nursing summaries, and discharge and transfer forms.

Minimum data set

Mandated by OBRA, the MDS is a federal regulatory form that must be filled out for every patient admitted to a long-term care facility. (See *Minimum Data Set form.*) The requirements for completion of the MDS vary with the type of admission.

For intermediate care patients, complete the MDS at these times:

▶ admission assessment—required by day 14
▶ quarterly review assessment—performed every 90 days
▶ annual assessment
▶ significant change in status assessment.

For skilled care Medicare Part A patients under the prospective payment system, Medicare mandates a more frequent schedule of assessments. This schedule is in addition to the OBRA schedule and requires completion at these times:

▶ 5-day assessment
▶ 14-day assessment
▶ 30-day assessment
▶ 60-day assessment
▶ 90-day assessment
▶ readmission or return assessment
▶ at the completion of skilled rehabilitation services, called an *Other Medicare Required Assessment.*

The RNAC is responsible for monitoring and coordinating these stringent assessment schedules.

Initially intended to be a primary source document for standardized assessments, the MDS has evolved into a tool for determining resource utilization groups (RUGs) or payment categories. In this capacity, surveyors and auditors require that information recorded on the MDS be obtained from information recorded elsewhere in the medical record. Each facility may have dif-

(Text continues on page 198.)

ChartWizard

Minimum Data Set form

Numeric Identifier_____

MINIMUM DATA SET (MDS) — *VERSION 2.0*
FOR NURSING HOME RESIDENT ASSESSMENT AND CARE SCREENING

BASIC ASSESSMENT TRACKING FORM

SECTION AA. IDENTIFICATION INFORMATION

1. RESIDENT NAME
Mary P. Klein
a. (First) b. (Middle Initial) c. (Last) d. (Jr/Sr)

2. GENDER 1. Male 2. Female — 2

3. BIRTHDATE
| 1 1 | - | 0 5 | - | 1 9 3 3 |
Month Day Year

4. RACE/ETHNICITY
1. American Indian/Alaskan Native
2. Asian/Pacific Islander
3. Black, not of Hispanic origin
4. Hispanic
5. White, not of Hispanic origin — 5

5. SOCIAL SECURITY AND MEDICARE NUMBERS [C in 1st box if non med. no.]
a. Social Security Number
| 0 5 0 | - | 5 0 | - | 5 0 0 0 |
b. Medicare number (or comparable railroad insurance number)

6. FACILITY PROVIDER NO.
a. State No.

b. Federal No.

7. MEDICAID NO. ["+" if pending, "N" if not a Medicaid recipient]

8. REASONS FOR ASSESSMENT
[Note—Other codes do not apply to this form]

a. Primary reason for assessment
1. Admission assessment (required by day 14)
2. Annual assessment
3. Significant change in status assessment
4. Significant correction of prior full assessment
5. Quarterly review assessment
10. Significant correction of prior quarterly assessment
0. *NONE OF ABOVE*
— 1

b. Codes for assessments required for Medicare PPS or the State
1. Medicare 5 day assessment
2. Medicare 30 day assessment
3. Medicare 60 day assessment
4. Medicare 90 day assessment
5. Medicare readmission/return assessment
6. Other state required assessment
7. Medicare 14 day assessment
8. Other Medicare required assessment
— 1

9. Signatures of Persons who Completed a Portion of the Accompanying Assessment or Tracking Form

I certify that the accompanying information accurately reflects resident assessment or tracking information for this resident and that I collected or coordinated collection of this information on the dates specified. To the best of my knowledge, this information was collected in accordance with applicable Medicare and Medicaid requirements. I understand that this information is used as a basis for ensuring that residents receive appropriate and quality care, and as a basis for payment from federal funds. I further understand that payment of such federal funds and continued participation in the government-funded health care programs is conditioned on the accuracy and truthfulness of this information, and that I may be personally subject to or may subject my organization to substantial criminal, civil, and/or administrative penalties for submitting false information. I also certify that I am authorized to submit this information by this facility on its behalf.

Signature and Title	Sections	Date
a. Sue Rayne, MSW	B,F	2/7/07
b. Sandra Landry, RN	C, D, E, G, H, I, JL	2/7/07
c. D.T. Arnold, Activities	N	2/7/07
d. Mary Jo Pope, RD	K	2/7/07
e. June Gold, PT	G3, G4, P1b, T	2/9/07
f. Jamie K. Kauffman, RN	M, O, P, Q	2/9/07
g.		
h.		
i.		
j.		
k.		
l.		

GENERAL INSTRUCTIONS

Complete this information for submission with all full and quarterly assessments (Admission, Annual, Significant Change, State or Medicare required assessments, or Quarterly Reviews, etc.)

⊙ = Key items for computerized resident tracking

☐ = When box blank, must enter number or letter a. ☐ = When letter in box, check if condition applies

MDS 2.0 September, 2000

(continued)

Minimum Data Set form (continued)

Resident   *Mary P. Klein*   Numeric Identifier _____

MINIMUM DATA SET (MDS) — VERSION 2.0
FOR NURSING HOME RESIDENT ASSESSMENT AND CARE SCREENING
BACKGROUND (FACE SHEET) INFORMATION AT ADMISSION

SECTION AB. DEMOGRAPHIC INFORMATION

1.	DATE OF ENTRY	Date the stay began. Note — Does not include readmission if record was closed at time of temporary discharge to hospital, etc. In such cases, use prior admission date

`0 2 - 0 2 - 2 0 0 7`
Month   Day   Year

2.	ADMITTED FROM (AT ENTRY)	1. Private home/apt. with no home health services 2. Private home/apt. with home health services 3. Board and care/assisted living/group home 4. Nursing home 5. Acute care hospital 6. Psychiatric hospital, MR/DD facility 7. Rehabilitation hospital 8. Other	**5**
3.	LIVED ALONE (PRIOR TO ENTRY)	0. No 1. Yes 2. In other facility	**0**
4.	ZIP CODE OF PRIOR PRIMARY RESIDENCE	`1 8 9 0 1`	
5.	RESIDENTIAL HISTORY 5 YEARS PRIOR TO ENTRY	(Check all settings resident lived in during 5 years prior to date of entry given in item AB1 above) Prior stay at this nursing home — a. Stay in other nursing home — b. Other residential facility—board and care home, assisted living, group home — c. MH/psychiatric setting — d. MR/DD setting — e. NONE OF ABOVE — f. ✓	
6.	LIFETIME OCCUPATION(S) [Put "/" between two occupations]	`T e a c h e r`	
7.	EDUCATION (Highest Level Completed)	1. No schooling 5. Technical or trade school 2. 8th grade/less 6. Some college 3. 9-11 grades 7. Bachelor's degree 4. High school 8. Graduate degree	**8**
8.	LANGUAGE	(Code for correct response) a. Primary Language 0. English 1. Spanish 2. French 3. Other b. If other, specify	**0**
9.	MENTAL HEALTH HISTORY	Does resident's RECORD indicate any history of mental retardation, mental illness, or developmental disability problem? 0. No 1. Yes	**0**
10.	CONDITIONS RELATED TO MR/DD STATUS	(Check all conditions that are related to MR/DD status that were manifested before age 22, and are likely to continue indefinitely) Not applicable—no MR/DD (Skip to AB11) — a. MR/DD with organic condition — b. Down's syndrome — c. Autism — d. Epilepsy — e. Other organic condition related to MR/DD — f. MR/DD with no organic condition —	
11.	DATE BACKGROUND INFORMATION COMPLETED	`0 2 - 0 3 - 2 0 0 7` Month Day Year	

SECTION AC. CUSTOMARY ROUTINE

1.	CUSTOMARY ROUTINE	(Check all that apply. If all information UNKNOWN, check last box only.)

(In year prior to DATE OF ENTRY to this nursing home, or year last in community if now being admitted from another nursing home)

CYCLE OF DAILY EVENTS

Stays up late at night (e.g., after 9 pm)	a. ✓
Naps regularly during day (at least 1 hour)	b.
Goes out 1+ days a week	c.
Stays busy with hobbies, reading, or fixed daily routine	d. ✓
Spends most of time alone or watching TV	e.
Moves independently indoors (with appliances, if used)	f.
Use of tobacco products at least daily	g.
NONE OF ABOVE	h.

EATING PATTERNS

Distinct food preferences	i.
Eats between meals all or most days	j. ✓
Use of alcoholic beverage(s) at least weekly	k.
NONE OF ABOVE	l.

ADL PATTERNS

In bedclothes much of day	m.
Wakens to toilet all or most nights	n. ✓
Has irregular bowel movement pattern	o.
Showers for bathing	p.
Bathing in PM	q. ✓
NONE OF ABOVE	r.

INVOLVEMENT PATTERNS

Daily contact with relatives/close friends	s.
Usually attends church, temple, synagogue (etc.)	t. ✓
Finds strength in faith	u.
Daily animal companion/presence	v. ✓
Involved in group activities	w. ✓
NONE OF ABOVE	x.
UNKNOWN—Resident/family unable to provide information	y.

SECTION AD. FACE SHEET SIGNATURES

SIGNATURES OF PERSONS COMPLETING FACE SHEET:

Sue Rayne, MSW

a. Signature of RN Assessment Coordinator   Date
Marie Smith, RNAC   `2/4/01`

I certify that the accompanying information accurately reflects resident assessment or tracking information for this resident and that I collected or coordinated collection of this information on the dates specified. To the best of my knowledge, this information was collected in accordance with applicable Medicare and Medicaid requirements. I understand that this information is used as a basis for ensuring that residents receive appropriate and quality care, and as a basis for payment from federal funds. I further understand that payment of such federal funds and continued participation in the government-funded health care programs is conditioned on the accuracy and truthfulness of this information, and that I may be personally subject to or may subject my organization to substantial criminal, civil, and/or administrative penalties for submitting false information. I also certify that I am authorized to submit this information by this facility on its behalf.

Signature and Title	Sections	Date
b.		
c.		
d.		
e.		
f.		
g.		

☐ = When box blank, must enter number or letter   ⓐ = When letter in box, check if condition applies

MDS 2.0   September, 2000

Minimum Data Set form *(continued)*

Resident _Mary P. Klein_   Numeric Identifier _____

MINIMUM DATA SET (MDS) — *VERSION 2.0*
FOR NURSING HOME RESIDENT ASSESSMENT AND CARE SCREENING
FULL ASSESSMENT FORM
(Status in last 7 days, unless other time frame indicated)

SECTION A. IDENTIFICATION AND BACKGROUND INFORMATION

1. RESIDENT NAME
Mary P. Klein
a. (First) b. (Middle Initial) c. (Last) d. (Jr/Sr)

2. ROOM NUMBER   `B 2 1 5`

3. ASSESSMENT REFERENCE DATE
a. Last day of MDS observation period
`0 2 - 0 7 - 2 0 0 7`
Month Day Year
b. Original (0) or corrected copy of form (enter number of correction)

4a. DATE OF REENTRY Date of reentry from most recent temporary discharge to a hospital in last 90 days (or since last assessment or admission if less than 90 days)
`_ _ - _ _ - _ _ _ _`
Month Day Year

5. MARITAL STATUS
1. Never married   3. Widowed   5. Divorced
2. Married   4. Separated   `2`

6. MEDICAL RECORD NO.   `1 2 1 / 0 5`

7. CURRENT PAYMENT SOURCES FOR N.H. STAY
(Billing Office to indicate; check all that apply in last 30 days)
Medicaid per diem `a.` | VA per diem `f.`
Medicare per diem `b. X` | Self or family pays for full per diem `g. X`
Medicare ancillary part A `c.` | Medicaid resident liability or Medicare co-payment `h.`
Medicare ancillary part B `d.` | Private insurance per diem (including co-payment) `i.`
CHAMPUS per diem `e.` | Other per diem `j.`

8. REASONS FOR ASSESSMENT
[Note—If this is a discharge or reentry assessment, only a limited subset of MDS items need be completed]
a. Primary reason for assessment
1. Admission assessment (required by day 14)
2. Annual assessment
3. Significant change in status assessment
4. Significant correction of prior full assessment
5. Quarterly review assessment
6. Discharged—return not anticipated
7. Discharged—return anticipated
8. Discharged prior to completing initial assessment
9. Reentry
10. Significant correction of prior quarterly assessment
0. NONE OF ABOVE   `1`
b. Codes for assessments required for Medicare PPS or the State
1. Medicare 5 day assessment
2. Medicare 30 day assessment
3. Medicare 60 day assessment
4. Medicare 90 day assessment
5. Medicare readmission/return assessment
6. Other state required assessment
7. Medicare 14 day assessment
8. Other Medicare required assessment   `1`

9. RESPONSIBILITY/ LEGAL GUARDIAN
(Check all that apply)
Legal guardian `a.` | Durable power attorney/financial `d.`
Other legal oversight `b.` | Family member responsible `e.`
Durable power of attorney/health care `c.` | Patient responsible for self `f. X`
| NONE OF ABOVE `g.`

10. ADVANCED DIRECTIVES
(For those items with supporting documentation in the medical record, check all that apply)
Living will `a. X` | Feeding restrictions `f.`
Do not resuscitate `b.` | Medication restrictions `g.`
Do not hospitalize `c.` | Other treatment restrictions `h.`
Organ donation `d.` | NONE OF ABOVE `i.`
Autopsy request `e.` |

SECTION B. COGNITIVE PATTERNS

1. COMATOSE (Persistent vegetative state/no discernible consciousness)
0. No   1. Yes   (If yes, skip to Section G)   `0`

2. MEMORY (Recall of what was learned or known)
a. Short-term memory OK—seems/appears to recall after 5 minutes
0. Memory OK   1. Memory problem   `1`
b. Long-term memory OK—seems/appears to recall long past
0. Memory OK   1. Memory problem   `0`

3. MEMORY/ RECALL ABILITY (Check all that resident was normally able to recall during last 7 days)
Current season `a. X` | That he/she is in a nursing home `d. X`
Location of own room `b.` |
Staff names/faces `c.` | NONE OF ABOVE are recalled `e.`

4. COGNITIVE SKILLS FOR DAILY DECISION-MAKING (Made decisions regarding tasks of daily life)
0. INDEPENDENT—decisions consistent/reasonable
1. MODIFIED INDEPENDENCE—some difficulty in new situations only
2. MODERATELY IMPAIRED—decisions poor; cues/supervision required
3. SEVERELY IMPAIRED—never/rarely made decisions   `2`

5. INDICATORS OF DELIRIUM—PERIODIC DISORDERED THINKING/ AWARENESS (Code for behavior in the last 7 days.) [Note: Accurate assessment requires conversations with staff and family who have direct knowledge of resident's behavior over this time].
0. Behavior not present
1. Behavior present, not of recent onset
2. Behavior present, over last 7 days appears different from resident's usual functioning (e.g., new onset or worsening)
a. EASILY DISTRACTED—(e.g., difficulty paying attention; gets sidetracked)   `1`
b. PERIODS OF ALTERED PERCEPTION OR AWARENESS OF SURROUNDINGS—(e.g., moves lips or talks to someone not present; believes he/she is somewhere else; confuses night and day)   `0`
c. EPISODES OF DISORGANIZED SPEECH—(e.g., speech is incoherent, nonsensical, irrelevant, or rambling from subject to subject; loses train of thought)   `0`
d. PERIODS OF RESTLESSNESS—(e.g., fidgeting or picking at skin, clothing, napkins, etc; frequent position changes; repetitive physical movements or calling out)   `0`
e. PERIODS OF LETHARGY—(e.g., sluggishness; staring into space; difficult to arouse; little body movement)   `0`
f. MENTAL FUNCTION VARIES OVER THE COURSE OF THE DAY—(e.g., sometimes better, sometimes worse; behaviors sometimes present, sometimes not)   `1`

6. CHANGE IN COGNITIVE STATUS Resident's cognitive status, skills, or abilities have changed as compared to status of 90 days ago (or since last assessment if less than 90 days)
0. No change   1. Improved   2. Deteriorated   `0`

SECTION C. COMMUNICATION/HEARING PATTERNS

1. HEARING (With hearing appliance, if used)
0. HEARS ADEQUATELY—normal talk, TV, phone
1. MINIMAL DIFFICULTY when not in quiet setting
2. HEARS IN SPECIAL SITUATIONS ONLY—speaker has to adjust tonal quality and speak distinctly
3. HIGHLY IMPAIRED/absence of useful hearing   `1`

2. COMMUNICATION DEVICES/ TECHNIQUES (Check all that apply during last 7 days)
Hearing aid, present and used `a. X`
Hearing aid, present and not used regularly `b.`
Other receptive comm. techniques used (e.g., lip reading) `c.`
NONE OF ABOVE `d.`

3. MODES OF EXPRESSION (Check all used by resident to make needs known)
Speech `a. X` | Signs/gestures/sounds `d.`
Writing messages to express or clarify needs `b.` | Communication board `e.`
American sign language or Braille `c.` | Other `f.`
| NONE OF ABOVE `g.`

4. MAKING SELF UNDERSTOOD (Expressing information content—however able)
0. UNDERSTOOD
1. USUALLY UNDERSTOOD—difficulty finding words or finishing thoughts
2. SOMETIMES UNDERSTOOD—ability is limited to making concrete requests
3. RARELY/NEVER UNDERSTOOD   `2`

5. SPEECH CLARITY (Code for speech in the last 7 days)
0. CLEAR SPEECH—distinct, intelligible words
1. UNCLEAR SPEECH—slurred, mumbled words
2. NO SPEECH—absence of spoken words   `1`

6. ABILITY TO UNDERSTAND OTHERS (Understanding verbal information content—however able)
0. UNDERSTANDS
1. USUALLY UNDERSTANDS—may miss some part/intent of message
2. SOMETIMES UNDERSTANDS—responds adequately to simple, direct communication
3. RARELY/NEVER UNDERSTANDS   `2`

7. CHANGE IN COMMUNICATION/ HEARING Resident's ability to express, understand, or hear information has changed as compared to status of 90 days ago (or since last assessment if less than 90 days)
0. No change   1. Improved   2. Deteriorated   `2`

☐ = When box blank, must enter number or letter   `a.` = When letter in box, check if condition applies

MDS 2.0 September, 2000

(continued)

Minimum Data Set form (continued)

Resident _Mary P. Klein_   Numeric Identifier _____

SECTION D. VISION PATTERNS

1.	VISION	(Ability to see in adequate light and with glasses if used)	
		0. *ADEQUATE*—sees fine detail, including regular print in newspapers/books 1. *IMPAIRED*—sees large print, but not regular print in newspapers/books 2. *MODERATELY IMPAIRED*—limited vision; not able to see newspaper headlines, but can identify objects 3. *HIGHLY IMPAIRED*—object identification in question, but eyes appear to follow objects 4. *SEVERELY IMPAIRED*—no vision or sees only light, colors, or shapes; eyes do not appear to follow objects	1
2.	VISUAL LIMITATIONS/DIFFICULTIES	Side vision problems—decreased peripheral vision (e.g., leaves food on one side of tray, difficulty traveling, bumps into people and objects, misjudges placement of chair when seating self)	a.
		Experiences any of following: sees halos or rings around lights; sees flashes of light; sees "curtains" over eyes	b.
		NONE OF ABOVE	c. X
3.	VISUAL APPLIANCES	Glasses; contact lenses; magnifying glass 0. No 1. Yes	1

SECTION E. MOOD AND BEHAVIOR PATTERNS

1.	INDICATORS OF DEPRESSION, ANXIETY, SAD MOOD	(Code for indicators observed in last 30 days, irrespective of the assumed cause) 0. Indicator not exhibited in last 30 days 1. Indicator of this type exhibited up to five days a week 2. Indicator of this type exhibited daily or almost daily (6, 7 days a week)	

VERBAL EXPRESSIONS OF DISTRESS

a.	Resident made negative statements—e.g., "Nothing matters; Would rather be dead; What's the use; Regrets having lived so long; Let me die"	O	h.	Repetitive health complaints—e.g., persistently seeks medical attention, obsessive concern with body functions	O
b.	Repetitive questions—e.g., "Where do I go; What do I do?"	O	i.	Repetitive anxious complaints/concerns (non-health related) e.g., persistently seeks attention/reassurance regarding schedules, meals, laundry, clothing, relationship issues	O
c.	Repetitive verbalizations—e.g., calling out for help, ("God help me")	O		**SLEEP-CYCLE ISSUES**	
d.	Persistent anger with self or others—e.g., easily annoyed, anger at placement in nursing home; anger at care received	O	j.	Unpleasant mood in morning	1
			k.	Insomnia/change in usual sleep pattern	O
				SAD, APATHETIC, ANXIOUS APPEARANCE	
e.	Self deprecation—e.g., "I am nothing; I am of no use to anyone"	O	l.	Sad, pained, worried facial expressions—e.g., furrowed brows	1
f.	Expressions of what appear to be unrealistic fears—e.g., fear of being abandoned, left alone, being with others	O	m.	Crying, tearfulness	1
			n.	Repetitive physical movements—e.g., pacing, hand wringing, restlessness, fidgeting, picking	O
g.	Recurrent statements that something terrible is about to happen—e.g., believes he or she is about to die, have a heart attack	O		**LOSS OF INTEREST**	
			o.	Withdrawal from activities of interest—e.g., no interest in long standing activities or being with family/friends	O
			p.	Reduced social interaction	O

2.	MOOD PERSISTENCE	One or more indicators of depressed, sad or anxious mood were not easily altered by attempts to "cheer up", console, or reassure the resident over last 7 days 0. No mood indicators 1. Indicators present, easily altered 2. Indicators present, not easily altered	2
3.	CHANGE IN MOOD	Resident's mood status has changed as compared to status of 90 days ago (or since last assessment if less than 90 days) 0. No change 1. Improved 2. Deteriorated	O

4.	BEHAVIORAL SYMPTOMS	(A) Behavioral symptom frequency in last 7 days 0. Behavior not exhibited in last 7 days 1. Behavior of this type occurred 1 to 3 days in last 7 days 2. Behavior of this type occurred 4 to 6 days, but less than daily 3. Behavior of this type occurred daily		
		(B) Behavioral symptom alterability in last 7 days 0. Behavior not present OR behavior was easily altered 1. Behavior was not easily altered	(A)	(B)
		a. WANDERING (moved with no rational purpose, seemingly oblivious to needs or safety)	O	O
		b. VERBALLY ABUSIVE BEHAVIORAL SYMPTOMS (others were threatened, screamed at, cursed at)	O	O
		c. PHYSICALLY ABUSIVE BEHAVIORAL SYMPTOMS (others were hit, shoved, scratched, sexually abused)	O	O
		d. SOCIALLY INAPPROPRIATE/DISRUPTIVE BEHAVIORAL SYMPTOMS (made disruptive sounds, noisiness, screaming, self-abusive acts, sexual behavior or disrobing in public, smeared/threw food/faces, hoarding, rummaged through others' belongings)	1	1
		e. RESISTS CARE (resisted taking medications/ injections, ADL assistance, or eating)	O	O

5.	CHANGE IN BEHAVIORAL SYMPTOMS	Resident's behavior status has changed as compared to status of 90 days ago (or since last assessment if less than 90 days) 0. No change 1. Improved 2. Deteriorated	O

SECTION F. PSYCHOSOCIAL WELL-BEING

1.	SENSE OF INITIATIVE/INVOLVEMENT	At ease interacting with others	a.
		At ease doing planned or structured activities	b. X
		At ease doing self-initiated activities	c.
		Establishes own goals	d.
		Pursues involvement in life of facility (e.g., makes/keeps friends; involved in group activities; responds positively to new activities; assists at religious services)	e.
		Accepts invitations into most group activities	f.
		NONE OF ABOVE	g.
2.	UNSETTLED RELATIONSHIPS	Covert/open conflict with or repeated criticism of staff	a.
		Unhappy with roommate	b.
		Unhappy with residents other than roommate	c.
		Openly expresses conflict/anger with family/friends	d.
		Absence of personal contact with family/friends	e.
		Recent loss of close family member/friend	f.
		Does not adjust easily to routines	g. X
		NONE OF ABOVE	h.
3.	PAST ROLES	Strong identification with past roles and life status	a.
		Expresses sadness/anger/empty feeling over lost roles/status	b.
		Resident perceives that daily routine (customary routine, activities) is very different from prior pattern in the community	c. X
		NONE OF ABOVE	d.

SECTION G. PHYSICAL FUNCTIONING AND STRUCTURAL PROBLEMS

1.	(A) ADL SELF-PERFORMANCE—(Code for resident's PERFORMANCE OVER ALL SHIFTS during last 7 days—Not including setup)	

0. *INDEPENDENT*—No help or oversight —OR— Help/oversight provided only 1 or 2 times during last 7 days
1. *SUPERVISION*—Oversight, encouragement or cueing provided 3 or more times during last 7 days —OR— Supervision (3 or more times) plus physical assistance provided only 1 or 2 times during last 7 days
2. *LIMITED ASSISTANCE*—Resident highly involved in activity; received physical help in guided maneuvering of limbs or other nonweight bearing assistance 3 or more times —OR—More help provided only 1 or 2 times during last 7 days
3. *EXTENSIVE ASSISTANCE*—While resident performed part of activity, over last 7-day period, help of following type(s) provided 3 or more times:
— Weight-bearing support
— Full staff performance during part (but not all) of last 7 days
4. *TOTAL DEPENDENCE*—Full staff performance of activity during entire 7 days
8. *ACTIVITY DID NOT OCCUR* during entire 7 days

(B) ADL SUPPORT PROVIDED—(Code for MOST SUPPORT PROVIDED OVER ALL SHIFTS during last 7 days; code regardless of resident's self-performance classification)		(A)	(B)
0. No setup or physical help from staff 1. Setup help only 2. One person physical assist 3. Two+ persons physical assist	8. ADL activity itself did not occur during entire 7 days	SELF-PERF	SUPPORT

			(A)	(B)
a.	BED MOBILITY	How resident moves to and from lying position, turns side to side, and positions body while in bed	3	3
b.	TRANSFER	How resident moves between surfaces—to/from: bed, chair, wheelchair, standing position (EXCLUDE to/from bath/toilet)	3	2
c.	WALK IN ROOM	How resident walks between locations in his/her room	2	2
d.	WALK IN CORRIDOR	How resident walks in corridor on unit	2	3
e.	LOCOMOTION ON UNIT	How resident moves between locations in his/her room and adjacent corridor on same floor. If in wheelchair, self-sufficiency once in chair	2	2
f.	LOCOMOTION OFF UNIT	How resident moves to and returns from off unit locations (e.g., areas set aside for dining, activities, or treatments). If facility has only one floor, how resident moves to and from distant areas on the floor. If in wheelchair, self-sufficiency once in chair	2	2
g.	DRESSING	How resident puts on, fastens, and takes off all items of street clothing, including donning/removing prosthesis	3	2
h.	EATING	How resident eats and drinks (regardless of skill). Includes intake of nourishment by other means (e.g., tube feeding, total parenteral nutrition)	1	1
i.	TOILET USE	How resident uses the toilet room (or commode, bedpan, urinal); transfer on/off toilet, cleanses, changes pad, manages ostomy or catheter, adjusts clothes	3	2
j.	PERSONAL HYGIENE	How resident maintains personal hygiene, including combing hair, brushing teeth, shaving, applying makeup, washing/drying face, hands, and perineum (EXCLUDE baths and showers)	3	2

MDS 2.0 September, 2000

Minimum Data Set form *(continued)*

Resident __Mary P. Klein__   Numeric Identifier _____

2.	BATHING	How resident takes full-body bath/shower, sponge bath, and transfers in/out of tub/shower (EXCLUDE washing of back and hair.) *Code for most dependent in self-performance and support* **(A) BATHING SELF-PERFORMANCE** codes appear below	(A)	(B)
		0. Independent—No help provided	**3**	**2**
		1. Supervision—Oversight help only		
		2. Physical help limited to transfer only		
		3. Physical help in part of bathing activity		
		4. Total dependence		
		8. Activity itself did not occur during entire 7 days *(Bathing support codes are as defined in Item 1, code B above)*		

3.	TEST FOR BALANCE (see training manual)	*(Code for ability during test in the last 7 days)* 0. Maintained position as required in test 1. Unsteady, but able to rebalance self without physical support 2. Partial physical support during test; or stands (sits) but does not follow directions for test 3. Not able to attempt test without physical help	
		a. Balance while standing	
		b. Balance while sitting—position, trunk control	0

4.	FUNCTIONAL LIMITATION IN RANGE OF MOTION (see training manual)	*(Code for limitations during last 7 days that interfered with daily functions or placed resident at risk of injury)* **(A) RANGE OF MOTION** **(B) VOLUNTARY MOVEMENT** 0. No limitation 0. No loss 1. Limitation on one side 1. Partial loss 2. Limitation on both sides 2. Full loss	(A)	(B)
		a. Neck	1	1
		b. Arm—Including shoulder or elbow	1	1
		c. Hand—Including wrist or fingers	0	0
		d. Leg—Including hip or knee	0	0
		e. Foot—Including ankle or toes	0	0
		f. Other limitation or loss	0	0

5.	MODES OF LOCOMOTION	*(Check all that apply during last 7 days)*	
		Cane/walker/crutch **a.** X Wheelchair primary mode of **d.** X locomotion	
		Wheeled self **b.** X	
		Other person wheeled **c.** X NONE OF ABOVE **e.**	

6.	MODES OF TRANSFER	*(Check all that apply during last 7 days)*	
		Bedfast all or most of time **a.** Lifted mechanically **d.**	
		Bed rails used for bed mobility or transfer **b.** X Transfer aid (e.g., slide board, trapeze, cane, walker, brace) **e.**	
		Lifted manually **c.** X NONE OF ABOVE **f.**	

7.	TASK SEGMENTA-TION	Some or all of ADL activities were broken into subtasks during last 7 days so that resident could perform them 0. No 1. Yes	

8.	ADL FUNCTIONAL REHABILITA-TION POTENTIAL	Resident believes he/she is capable of increased independence in at least some ADLs **a.** 1	1
		Direct care staff believe resident is capable of increased independence in at least some ADLs **b.** X	
		Resident able to perform tasks/activity but is very slow **c.**	
		Difference in ADL Self-Performance or ADL Support, comparing mornings to evenings **d.** X	
		NONE OF ABOVE **e.**	

9.	CHANGE IN ADL FUNCTION	Resident's ADL self-performance status has changed as compared to status of 90 days ago (or since last assessment if less than 90 days) 0. No change 1. Improved 2. Deteriorated	0

SECTION H. CONTINENCE IN LAST 14 DAYS

1. CONTINENCE SELF-CONTROL CATEGORIES
(Code for resident's PERFORMANCE OVER ALL SHIFTS)

0. CONTINENT—Complete control *[includes use of indwelling urinary catheter or ostomy device that does not leak urine or stool]*

1. USUALLY CONTINENT—BLADDER, incontinent episodes once a week or less; BOWEL, less than weekly

2. OCCASIONALLY INCONTINENT—BLADDER, 2 or more times a week but not daily; BOWEL, once a week

3. FREQUENTLY INCONTINENT—BLADDER, tended to be incontinent daily, but some control present (e.g., on day shift); BOWEL, 2-3 times a week

4. INCONTINENT—Had inadequate control BLADDER, multiple daily episodes; BOWEL, all (or almost all) of the time

a.	BOWEL CONTI-NENCE	Control of bowel movement, with appliance or bowel continence programs, if employed	2
b.	BLADDER CONTI-NENCE	Control of urinary bladder function (if dribbles, volume insufficient to soak through underpants), with appliances (e.g., foley) or continence programs, if employed	2
2.	BOWEL ELIMINATION PATTERN	Bowel elimination pattern regular—at least one movement every three days **a.** Diarrhea **c.** X Fecal impaction **d.** Constipation **b.** NONE OF ABOVE **e.**	

MDS 2.0 September, 2000

3.	APPLIANCES AND PROGRAMS	Any scheduled toileting plan **a.** X Did not use toilet room/commode/urinal **f.**	
		Bladder retraining program **b.** Pads/briefs used **g.** X	
		External (condom) catheter **c.** Enemas/irrigation **h.**	
		Indwelling catheter **d.** Ostomy present **i.**	
		Intermittent catheter **e.** NONE OF ABOVE **j.**	
4.	CHANGE IN URINARY CONTINENCE	Resident's urinary continence has changed as compared to status of 90 days ago (or since last assessment if less than 90 days) 0. No change 1. Improved 2. Deteriorated	

SECTION I. DISEASE DIAGNOSES

Check only those diseases that have a relationship to current ADL status, cognitive status, mood and behavior status, medical treatments, nursing monitoring, or risk of death. (Do not list inactive diagnoses.)

1.	DISEASES	*(If none apply, CHECK the NONE OF ABOVE box)*	

ENDOCRINE/METABOLIC/NUTRITIONAL	Hemiplegia/Hemiparesis	**v.** X
	Multiple sclerosis	**w.**
Diabetes mellitus **a.**	Paraplegia	**x.**
Hyperthyroidism **b.**	Parkinson's disease	**y.**
Hypothyroidism **c.**	Quadriplegia	**z.**
HEART/CIRCULATION	Seizure disorder	**aa.**
Arteriosclerotic heart disease (ASHD) **d.**	Transient ischemic attack (TIA)	**bb.**
Cardiac dysrhythmias **e.**	Traumatic brain injury	**cc.**
Congestive heart failure **f.**	**PSYCHIATRIC/MOOD**	
Deep vein thrombosis **g.**	Anxiety disorder	**dd.**
Hypertension **h.** X	Depression	**ee.** X
Hypotension **i.**	Manic depression (bipolar disease)	**ff.**
Peripheral vascular disease **j.**	Schizophrenia	**gg.**
Other cardiovascular disease **k.**	**PULMONARY**	
MUSCULOSKELETAL	Asthma	**hh.**
Arthritis **l.** X	Emphysema/COPD	**ii.**
Hip fracture **m.**	**SENSORY**	
Missing limb (e.g., amputation) **n.**	Cataracts	**jj.**
Osteoporosis **o.**	Diabetic retinopathy	**kk.**
Pathological bone fracture **p.**	Glaucoma	**ll.**
NEUROLOGICAL	Macular degeneration	**mm.**
Alzheimer's disease **q.**	**OTHER**	
Aphasia **r.**	Allergies	**nn.** X
Cerebral palsy **s.**	Anemia	**oo.**
Cerebrovascular accident (stroke) **t.** X	Cancer	**pp.**
Dementia other than Alzheimer's disease **u.**	Renal failure	**qq.**
	NONE OF ABOVE	**rr.**

2.	INFECTIONS	*(If none apply, CHECK the NONE OF ABOVE box)*	

Antibiotic resistant infection (e.g., Methicillin resistant staph) **a.**	Septicemia	**g.**
	Sexually transmitted diseases	**h.**
Clostridium difficile (c. diff.) **b.**	Tuberculosis	**i.**
Conjunctivitis **c.**	Urinary tract infection in last 30 days	**j.**
HIV infection **d.**	Viral hepatitis	**k.**
Pneumonia **e.**	Wound infection	**l.**
Respiratory infection **f.**	NONE OF ABOVE	**m.**

3.	OTHER CURRENT OR MORE DETAILED DIAGNOSES AND ICD-9 CODES	a. *Gait Dysfunction* 781.2	
		b. ____ ___._	
		c. ____ ___._	
		d. ____ ___._	
		e. ____ ___._	

SECTION J. HEALTH CONDITIONS

1.	PROBLEM CONDITIONS	*(Check all problems present in last 7 days unless other time frame is indicated)*	

INDICATORS OF FLUID STATUS	Dizziness/Vertigo	**f.**
Weight gain or loss of 3 or more pounds within a 7 day period **a.**	Edema	**g.**
	Fever	**h.**
	Hallucinations	**i.**
Inability to lie flat due to shortness of breath **b.**	Internal bleeding	**j.**
	Recurrent lung aspirations in last 90 days	**k.**
Dehydrated; output exceeds input **c.**	Shortness of breath	**l.**
	Syncope (fainting)	**m.**
Insufficient fluid; did NOT consume all/almost all liquids provided during last 3 days **d.**	Unsteady gait	**n.** X
	Vomiting	**o.**
OTHER	NONE OF ABOVE	**p.**
Delusions **e.**		

(continued)

Minimum Data Set form *(continued)*

Resident _Mary P. Klein_

Numeric Identifier _____

2.	PAIN SYMPTOMS	(Code the highest level of pain present in the last 7 days)	
		a. FREQUENCY with which resident complains or shows evidence of pain 0. No pain *(skip to J4)* 1. Pain less than daily 2. Pain daily	**1**
		b. INTENSITY of pain 1. Mild pain 2. Moderate pain 3. Times when pain is horrible or excruciating	
3.	PAIN SITE	(If pain present, check all sites that apply in last 7 days)	
		Back pain — a. Bone pain — b. Chest pain while doing usual activities — c. Headache — d. Hip pain — e.	Incisional pain — f. **X** Joint pain (other than hip) — g. Soft tissue pain (e.g., lesion, muscle) — h. Stomach pain — i. Other — j.
4.	ACCIDENTS	(Check all that apply) Fell in past 30 days — a. **X** Fell in past 31-180 days — b.	Hip fracture in last 180 days — c. Other fracture in last 180 days — d. e.
5.	STABILITY OF CONDITIONS	Conditions/diseases make resident's cognitive, ADL, mood or behavior patterns unstable—(fluctuating, precarious, or deteriorating) — a. Resident experiencing an acute episode or a flare-up of a recurrent or chronic problem — b. End-stage disease, 6 or fewer months to live — c. NONE OF ABOVE — d. **X**	

SECTION K. ORAL/NUTRITIONAL STATUS

1.	ORAL PROBLEMS	Chewing problem — a. Swallowing problem — b. Mouth pain — c. NONE OF ABOVE — d.	
2.	HEIGHT AND WEIGHT	Record (a.) height in inches and (b.) weight in pounds. Base weight on most recent measure in last 30 days; measure weight consistently in accord with standard facility practice—e.g., in a.m. after voiding, before meal, with shoes off, and in nightclothes a. HT (in.) **6 6** b. WT (lb.) **1 7 0**	
3.	WEIGHT CHANGE	a. Weight loss—5 % or more in last 30 days; or 10 % or more in last 180 days 0. No 1. Yes — **0** b. Weight gain—5 % or more in last 30 days; or 10 % or more in last 180 days 0. No 1. Yes — **0**	
4.	NUTRITIONAL PROBLEMS	Complains about the taste of many foods — a. Regular or repetitive complaints of hunger — b.	Leaves 25% or more of food uneaten at most meals — c. NONE OF ABOVE — d. **X**
5.	NUTRITIONAL APPROACHES	(Check all that apply in last 7 days) Parenteral/IV — a. Feeding tube — b. Mechanically altered diet — c. Syringe (oral feeding) — d. Therapeutic diet — e.	Dietary supplement between meals — f. Plate guard, stabilized built-up utensil, etc. — g. On a planned weight change program — h. NONE OF ABOVE — i.
6.	PARENTERAL OR ENTERAL INTAKE	(Skip to Section L if neither 5a nor 5b is checked) a. Code the proportion of total calories the resident received through parenteral or tube feedings in the last 7 days 0. None 3. 51% to 75% 1. 1% to 25% 4. 76% to 100% 2. 26% to 50% b. Code the average fluid intake per day by IV or tube in last 7 days 0. None 3. 1001 to 1500 cc/day 1. 1 to 500 cc/day 4. 1501 to 2000 cc/day 2. 501 to 1000 cc/day 5. 2001 or more cc/day	

SECTION L. ORAL/DENTAL STATUS

1.	ORAL STATUS AND DISEASE PREVENTION	Debris (soft, easily movable substances) present in mouth prior to going to bed at night — a. Has dentures or removable bridge — b. **X** Some/all natural teeth lost—does not have or does not use dentures (or partial plates) — c. Broken, loose, or carious teeth — d. Inflamed gums (gingiva); swollen or bleeding gums; oral abscesses; ulcers or rashes — e. Daily cleaning of teeth/dentures or daily mouth care—by resident or staff — f. **X** NONE OF ABOVE — g.	

SECTION M. SKIN CONDITION

			Number at Stage
1.	ULCERS (Due to any cause)	(Record the number of ulcers at each ulcer stage—regardless of cause. If none present at a stage, record "0" (zero). Code all that apply during last 7 days. Code 9 = 9 or more.) [Requires full body exam.]	
		a. Stage 1. A persistent area of skin redness (without a break in the skin) that does not disappear when pressure is relieved.	**1**
		b. Stage 2. A partial thickness loss of skin layers that presents clinically as an abrasion, blister, or shallow crater.	**0**
		c. Stage 3. A full thickness of skin is lost, exposing the subcutaneous tissues - presents as a deep crater with or without undermining adjacent tissue.	**0**
		d. Stage 4. A full thickness of skin and subcutaneous tissue is lost, exposing muscle or bone.	**0**
2.	TYPE OF ULCER	(For each type of ulcer, code for the highest stage in the last 7 days using scale in item M1—i.e., 0=none; stages 1, 2, 3, 4) a. Pressure ulcer—any lesion caused by pressure resulting in damage of underlying tissue	**1**
		b. Stasis ulcer—open lesion caused by poor circulation in the lower extremities	**0**
3.	HISTORY OF RESOLVED ULCERS	Resident had an ulcer that was resolved or cured in LAST 90 DAYS 0. No 1. Yes	**0**
4.	OTHER SKIN PROBLEMS OR LESIONS PRESENT	(Check all that apply during last 7 days) Abrasions, bruises — a. **X** Burns (second or third degree) — b. Open lesions other than ulcers, rashes, cuts (e.g., cancer lesions) — c. Rashes—e.g., intertrigo, eczema, drug rash, heat rash, herpes zoster — d. Skin desensitized to pain or pressure — e. Skin tears or cuts (other than surgery) — f. Surgical wounds — g. NONE OF ABOVE — h.	
5.	SKIN TREATMENTS	(Check all that apply during last 7 days) Pressure relieving device(s) for chair — a. **X** Pressure relieving device(s) for bed — b. Turning/repositioning program — c. Nutrition or hydration intervention to manage skin problems — d. **X** Ulcer care — e. Surgical wound care — f. Application of dressings (with or without topical medications) other than to feet — g. Application of ointments/medications (other than to feet) — h. Other preventative or protective skin care (other than to feet) — i. **X** NONE OF ABOVE — j.	
6.	FOOT PROBLEMS AND CARE	(Check all that apply during last 7 days) Resident has one or more foot problems—e.g., corns, calluses, bunions, hammer toes, overlapping toes, pain, structural problems — a. Infection of the foot—e.g., cellulitis, purulent drainage — b. Open lesions on the foot — c. Nails/calluses trimmed during last 90 days — d. **X** Received preventative or protective foot care (e.g., used special shoes, inserts, pads, toe separators) — e. Application of dressings (with or without topical medications) — f. NONE OF ABOVE — g.	

SECTION N. ACTIVITY PURSUIT PATTERNS

1.	TIME AWAKE	(Check appropriate time periods over last 7 days) Resident awake all or most of time (i.e., naps no more than one hour per time period) in the: Morning — a. **X** Afternoon — b.	Evening — c. NONE OF ABOVE — d.
		(If resident is comatose, skip to Section O)	
2.	AVERAGE TIME INVOLVED IN ACTIVITIES	(When awake and not receiving treatments or ADL care) 0. Most—more than 2/3 of time 2. Little—less than 1/3 of time 1. Some—from 1/3 to 2/3 of time 3. None	**2**
3.	PREFERRED ACTIVITY SETTINGS	(Check all settings in which activities are preferred) Own room — a. Day/activity room — b. Inside NH/off unit — c.	Outside facility — d. NONE OF ABOVE — e.
4.	GENERAL ACTIVITY PREFERENCES (adapted to resident's current abilities)	(Check all PREFERENCES whether or not activity is currently available to resident) Cards/other games — a. Crafts/arts — b. Exercise/sports — c. Music — d. **X** Reading/writing — e. Spiritual/religious activities — f. **X**	Trips/shopping — g. Walking/wheeling outdoors — h. Watching TV — i. **X** Gardening or plants — j. Talking or conversing — k. Helping others — l. NONE OF ABOVE — m.

MDS 2.0 September, 2000

Minimum Data Set form *(continued)*

Resident _Mary P. Klein_   Numeric Identifier _____

5.	PREFERS CHANGE IN DAILY ROUTINE	Code for resident preferences in daily routines 0. No change 1. Slight change 2. Major change	
		a. Type of activities in which resident is currently involved	0
		b. Extent of resident involvement in activities	0

SECTION O. MEDICATIONS

1.	NUMBER OF MEDICA-TIONS	*(Record the number of different medications used in the last 7 days; enter "0" if none used)*	07
2.	NEW MEDICA-TIONS	*(Resident currently receiving medications that were initiated during the last 90 days)* 0. No 1. Yes	0
3.	INJECTIONS	*(Record the number of DAYS injections of any type received during the last 7 days; enter "0" if none used)*	0
4.	DAYS RECEIVED THE FOLLOWING MEDICATION	*(Record the number of DAYS during last 7 days; enter "0" if not used. Note—enter "1" for long-acting meds used less than weekly)*	

a. Antipsychotic	0	d. Hypnotic	0
b. Antianxiety	3	e. Diuretic	0
c. Antidepressant	7		

SECTION P. SPECIAL TREATMENTS AND PROCEDURES

1.	SPECIAL TREAT-MENTS, PROCE-DURES, AND PROGRAMS	a. SPECIAL CARE—*Check treatments or programs received during the last 14 days*	

TREATMENTS			Ventilator or respirator	l.	
Chemotherapy	a.		**PROGRAMS**		
Dialysis	b.		Alcohol/drug treatment program	m.	
IV medication	c.				
Intake/output	d.		Alzheimer's/dementia special care unit	n.	
Monitoring acute medical condition	e.		Hospice care	o.	
Ostomy care	f.		Pediatric unit	p.	
Oxygen therapy	g.		Respite care	q.	
Radiation	h.		Training in skills required to return to the community (e.g., taking medications, house work, shopping, transportation, ADLs)	r.	
Suctioning	i.				
Tracheostomy care	j.				
Transfusions	k.		NONE OF ABOVE	s.	X

b. THERAPIES - *Record the number of days and total minutes each of the following therapies was administered (for at least 15 minutes a day) in the last 7 calendar days (Enter 0 if none or less than 15 min. daily)*
[Note—count only post admission therapies]
(A) = # of days administered for 15 minutes or more
(B) = total # of minutes provided in last 7 days

	DAYS (A)	MIN (B)
a. Speech - language pathology and audiology services	3	05
b. Occupational therapy	0	20
c. Physical therapy	4	20
d. Respiratory therapy	0	
e. Psychological therapy (by any licensed mental health professional)	1	30

2.	INTERVEN-TION PROGRAMS FOR MOOD, BEHAVIOR, COGNITIVE LOSS	**(Check all interventions or strategies used in last 7 days—no matter where received)**	
		Special behavior symptom evaluation program	a. X
		Evaluation by a licensed mental health specialist in last 90 days	b. X
		Group therapy	c.
		Resident-specific deliberate changes in the environment to address mood/behavior patterns—e.g., providing bureau in which to rummage	d.
		Reorientation—e.g., cueing	e.
		NONE OF ABOVE	f.

3.	NURSING REHABILITA-TION/ RESTOR-ATIVE CARE	*Record the NUMBER OF DAYS each of the following rehabilitation or restorative techniques or practices was provided to the resident for more than or equal to 15 minutes per day in the last 7 days (Enter 0 if none or less than 15 min. daily)*	

a. Range of motion (passive)	0	f. Walking	0
b. Range of motion (active)	0	g. Dressing or grooming	5
c. Splint or brace assistance	0	h. Eating or swallowing	0
TRAINING AND SKILL PRACTICE IN:		i. Amputation/prosthesis care	0
d. Bed mobility	0	j. Communication	0
e. Transfer	0	k. Other	0

4.	DEVICES AND RESTRAINTS	*(Use the following codes for last 7 days:)* 0. Not used 1. Used less than daily 2. Used daily	
		Bed rails	
		a. — Full bed rails on all open sides of bed	0
		b. — Other types of side rails used (e.g., half rail, one side)	2
		c. Trunk restraint	0
		d. Limb restraint	0
		e. Chair prevents rising	0
5.	HOSPITAL STAY(S)	Record number of times resident was admitted to hospital with an overnight stay in last 90 days (or since last assessment if less than 90 days). *(Enter 0 if no hospital admissions)*	01
6.	EMERGENCY ROOM (ER) VISIT(S)	Record number of times resident visited ER without an overnight stay in last 90 days (or since last assessment if less than 90 days). *(Enter 0 if no ER visits)*	01
7.	PHYSICIAN VISITS	In the LAST 14 DAYS (or since admission if less than 14 days in facility) how many days has the physician (or authorized assistant or practitioner) examined the resident? *(Enter 0 if none)*	02
8.	PHYSICIAN ORDERS	In the LAST 14 DAYS (or since admission if less than 14 days in facility) how many days has the physician (or authorized assistant or practitioner) changed the resident's orders? Do not include order renewals without change. *(Enter 0 if none)*	02
9.	ABNORMAL LAB VALUES	Has the resident had any abnormal lab values during the last 90 days (or since admission)? 0. No 1. Yes	1

SECTION Q. DISCHARGE POTENTIAL AND OVERALL STATUS

1.	DISCHARGE POTENTIAL	a. Resident expresses/indicates preference to return to the community 0. No 1. Yes	1
		b. Resident has a support person who is positive towards discharge 0. No 1. Yes	1
		c. Stay projected to be of a short duration— discharge projected within 90 days (do not include expected discharge due to death) 0. No 2. Within 31-90 days 1. Within 30 days 3. Discharge status uncertain	2
2.	OVERALL CHANGE IN CARE NEEDS	Resident's overall self sufficiency has changed significantly as compared to status of 90 days ago (or since last assessment if less than 90 days) 0. No change 1. Improved—receives fewer supports, needs less restrictive level of care 2. Deteriorated—receives more support	0

SECTION R. ASSESSMENT INFORMATION

1.	PARTICIPA-TION IN ASSESS-MENT	a. Resident: 0. No 1. Yes	1
		b. Family: 0. No 1. Yes 2. No family	1
		c. Significant other: 0. No 1. Yes 2. None	1

2. SIGNATURE OF PERSON COORDINATING THE ASSESSMENT:

Marie Smith, RNAC

a. Signature of RN Assessment Coordinator (sign on above line)

b. Date RN Assessment Coordinator signed as complete

02	-	10	-	2007
Month		Day		Year

MDS 2.0 September, 2000

(continued)

Minimum Data Set form *(continued)*

Resident _Mary P. Klein_   Numeric Identifier _____

SECTION T. THERAPY SUPPLEMENT FOR MEDICARE PPS

1.	SPECIAL TREAT-MENTS AND PROCE-DURES	**a. RECREATION THERAPY**—*Enter number of days and total minutes of recreation therapy administered (for at least 15 minutes a day) in the last 7 days (Enter 0 if none)*	

		DAYS (A)	MIN (B)
(A) = # of days administered for 15 minutes or more		**O**	
(B) = total # of minutes provided in last 7 days			

Skip unless this is a Medicare 5 day or Medicare readmission/return assessment.

b. ORDERED THERAPIES— Has physician ordered any of following therapies to begin in FIRST 14 days of stay—physical therapy, occupational therapy, or speech pathology service?
  0. No   1. Yes   **1**

If not ordered, skip to item 2

c. Through day 15, provide an estimate of the number of days when at least 1 therapy service can be expected to have been delivered.   **11**

d. Through day 15, provide an estimate of the number of therapy minutes (across the therapies) that can be expected to be delivered?   **450**

2.	WALKING WHEN MOST SELF SUFFICIENT	*Complete item 2 if ADL self-performance score for TRANSFER (G.1.b.A) is 0,1,2, or 3 AND at least one of the following are present:*

- Resident received physical therapy involving gait training (P.1.b.c)
- Physical therapy was ordered for the resident involving gait training (T.1.b)
- Resident received nursing rehabilitation for walking (P.3.f)
- Physical therapy involving walking has been discontinued within the past 180 days

Skip to item 3 if resident did not walk in last 7 days

(FOR FOLLOWING FIVE ITEMS, BASE CODING ON THE EPISODE WHEN THE RESIDENT WALKED THE FARTHEST WITHOUT SITTING DOWN. INCLUDE WALKING DURING REHABILITATION SESSIONS.)

a. Furthest distance walked without sitting down during this episode.   **2**

0. 150+ feet	3. 10-25 feet
1. 51-149 feet	4. Less than 10 feet
2. 26-50 feet	

b. Time walked without sitting down during this episode.   **2**

0. 1-2 minutes	3. 11-15 minutes
1. 3-4 minutes	4. 16-30 minutes
2. 5-10 minutes	5. 31+ minutes

c. Self-Performance in walking during this episode.   **2**

0. *INDEPENDENT*—No help or oversight
1. *SUPERVISION*—Oversight, encouragement or cueing provided
2. *LIMITED ASSISTANCE*—Resident highly involved in walking; received physical help in guided maneuvering of limbs or other nonweight bearing assistance
3. *EXTENSIVE ASSISTANCE*—Resident received weight bearing assistance while walking

d. Walking support provided associated with this episode (code regardless of resident's self-performance classification).   **1**

0. No setup or physical help from staff
1. Setup help only
2. One person physical assist
3. Two+ persons physical assist

e. Parallel bars used by resident in association with this episode.

  0. No   1. Yes

3.	CASE MIX GROUP	Medicare	State

MDS 2.0 September, 2000

Minimum Data Set form *(continued)*

SECTION V. RESIDENT ASSESSMENT PROTOCOL SUMMARY   Numeric Identifier _____

Resident's Name: *Mary P. Klein* | Medical Record No.:

1. Check if RAP is triggered.

2. For each triggered RAP, use the RAP guidelines to identify areas needing further assessment. Document relevant assessment information regarding the resident's status.

   • Describe:
   — Nature of the condition (may include presence or lack of objective data and subjective complaints).
   — Complications and risk factors that affect your decision to proceed to care planning.
   — Factors that must be considered in developing individualized care plan interventions.
   — Need for referrals/further evaluation by appropriate health professionals.

   • Documentation should support your decision-making regarding whether to proceed with a care plan for a triggered RAP and the type(s) of care plan interventions that are appropriate for a particular resident.

   • Documentation may appear anywhere in the clinical record (e.g., progress notes, consults, flowsheets, etc.).

3. Indicate under the Location of RAP Assessment Documentation column where information related to the RAP assessment can be found.

4. For each triggered RAP, indicate whether a new care plan, care plan revision, or continuation of current care plan is necessary to address the problem(s) identified in your assessment. The Care Planning Decision column must be completed within 7 days of completing the RAI (MDS and RAPs).

A. RAP PROBLEM AREA	(a) Check if triggered	Location and Date of RAP Assessment Documentation	(b) Care Planning Decision—check if addressed in care plan
1. DELIRIUM			
2. COGNITIVE LOSS			
3. VISUAL FUNCTION			
4. COMMUNICATION	X	2/5/07 Progress notes	X
5. ADL FUNCTIONAL/ REHABILITATION POTENTIAL	X	2/6/07 Progress notes	X
6. URINARY INCONTINENCE AND INDWELLING CATHETER			
7. PSYCHOSOCIAL WELL-BEING			
8. MOOD STATE	X	2/6/07 Progress notes	X
9. BEHAVIORAL SYMPTOMS	X	2/6/07 Progress notes	X
10. ACTIVITIES	X	2/5/07 Progress notes	X
11. FALLS	X	2/6/07 Progress notes	X
12. NUTRITIONAL STATUS			
13. FEEDING TUBES			
14. DEHYDRATION/FLUID MAINTENANCE			
15. DENTAL CARE			
16. PRESSURE ULCERS			
17. PSYCHOTROPIC DRUG USE			
18. PHYSICAL RESTRAINTS			

B. *Marie Smith, RNAC*   2. 02-11-2007 Month Day Year
1. Signature of RN Coordinator for RAP Assessment Process

  Jamie K. Kauffman, RN   4. 02-11-2007 Month Day Year
3. Signature of Person Completing Care Planning Decision

MDS 2.0 September, 2000

ferent types of methods or forms for recording this information, but an electronic medical record where daily notes automatically record into the MDS is the most efficient process.

HELPFUL HINTS FOR COMPLETING THE MDS

It's important for you to recognize that data recorded on the MDS requires information from specific time periods. For example, section G, Physical functioning and structural problems, has a look-back period of 7 days, where section E, Mood and behavior patterns, has a look-back period of 30 days. All look-back periods are determined by the assessment reference date that's recorded in section A3 of the MDS; the RNAC is responsible for determining this date.

It's also your responsibility to ensure that the scores recorded within the MDS are consistent between sections. For example, if you record aphasia in section I, Disease diagnoses, the symptoms should correspond to the coding in section C, Communication/Hearing patterns. You should also mark and grade sections C4, Making self understood, and C6, Ability to understand others, appropriately.

If you record the performance of physical therapy, occupational therapy, or speech therapy in Section P, Special treatments and procedures, be sure to record that either the patient or the direct care staff believe that the patient is capable of increased independence. Also ensure that the diagnosis listed in section I, Disease diagnoses, accurately reflects the reason for rehabilitation services.

Pay particular attention to accurately scoring the late-loss ADLs (bed mobility, toileting, eating, and transfers). These scores impact directly on all RUG payment categories. Many facilities have developed specific ADL forms that capture daily information on function, including a patient's self-performance code and a code recording the amount of ADL support provided by the staff.

Resident assessment protocols

Another federally mandated form, the resident assessment protocols (RAP) summary lists identified problems and documents the existence of a corresponding care plan. For example, if the patient has a stage 2 pressure ulcer documented in the MDS, the RAP summary should indicate the need for a care plan to treat the pressure ulcer.

Care plans

Each patient in a long-term care facility must have a documented interdisciplinary care plan. The care plan must include a problem list (to include items identified on the RAP summary), a measurable goal for each problem identified, and individualized approaches that will be used to attain those goals.

When a patient is admitted to a long-term care facility, the health care team will commonly utilize an interim care plan (which should be in place within 24 hours of admission) until there's an interdisciplinary care conference regarding the patient. Usual standards require that the interdisciplinary care plan be completed within 7 days of the completion of the MDS, and a documented review of the plan completed every 3 months, as a patient's condition changes, or when unplanned events such as a fall occur.

PASARR

The PASARR screens for mental illness, mental retardation, and other related conditions that may affect ADL functioning. Federal statutes require the completion of the PASARR form on or prior to admission to a long-term care facility, and it's usually the responsibility of a social worker or the admissions director.

Initial nursing assessment

The initial nursing assessment must be performed and documented for all patients admitted to a long-term care facility. Many facilities have forms that cue staff on obtaining and documenting complete assessment information; however, in general, if you utilize the topic categories of the MDS, you'll perform a comprehensive assessment. Among the areas that you'll assess are cognitive function; communication and hearing patterns (note if a hearing aid is present); vision (note if visual appliances are necessary); mood and behavior; psychosocial well-being; physical functioning and structural problems; continence; disease processes, including system assessments, vital signs, height, and weight; health conditions; oral, dental, and nutritional status (be sure to note if dentures are present); and skin conditions.

Other assessment forms

In addition to the initial nursing assessment, you'll commonly use other forms to collect patient information, such as pain assessment and restraint assessment forms. Certain risk assessment forms can help to quantify a patient's risk for falls and skin breakdown. (See *Braden scale for predicting pressure sore risk,* pages 200 and 201. See also *Fall assessment and action plan,* page 202.)

Nursing summaries

Some states require a monthly summary; others don't. In general, you must perform an assessment of all interventions and treatments periodically and adjust the care plan accordingly. Follow your facility policy for the frequency of these assessments.

Discharge and transfer forms

When the facility discharges a patient to home or another institution, you must document the reason for the discharge, the patient's destination, his mode of transportation, and the person or staff member accompanying him, if appropriate. The Joint Commission's 2007 National Patient Safety Goals require facilities to implement a standardized approach to "hand-off" communications, in which one care provider gives a full and accurate report of the patient to the next care provider. During the hand-off, the providers also must have an opportunity to ask and respond to questions.

If the patient is transferred home, be sure to review medications, providing an up-to-date comprehensive list of medications to the patient. Review all treatments and instructions with the patient or responsible caregiver and document their understanding. Also document all patient and family or caregiver teaching.

If a patient is transferred to the hospital, a transfer form is generally required. In addition, be sure to document your "hand-off" communication with the receiving provider as well as all equipment and devices sent with the patient, such as a walker, dentures, or hearing aids. If these items are lost while in the hospital, this documentation may save the long-term care facility the expense of replacing the items. (See *Transfer and personal belongings form,* pages 203 and 204.)

(Text continues on page 205.)

ChartWizard

Braden scale for predicting pressure sore risk

The Braden scale, shown below, is the most reliable of several existing instruments for assessing the older patient's risk of developing pressure ulcers. The lower the score, the greater the risk.

Patient's name _Kevin Lawson_   Evaluator's name _Joan Norris, RN_

SENSORY PERCEPTION Ability to respond meaningfully to pressure-related discomfort	**1. Completely limited:** Unresponsive (does not moan, flinch, or grasp) to painful stimuli because of diminished level of consciousness or sedation OR Limited ability to feel pain over most of body surface	**2. Very limited:** Responds only to painful stimuli; cannot communicate discomfort except by moaning or restlessness OR Has a sensory impairment that limits the ability to feel pain or discomfort over half of body
MOISTURE Degree to which skin is exposed to moisture	**1. Constantly moist:** Skin is kept moist almost constantly by perspiration, urine, and so forth; dampness is detected every time patient is moved or turned	**2. Very moist:** Skin is often but not always moist; linen must be changed at least once per shift
ACTIVITY Degree of physical activity	**1. Bedfast:** Confined to bed	**2. Chairfast:** Ability to walk severely limited or nonexistent; cannot bear own weight and must be assisted into chair or wheelchair
MOBILITY Ability to change and control body position	**1. Completely immobile:** Does not make even slight changes in body or extremity position without assistance	**2. Very limited:** Makes occasional slight changes in body or extremity position but unable to make frequent or significant changes independently
NUTRITION Usual food intake pattern	**1. Very poor:** Never eats a complete meal; rarely eats more than one-third of any food offered; eats two servings or less of protein (meat or dairy products) per day; takes fluids poorly; does not take a liquid dietary supplement OR Is NPO or maintained on clear liquids or I.V. fluids for more than 5 days	**2. Probably inadequate:** Rarely eats a complete meal and generally eats only about half of any food offered; protein intake includes only three servings of meat or dairy products per day; occasionally will take a dietary supplement OR Receives less than optimum amount of liquid diet or tube feeding
FRICTION AND SHEAR	**1. Problem:** Requires moderate to maximum assistance in moving; complete lifting without sliding against sheets is impossible; frequently slides down in bed or chair, requiring frequent repositioning with maximum assistance; spasticity, contractures, or agitation leads to almost constant friction	**2. Potential problem:** Moves feebly or requires minimum assistance; during a move, skin probably slides to some extent against sheets, chair restraints, or other devices; maintains relatively good position in chair or bed most of the time but occasionally slides down

Date of assessment ___2/18/07___

3. Slightly limited: Responds to verbal commands but cannot always communicate discomfort or need to be turned OR Has some sensory impairment that limits ability to feel pain or discomfort in one or two extremities	**4. No impairment:** Responds to verbal commands; has no sensory deficit that would limit ability to feel or voice pain or discomfort	3
3. Occasionally moist: Skin is occasionally moist, requiring an extra linen change approximately once per day	**4. Rarely moist:** Skin is usually dry; linen requires changing only at routine intervals	3
3. Walks occasionally: Walks occasionally during day, but for very short distances, with or without assistance; spends majority of each shift in bed or chair	**4. Walks frequently:** Walks outside the room at least twice per day and inside room at least once every 2 hours during waking hours	4
3. Slightly limited: Makes frequent though slight changes in body or extremity position independently	**4. No limitations:** Makes major and frequent changes in position without assistance	4
3. Adequate: Eats more than half of most meals; eats four servings of protein (meat, dairy products) each day; occasionally will refuse a meal, but will usually take a supplement if offered OR Is on a tube feeding or total parenteral nutrition regimen that probably meets most nutritional needs	**4. Excellent:** Eats most of every meal and never refuses a meal; usually eats four or more servings of meat and dairy products; occasionally eats between meals; does not require supplementation	4
3. No apparent problem: Moves in bed and in chair independently and has sufficient muscle strength to lift up completely during move; maintains good position in bed or chair at all times		3
	TOTAL SCORE	21

ChartWizard

Fall assessment and action plan

This standardized assessment tool can help you evaluate your patient's risk for falls and plan preventive measures if needed.

Does the patient have problems with:

ISSUE	ASSESSMENT	ACTION
Comfort ● Pain	greater than or equal to 3 ___ Yes ✓ No	___ Notify practitioner of pain level. ___ Offer thermal modalities 4x/day while awake. ___ Tailor pain medication schedule to wake-up time/therapy schedule/HS. ___ Reposition as needed.
Elimination ● Incontinence	✓ Yes ___ No	✓ Time void q2 hours while awake and q4 hours at night as needed. ✓ Initiate bowel program. ✓ Restrict fluids after 1900 hours unless contraindicated. ✓ Place commode at bedside on dominant side. ✓ Orient to call bell and location of bathroom/bathroom safety.
Tubings ● I.V.s ● Chest tubes ● Urinary catheter	✓ Yes ___ No ___ Yes ✓ No ___ Yes ✓ No	✓ Position tube and pole for safety. ✓ Verbal reminder to patient. ___ Use leg bag during waking hours.
Mobility ● Unsteady gait; poor balance	___ Yes ✓ No	___ Physical assistance required at all times. ___ Consult physical therapy if appropriate.
● Transfer	greater than or equal to min assist ___ Yes ✓ No	___ Ensure at least one bottom side rail is down on dominant side. ___ Ensure top two side rails are up to help with transfers. ___ Ensure appropriate number of staff available for transfer. ___ Place sign "CALL AND WAIT FOR ASSISTANCE" IN BATHROOM.
● Limited endurance	✓ Yes ___ No	✓ Schedule rest periods in daily activity schedule.
● Orthostatic hypotension	✓ Yes ___ No	✓ Instruct in gradual position change.
Mental status ● Cognitive deficit present	✓ Yes ___ No	✓ 24-hour usage of bed/chair alarm. ✓ Time void q2 hours while awake and q4 hours at night as needed. ✓ Implement appropriate seating device. ✓ Track and document behavioral patterns. ✓ Provide appropriate diversional activities. ✓ Orient to environment. ✓ Check medication list.
Communication barrier ● Non-English Speaking	___ Yes ✓ No	___ Arrange for interpreter. ___ Ask for help from family if appropriate.
● Unable to make needs known	___ Yes ✓ No	___ Use picture/communication board.
● Hearing deficit	✓ Yes ___ No	___ Ensure hearing aid is present and functional. ___ Use amplification devices.
● Visual deficit	___ Yes ✓ No	___ Clear pathways and ensure ambulation aids are close to patient. ___ Orient to environment.
Medications ● Cardiovascular	✓ Yes ___ No	✓ If cardiovascular meds used and symptoms or dizziness present, check orthostatic blood pressure and heart rate. Call practitioner if needed.
● Psychoactive/sleep	___ Yes ✓ No	___ If psychoactive/sleep meds used and symptoms or dizziness present, notify practitioner of side effects, check orthostatic blood pressure.
● Diuretics	___ Yes ✓ No	___ If diuretics used, time void q2 hours while awake and q4 hours at night as needed.
● Anesthetic (1st 24hr. post-op)	___ Yes ✓ No	___ If 1st 24 hr. post-op, physical assistance provided at all times.
● Anticoagulants	___ Yes ✓ No	___ If anticoagulants used, implement Anticoagulant Therapy Protocol.

Above action plan reviewed and implemented:

DATE _1/9/07_ TIME _0800_ NAME _J. Kuka, RN_

DATE _1/9/07_ TIME _1600_ NAME _H. Cane, RN_

DATE _1/10/07_ TIME _2400_ NAME _P. Seria, RN_

Adapted with permission from Abington Memorial Hospital Department of Nursing, Abington, Pa.

ChartWizard

Transfer and
personal belongings form

Patients in long-term care facilities may be admitted to the hospital, discharged to home, or transferred to other facilities. The forms below are used during this process.

1. PATIENT'S LAST NAME	FIRST NAME	MI	2. SEX	3. Hospital I.D.
Clark	Robert	T	Male	12345678

4. PATIENT'S ADDRESS (Street, City, State, Zip Code)	5. DATE OF BIRTH	6. RELIGION
1 Wise street Springhouse, PA 19411	2-8-35	unknown

7. DATE OF THIS TRANSFER	8. FACILITY NAME AND ADDRESS TRANSFERRING TO	9. PHYSICIAN IN CHARGE AT TIME OF TRANSFER
1/29/01	Seniors Care Facility 22 Elderly Way Phila., PA	Dr. Nicholas

9. Will this physician care for patient after admission to new facility? ☐ YES ☒ NO

10. DATES OF STAY AT FACILITY TRANSFERRING FROM

ADMISSION 12/14/06   DISCHARGE 1/29/01

11. PAYMENT SOURCE FOR CHARGES TO PATIENT

A. ☒ SELF OR FAMILY
B. ☐ PRIVATE INSURANCE
C. ☐ BLUE CROSS BLUE SHIELD
D. ☐ EMPLOYER OR UNION
E. ☐ PUBLIC AGENCY (Give name)
F. ☐ OTHER (Explain)

12-A. NAME AND ADDRESS OF FACILITY TRANSFERRING FROM

Community Hospital   3000 Medical Way, Phila., PA

12-B. NAMES AND ADDRESSES OF ALL HOSPITALS AND EXTENDED CARE FACILITIES FROM WHICH PATIENT WAS DISCHARGED IN PAST 60 DAYS.

13. CLINIC APPOINTMENT DATE TIME CLINIC APPOINTMENT CARD ATTACHED	14. DATE OF LAST PHYSICAL EXAMINATION
	1/26/01

15. RELATIVE OR GUARDIAN: Name Katherine Clark   Address 1 Wise Street Springhouse, PA 19411   Phone number 1-215-999-9000

16. DIAGNOSES AT TIME OF TRANSFER
(a) Primary ℞ CVA
(b) Secondary IDDM

EMPLOYMENT RELATED:
☐ YES
☒ NO

VITALS AT TIME OF TRANSFER
T 98°   P 68   R 20   B/P 140/82

ADVANCE DIRECTIVES ☐ YES ☒ NO ☐ COPY ATTACHED
CODE STATUS   Full code

CHECK ALL THAT APPLY

Disabilities
☐ Amputation
☒ Paralysis Ⓛ side
☐ Contracture
☐ Pressure Ulcer

Impairments
☐ Mental

☒ Speech
☐ Hearing
☒ Vision
☐ Sensation

Incontinence
☒ Bladder
☒ Bowel
☒ Saliva

Activity Tolerance Limitations
☐ None
☒ Moderate
☐ Severe

Patient knows diagnosis?
☒ Yes
☐ No

Potential for Rehabilitation
☐ Good
☒ Fair
☐ Poor

IMPORTANT MEDICAL INFORMATION
(State allergies if any)
PCN

DIET, DRUGS, AND OTHER THERAPY at time of discharge
-Mechanical soft diet (2,000 cal)
-Magace 4 tabs q6h
-Lasix 40 mg P.O. b.i.d.
-Aspirin 81 mg P.O. daily.
-Humulin ⁷⁰/₃₀ 20 units q a.m. & at bedtime.
-Sliding scale coverage BG less than 40 greater than 400
-Call Dr. Nicholas, BG 200-250:2units 301-350:4units
251-300:3units 351-400:5units Humulin R
(Practitioner, please sign below)

SUGGESTIONS FOR ACTIVE CARE

BED
Position in good body alignment and change position every 2 hrs.
Avoid flat supine position
Prone position 2 time/day as tolerated.

SITTING
4 hr 3 times/day

WEIGHT BEARING
☐ Full
☒ Partial
☐ None
on_____leg

EXERCISES
Range of motion 3 times/day.
to Ⓛ extremities by
☐ patient ☐ nurse ☐ family
Stand 3 min. 2 times/day.

LOCOMOTION
Walk unable times/day.

SOCIAL ACTIVITIES
Encourage (☒ group ☐ individual) activities
(☒ within ☐ outside) home.
Transportation: ☒ Ambulance ☐ Car
☐ Car for handicapped ☐ Bus

Signature of Physician or Nurse   John Brown, RN   Date   1 / 29 / 01

(continued)

Transfer and personal belongings form (continued)

Any articles of clothing or other belongings left at the hospital will be held for 30 days after discharge. Items remaining after this period will be disposed of by the hospital.

COMMENTS

Date: 1/29/01		
Initials: RC		
VALUABLES DESCRIBE		
Wallet:	✔	1 brown leather wallet
Money (Amount): $25.00	✔	1-$20.00 bill 5 $1 bills
Watch:		
Jewelry:		
Glasses/Contacts: Glasses	✔	Wire rim-gold
Hearing Aids:		
Dentures:	✔	
Partial		
Complete	✔	Container labeled
Keys		
ARTICLE DESCRIBE		
Ambulatory Aids:		
Cane, Walker, Etc.		
Bedclothes	✔	1 pair plaid pajamas
Belt		
Dress		
Outer Wear		
Pants		
Pocketbook		
Shirt		
Shoes		
Sweater		
Undergarments		
Other		

All belongings were sent home with patient's family: YES   (NO)

Patient's Signature ___Bob Clark___

Witnessed by Hospital Personnel ___Mary Jones, RN___

Documentation guidelines

In a long-term care facility, consider the following points when updating your records:

▶ When writing nursing summaries, be sure to address all specific patient problems noted in the care plan.

▶ When writing progress notes, confirm that the patient's progress is being evaluated and reevaluated continually in relation to the goals or outcomes defined in the care plan. If the patient's goals aren't met, this also needs to be addressed. Any additional actions should be described and documented.

▶ Record transfers and discharges according to facility protocol.

▶ Document changes in the patient's condition and report them to the practitioner and the family as soon as possible, but within 24 hours.

▶ Document any follow-up interventions or other measures implemented in response to a reported change in the patient's condition.

▶ Keep a record of visits from family or friends and of phone calls about the patient.

▶ If an incident occurs, such as a fall or a treatment error, fill out an incident report and write follow-up notes for at least 48 hours after the incident (or follow your facility's policy).

▶ During the first week of residence, keep detailed records on each shift (or follow your facility's policy).

▶ Keep reimbursement issues in mind when documenting. For a facility to qualify for payment, its records must clearly reflect the level of care given to the patient.

▶ Be certain that your records accurately reflect any skilled service that the patient receives.

▶ Always record a practitioner's verbal and telephone orders, and make sure that the practitioner countersigns these orders within the time frames specified by state regulations and facility policy.

▶ Document practitioner and professional consult visits to the patient.

Selected references

Alexander, B.J., et al. "Methods of Pain Assessment in Residents of Long-Term Care Facilities: A Pilot Study," *Journal of the American Medical Directors Association* 6(2):137-43, March-April 2005.

Buhr, G.T., and White, H.K. "Quality Improvement Initiative for Chronic Pain Assessment and Management in the Nursing Home: A Pilot Study," *Journal of the American Medical Directors Association* 7(4):246-53, May 2006.

Crutchfield, D. "Impact of Medicare Part D on Long-Term Care," *Managed Care* 15(7 Suppl 3): 28-30, July 2006.

Del Rio, R.A., et al. "The Accuracy of Minimum Data Set Diagnoses in Describing Recent Hospitalization at Acute Care Facilities," *Journal of the American Medical Directors Association* 7(4): 212-8, May 2006.

Doran, D.M., et al. "Nursing-Sensitive Outcomes Data Collection in Acute Care and Long-Term Care Settings," *Nursing Research* 55(2 Suppl): S75-81, March-April 2006.

Dougherty, M., and Mitchell, S. "Getting Better Data from the MDS. Improving Diagnostic Data Reporting in Long-Term Care Facilities," *Journal of American Health Information Management Association* 75(10):28-33, November-December 2004.

Loeb, M., et al. "Effect of a Clinical Pathway to Reduce Hospitalizations in Nursing Home Residents with Pneumonia: A Randomized Controlled Trial," *JAMA* 295(21):2503-10, June 2006.

Simonson, W. "Medicare Part D in Long-Term Care: Special Consideration for the Vulnerable Elderly Nursing Facility Resident," *Managed Care Interface* 19(6):21, 23, June 2006.

Vu, M.Q., et al. "Falls in the Nursing Home: Are They Preventable?" *Journal of the American Medical Directors Association* 7(3 Suppl):S53-8, March 2006.

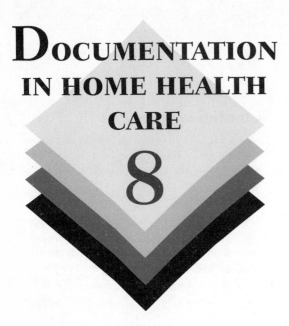

DOCUMENTATION IN HOME HEALTH CARE

8

As with hospitals, rehabilitation centers, and long-term care facilities, state and federal laws and agencies regulate home health care agencies. These regulatory standard bearers require home health care agencies to provide accurate, complete documentation and a high level of care. If a home health care agency fails to meet these regulatory standards, it jeopardizes its licensure, accreditation, and reimbursement.

Accreditation and quality improvement programs are available through the Foundation for Hospice and Homecare, The Joint Commission (using the ORYX continuous quality improvement standards), and the American Nurses Association (ANA), which uses the ANA Standards of Home Care Nursing Practice. The nursing process forms the basis of these standards.

Another accrediting body, the Community Health Accreditation Program (CHAP) began accrediting home health care agencies in 1965. CHAP specializes in home health and community health care, and CHAP accreditation means the agency meets or exceeds Medicare standards.

In many cases, obtaining state licensure hinges on having accreditation and adhering to Medicare and Medicaid regulations administered by the Centers for Medicare and Medicaid Services (CMS) and its agencies and carriers.

▶ Home health care growth

Recent trends have contributed to the growth of the home health care industry, including the development of a prospective payment system (PPS) for home health care agencies, improved utilization review, greater patient diversity, and more affordable support services.

Prospective payment system

The Balanced Budget Act of 1997, which required the development of a PPS for Medicare home health care services, was implemented in October 2000 and marked a turning point in home health care coverage. Under this system, Medicare pays home health care agencies a predetermined base payment, which is then adjusted for the health care needs and conditions of the patient. This system helps to ensure appropriate reimbursements for quality, efficient home health care.

Utilization review

Managed care organizations have identified sophisticated methods of performing utilization review, including the use of the Outcome and Assessment Information Set (OASIS). This has caused a decrease in the average length of a patient's hospitalization, which means that patients are typically sicker and more reliant on home health care after discharge.

Patient diversity

Traditionally, homebound Medicare recipients have constituted the major portion of the home health care caseload. Agencies, however, have expanded services to new populations, representing all age groups and a variety of medical conditions. This has led to the emergence of home health care subspecialties, such as home infusion agencies and high-tech cancer-related home health care, including stem cell transplants. These agencies may be offshoots of parent organizations or stand-alone agencies. (See *The hospice alternative*, page 208.)

Support services

Government and private insurance payers are expanding their coverage of home health care because support services in the home and community cost less than institutional care. As a result, the availability of home health care is increasing. In the future, the home health care industry may become the primary supplier of health care in the United States.

Standardized and required documents

In the home health care setting, the nurse is more responsible for ensuring reimbursement payments than in any other health care setting. Your agency's success or failure virtually depends on your documentation skills because home health care agencies are paid prospectively, meaning they receive two payments of a preset amount of money based on the documentation of the initial nursing assessment. If the patient's care requires more than the preset reimbursement level, the agency is responsible for covering the difference in cost. For this reason, home health care organizations have a tightly structured documentation system.

As a home health care nurse, you're bound by all the controls imposed by the professional standards and nurse practice acts that govern nurses in all other settings. In addition, every home health care agency has its own standards, requirements, and forms to be used when documenting a patient's care. Naturally, you'll want to be familiar with your agency's requirements and follow them to the best of your ability. For the most part, however, you'll find that all agencies and payers require certain types of documentation, even if they use different forms to report the information.

ChartWizard

The hospice alternative

Many home health care agencies provide hospice care services. Hospice programs provide palliative care to the terminally ill in homes and hospitals.

MEDICARE COVERAGE

Since 1983, patients who have met specific admission criteria can qualify for the hospice Medicare benefit instead of the traditional Medicare benefit, allowing greater freedom to choose the hospice alternative for terminal care. The patient receives noncurative medical and support services not otherwise covered by Medicare.

Medicare coverage for hospice care is available if:

▶ The patient is eligible for Medicare Part A, which covers skilled nursing home and hospital care. People eligible for Medicare are those age 65 or older, long-term disabled patients, and people with end-stage renal disease.

▶ The patient's physician and the hospice medical director certify that the patient is terminally ill with a life expectancy of 6 months or less if the disease runs its natural course.

▶ The patient signs a statement indicating that he is choosing hospice care instead of the routine Medicare-covered benefits for his terminal illness. (Medicare will still pay for covered benefits for health issues unrelated to the terminal illness.)

▶ The patient receives care from a Medicare-approved hospice program.

A Medicare-approved hospice will usually provide care in the patient's home. The hospice team and the patient's physician establish a care plan for medical and support services for the management of a terminal illness.

A patient without coverage for hospice benefits may be eligible for free or reduced-cost care through local programs or foundations. Alternatively, a patient may pay privately for hospice services.

UNDERSTANDING AND ACCEPTANCE OF TREATMENT

With hospice care, the patient and primary caregiver must complete documentation indicating their understanding of hospice care. The patient and caregiver must sign an informed consent form that outlines everyone's responsibilities. They must also sign a form indicating their understanding and acceptance of the role of the primary caregiver. The form below is an example of this type of document.

REEDSVILLE HOME HEALTH AND HOSPICE ACCEPTANCE OF PRIMARY CAREGIVER ROLE

I've been offered the opportunity to ask questions regarding the Hospice program and Hospice care of this patient. I understand that the Hospice program provides palliative, or comfort, measures and services, but not aggressive, invasive, or life-sustaining procedures.

I also understand that the Hospice concept of care is based upon the active participation of a primary care person who isn't provided through the Hospice benefit, who is and will be willing to assist this patient with personal care and with activities of daily living as well as with safety precautions when Hospice personnel aren't scheduled to be in the home. I accept the responsibility of being primary caregiver, and I agree to make appropriate arrangements to provide this role to this patient.

If, for any reason, I'm unable to serve in this capacity at a time as deemed necessary for the safety and care of this patient, I agree to make other arrangements to fulfill the responsibilities of primary caregiver, which are acceptable to Reedsville Home Health and Hospice. I further understand that Reedsville Home Health and Hospice will assist in making the arrangements, but that I'll be financially responsible for any costs associated with them.

Name of Patient: _Joan Powell_

Signature of Patient: _Joan Powell_

Date: _1/17/07_

Name of primary caregiver: _Joseph Powell_

Date: _1/17/07_

Signature of primary caregiver: _Joseph Powell_

Relationship: _husband_

Witness: _Cathy Melvin, RN_

Date: _1/17/07_

The areas in which you'll need to ensure accurate and complete documentation typically include the referral for home health care, Medicare and Medicaid forms, assessment (including the OASIS-B1), nursing care plan, medical update, progress notes, nursing summaries, patient or caregiver teaching, recertification, discharge summary, and referral to community resources.

Referral forms

Before you begin caring for a patient in his home, your agency will verify that the patient qualifies for home health care. To do this, the following criteria are evaluated:

▶ *clinical criteria*—skilled care needed, appropriately prescribed therapy that can be done in the home, caregiver available to assist the patient

▶ *technical criteria (patient or caregiver)*—senses intact, ability to learn and follow procedures, ability to recognize complications and initiate emergency medical procedures

▶ *environmental criteria*—access to a telephone, electricity, and water; clean living environment

▶ *financial criteria*—verification of insurance coverage, full knowledge of copayment or out-of-pocket expenses, agreement to comply with the conditions of participation.

The referral form is then used to make sure that the agency can provide the services the patient needs before it agrees to take the new case. (See *Using a referral form for home care,* pages 210 and 211.)

Medicare and Medicaid forms

By mandate in 1985, CMS required home health care agencies to standardize and update their record keeping and documentation methods. Since the implementation of OASIS, the collection of specific data elements is required. For each qualified Medicare or Medicaid recipient, the agency must complete a Home Health Certification and Plan of Care form (Form 485) and submit it for approval every 60 days. (See *Certifying home health care needs,* page 212.) A Medical Update and Patient Information form (Form 486) is completed to obtain recertification for additional home care or whenever Medicare requests it. (See *Providing updated medical and patient information,* page 213.)

These data elements allow Medicare reviewers, also known as fiscal intermediaries, to evaluate each claim in accordance with the criteria for coverage. Medicare will provide no payment unless the required forms are properly completed, signed, dated, and submitted within preset timelines and before billing for reimbursement. Nurses assigned to the patient usually complete these forms; however, some agencies utilize an admission team for this purpose. The data are usually filed after completing a comprehensive nursing assessment and devising a suitable care plan. The nurse and the attending physician must sign these forms.

The federal government receives all OASIS-related data electronically, which allows for quicker reimbursement. However, claim audits by fiscal intermediaries and other government agencies, such as the Office of the Inspector General, can slow down the reimbursement process.

To meet Medicare's criteria for home health care reimbursement, the patient must meet all of these conditions:

▶ He must be confined to his home.

▶ He must need skilled services.

▶ He must need those skilled services on an intermittent basis.

(Text continues on page 214.)

ChartWizard

Using a referral form for home care

Also called an *intake form,* a referral form is used to document a new patient's needs when you begin your evaluation. Use the sample below as a guide.

Date of referral: _1/17/07_   Branch: _North_   Chart #: _97-413_   H ✓

Info taken by: _Beth Isham, RN_   Admit date: _1/18/07_

Patient's name: _Geraldine Rush_

Address: _66 Newton St._

City: _Burlington_   State: _VT_   Zip: _05402_

Phone: _(802) 123-4567_   Date of birth: _4/3/34_

Primary caregiver name & phone number: _husband (Dennis)   (802) 123-4567_

Insurance name: _Medicare_   Ins. #: _123-45-6789_

Is this a managed care policy (HMO)? _no_

Primary Dx: (Code _162.5_) _lung cancer_   Date: _12/11/04_

(Code _877_) _pressure ulcer (coccyx)_   Date: _3/13/06_

(Code _714.0_) _rheumatoid arthritis_   Date: _1990s_

Procedures: (Code _86.28_) _ulcer care_   Date: _3/14/06_

Referral source: _J. Silva, hospital SW_   Phone: _765-2813_

Doctor name & phone #: _Frank Crabbe_   Phone: _765-4321_

Doctor address: _9073 Parkway Drive, Burlington_

Hospital: _University Hospital_   Admit: _1/1/07_   Discharge: _1/16/07_

Functional limitations: _Pain management, nonambulatory, poor fine motor skills 2° rheumatoid arthritis_

ORDERS/SERVICES: (specify amount, frequency, and duration)

(SN:) _SN visits 3x per week and p.r.n. x 2 months_

(AL:) _CNA visits daily 5 days per week x 2 months_

(PT, OT), ST: _PT and OT evaluations and visits 2-3 x per week and p.r.n. x 2 months_

(MSW:) _MSW evaluation and weekly visits x 2 months_

Spiritual coordinator: _Rev. Carlson, St. Paul's Lutheran Church_

Counselor: _JoAnne Knowton, MSW_

Volunteer: _Rosalie Marshall (niece) will provide care on weekends_

Other services provided: _shopping, laundry, meal prep_

Goals: _wound care, pain management, terminal care at home_

Equipment: _Needs commode, hospital bed, bedpan, Hoyer lift, side rail w/c_

Company & phone number: _Scott Medical Equipment   765-9931_

Safety measures: _side rails up X 2_   Nutritional req _diet as tolerated_

FUNCTIONAL LIMITATIONS: (Circle applicable)   ACTIVITIES PERMITTED: (Circle applicable)

1. Amputation	5. Paralysis	9.Legally blind	1. Complete bed rest 6. Partial wgt bearing (A) Wheelchair
2. Bowel/Bladder	(6) Endurance	A. Dyspnea with	2. Bed rest BRP 7. Independent at home B. Walker
3. Contracture	(7) Ambulation	minimal exer	3. Up as tolerated 8. Crutches C. No restriction
4. Hearing	8. Speech	(B) Other _RA_	(4) Transfer bed/chair 9. Cane D. Other -specify

Accessibility to bath: Y - (N)   Shower   Y - (N)   Bathroom   Y - (N)   Exit (Y) - N

Mental status: (Circle)   Oriented   Comatose   Forgetful   (Depressed)   Disoriented   Lethargic   Agitated   Other

Using a referral form for home care *(continued)*

Allergies: _____ none known _____
• Hospice appropriate meds   • Med company: _____ Walker Pharmacy _____

MEDICATIONS:
morphine sulfate liq. 20 mg/ml 40 mg P.O. q6h p.r.n. pain
Compazine 10 mg P.O. or P.R. q4-6h p.r.n. n/v
Colace   200 mg P.O. daily p.r.n. constipation
Benadryl 25 – 50 mg P.O. at bedtime p.r.n. sleeplessness

Living will   Yes ✓   No _____   Obtained _____   Family to mail to office
Guardian, POA, or responsible person: _____ husband _____
Address & phone number: _____ same _____
Other family members: _____
ETOH: _____ 0 _____ Drug use: _____ 0 _____ Smoker: _____ 2 ppd x 40 years; quit 2 yrs ago _____
History: _____ Other than problems associated with arthritis, was in general good health until 12/04, Dx: lung CA – husband cared for at home until 1/1/07.

Social history (place of birth, education, jobs, retirement, etc.): _____ Born & raised in Toronto, became U.S. citizen when married in 1955. 2 yrs. college – majored in music. Retired church organist.

ADMISSION NOTES: VS: T 98.4° P.O. AP 86   RR 18   BP 140/72
Lungs: decreased breath sounds LLL   Extremities: cool to touch; pedal pulses present
Wgt: _____ 118 _____   Recent wgt loss/gain of _____ 40 lb over 6 months _____
Admission narrative: _____ Visit made to pt/husband in hospital before discharge. Both have been told that she is failing rapidly, and would like her to return home with Hospice services. Niece willing to help 2 days/week. Pt apprehensive; husband blames himself for the coccygeal pressure ulcer which developed under his care.
Psychosocial issues: _____ Pt has always cared for husband. Describes self as depressed that she is no longer able to do so; worries who will care for him after she dies.
Environmental concerns: _____ Need smoke detectors

Are there any cultural or spiritual customs or beliefs of which we should be aware before providing Hospice services? _____ Pt would like Holy Communion just before death (and weekly)
Funeral home: _____ not yet chosen _____   Contact made: Yes _____ X _____ No _____

DIRECTIONS: _____ Corner Newton & Elm; duplex, white with green trim. Door on (L) says 66. Bell broken – knock loudly.

Agency representative signature: _____ Beth Isham, RN _____   Date: _____ 1/18/07 _____
                                       Home Care Supervisor

Certifying home health care needs

The Home Health Certification and Plan of Care form (also known as Form 485) is the official form required by Medicare to authorize coverage for home care. To maintain Medicare coverage, this form must be updated and resubmitted every 60 days.

Department of Health and Human Services
Health Care Financing Administration

Form Approved
OMB No. 0938-0357

HOME HEALTH CERTIFICATION AND PLAN OF CARE

1. Patient's HI Claim No.	2. Start Of Care Date	3. Certification Period	4. Medical Record No.	5. Provider No.
111-111	1/8/07	From: 1/8/07 To: 3/8/07	78-9101	11-1213

6. Patient's Name and Address
Mary Long
2218 Central Ave.
Wichita, Kansas

7. Provider's Name, Address and Telephone Number
Home Health Agency
301 Main Street
Wichita, Kansas

8. Date of Birth 06/04/33	9. Sex ☐ M ☑ F

10. Medications: Dose/Frequency/Route (N)ew (C)hanged
digoxin 0.125 mg P.O. daily; Lasix 20 mg P.O. daily; warfarin 5 mg P.O. daily; Capoten 12.5 mg b.i.d.; Proventil 2 puffs q.i.d./p.r.n.; MVI one P.O. daily; FeSO4 325 mg daily; Ex-Strength Tylenol 500 mg q4h p.r.n.; albuterol 0.5 ml with 3 ml NSS via nebulizer b.i.d.; aspirin 325 mg 1 P.O. daily

11. ICD-9-CM	Principal Diagnosis	Date
4-27-31	atrial fibrillation	12/20/06

12. ICD-9-CM	Surgical Procedure	Date
0000	gastrostomy tube insertion	1/2/07

13. ICD-9-CM	Other Pertinent Diagnoses	Date
4280	heart failure	12/31/06
496	chronic airway obstruction	11/29/06

14. DME and Supplies
Gastrostomy tube supplies, cane

15. Safety Measures:
Prevent falls

16. Nutritional Req. Magnacal 80 ml/hr

17. Allergies: NKA

18.A. Functional Limitations

1	Amputation	5	☑ Paralysis	9	Legally Blind
2	Bowel/Bladder (Incontinence)	6	☑ Endurance	A	Dyspnea With Minimal Exertion
3	Contracture	7	Ambulation	B	Other (Specify)
4	Hearing	8	Speech		

18.B. Activities Permitted

1	Complete Bedrest	6	Partial Weight Bearing	A	Wheelchair
2	Bedrest BRP	7	Independent At Home	B	Walker
3	☑ Up As Tolerated	8	Crutches	C	No Restrictions
4	Transfer Bed/Chair	9	☑ Cane	D	Other (Specify)
5	Exercises Prescribed				

19. Mental Status:

1	☑ Oriented	3	Forgetful	5	Disoriented	7	Agitated
2	Comatose	4	Depressed	6	Lethargic	8	Other

20. Prognosis:

1	Poor	2	Guarded	3	Fair	4	☑ Good	5	Excellent

21. Orders for Discipline and Treatments (Specify Amount/Frequency/Duration)
RN: Assess heart failure, effects of digoxin, monitor complaints of arthritis pain control; monitor gastrostomy tube site, instruct and assist the patient with gastrostomy feedings and tube care. Draw blood as ordered by MD. AIDE: 2-3wk; assist with personal care and ADLs.

22. Goals/Rehabilitation Potential/Discharge Plans
1. Patient will be free from complications related to heart failure and medication regimen by 3/8/07.
2. Patient will demonstrate independence with gastrostomy care and feedings by 3/8/07.
3. Patient will experience sufficient pain control by 3/8/07 as evidenced by verbalization of pain less than 1 on a scale of 0 = 5 (with 0 indicating no pain and 5 indicating the worst pain imaginable).
4. Discharge when medically stable.
5. Rehab potential is good.

23. Nurse's Signature and Date of Verbal SOC Where Applicable: N. Smith, RN 1/8/07	25. Date HHA Received Signed POT 1/8/07

24. Physician's Name and Address
M. Raser, MD
555 Main St.
Wichita, Kansas

26. ☑ I certify/recertify that this patient is confined to his/her home and needs intermittent skilled nursing care, physical therapy and/or speech therapy or continues to need occupational therapy. The patient is under my care, and I have authorized the services on this plan of care and will periodically review the plan.

27. Attending Physician's Signature and Date Signed
M. Raser, MD 1/8/07

28. Anyone who misrepresents, falsifies, or conceals essential information required for payment of Federal funds may be subject to fine, imprisonment, or civil penalty under applicable Federal laws.

Form HCFA-485 (C-4) (02-94) (Print Aligned)   **PROVIDER**

ChartWizard

Providing updated medical and patient information

To continue providing reimbursable skilled nursing care to a patient at home, Medicare requires that the home health care agency submit a Medical Update and Patient Information form (also known as Form 486) after the first 60 days of home care. A sample of this form appears below.

Department of Health and Human Services
Health Care Financing Administration

Form Approved
OMB No. 0938-0357

MEDICAL UPDATE AND PATIENT INFORMATION

1. Patient's HI Claim No.	2. SOC Date	3. Certification Period	4. Medical Record No.	5. Provider No.
48-7850	07/08/06	From: 11/08/06 To: 01/07/07	75-4099	98-7654

6. Patient's Name and Address
James Dole, 412 Main Street, Newark, NJ

7. Provider's Name
Home Health Agency

8. Medicare Covered: ☑Y ☐N | 9. Date Physician Last Saw Patient: *10/24/06* | 10. Date Last Contacted Physician: *10/25/06*

11. Is the Patient Receiving Care in an 1861 (J)(1) Skilled Nursing Facility or Equivalent? ☐Y ☑N ☐ Do Not Know

12. ☐ Certification ☑ Recertification ☐ Modified

13. Dates of Last Inpatient Stay: Admission *06/31/06* Discharge *07/05/06* | 14. Type of Facility: *A*

15. Updated information: New Orders/Treatments/Clinical Facts/Summary from Each Discipline

Discipline	Visits (this bill)	Frequency and duration	Treatment codes	Total visits projected this cert.
SN	00	2 times a week X 3 weeks	A1	06
Aide	00	3 times a week X 4 weeks	A6	12

SN: A&O x 3. Skin warm, dry, pale, slight dyspnea noted with activity. Trace bilat. pedal edema, lungs clear. No complaints. Improved and increased feeling of well-being demonstrated. Peg tube patent and functioning well. Correctly demonstrates checking for residual, peg tube site care.
Aide: pt seen 3x/wk. Increased difficulty ambulating. Expressed feelings of despair and hopelessness associated with physical condition.

16. Functional Limitations (Expand From 485 and Level of ADL) Reason Homebound/Prior Functional Status *Interaction between pt and daughter who wants pt to strive to live. Pt increasingly fearful of institutional care. Pt agrees to join gastrostomy support group. CCSW to facilitate. Needs more encouragement to perform ADLs. Daughter more involved with care.*

17. Supplementary Plan of Care on File from Physician Other than Referring Physician: (If Yes, Please Specify Giving Goals/Rehab. Potential/Discharge Plan) ☐Y ☐N

18. Unusual Home/Social Environment *N/A*

19. Indicate Any Time When the Home Health Agency Made a Visit and Patient was Not Home and Reason Why if Ascertainable

20. Specify Any Known Medical and/or Non-Medical Reasons the Patient Regularly Leaves Home and Frequency of Occurrence

21. Nurse or Therapist Completing or Reviewing Form
M. Hoffner, RN

Date (Mo., Day, Yr.)
2/14/07

Form HCFA-486 (C3) (02-94) (Print Aligned)   **PROVIDER**

ChartWizard

Physician's telephone orders

Home health nurses rely heavily on the use of telephone orders. The agency must make sure that its nurses follow guidelines established by the Centers for Medicare and Medicaid Services for taking and documenting these orders. Below is an example of a form used by one agency to fulfill documentation requirements. The physician must sign the order within 48 hours.

Facility name		Address	
Suburban Home Health Agency		123 Main Street, Phila. PA 19111	
Last name	**First name**	**Attending physician**	**Admission no.**
Smith	Kevin	Baker	147–111–471

Date ordered	Date discontinued	ORDERS
2/18/07	2/21/07	Tylenol 650 mg P.O. q6h p.r.n. Temp greater than 101° F

Signature of nurse receiving order	Time	Signature of physician	Date
Mary Reo, RN	1820		

▶ The care he needs must be reasonable and medically necessary.

▶ He must be under a physician's care.

In addition, home health care nurses must document a physician's telephone orders. The CMS has established guidelines for taking and documenting these orders. Some agencies develop their own forms to fulfill these requirements. (See *Physician's telephone orders*.)

Agency assessment and OASIS forms

When a patient is referred to a home health care agency, the agency must complete a thorough and specific assessment of the patient's:

▶ physical status

▶ nutritional status

▶ mental and emotional status

▶ home environment in relation to safety and supportive services and groups, such as his family, neighbors, and community

▶ knowledge of his disease or current condition, prognosis, and treatment plan

▶ potential for complying with the treatment plan.

This information must be charted on a patient assessment form. CMS's "Conditions of Participation for Home Health Agencies" requires that Medicare-certified agencies complete a comprehensive assessment of home health care patients using the most recently re-vised version of the OASIS, the OASIS-B1.

Medicare has tied reimbursement to the OASIS; therefore, all patients over age 18, ex-cluding women receiving maternal-child ser-vices, must have an OASIS evaluation. OASIS regulations require the nurse to complete an as-sessment and the agency to transmit that assess-ment and other data within strict time frames.

Patient assessment must be completed:
▶ within 5 days of the initiation of care and at 60 days and 120 days (if needed)
▶ when the patient is transferred to another agency
▶ when the patient is discharged from home care
▶ when there's a significant change in the pa-tient's condition.

The OASIS forms were developed specifically to measure outcomes for adults who receive home health care. Using this instrument, you'll collect data to measure changes in your patient's health status over time. Typically, you'll collect OASIS data when a patient starts home health care, at the 60-day recertification point, and when the patient is discharged or transferred to another facility, such as a hospital or subacute care facility. (See *Using the OASIS-B1 form,* pages 216 to 231.)

Care plan

As in any health care setting, the nursing pro-cess forms the basis for developing the care plan. However, because the patient's care occurs in the home—usually with family participa-tion—you have less control than you would in an institutional setting. The patient and his family become the decision makers in many aspects and have greater control of the situation. You should address these factors realistically when developing the care plan. Remember that you're a guest in the patient's home; you may need to adjust your interventions, patient goals, and teaching accordingly.

Many agencies use the Home Health Certifi-cation and Plan of Care form as the patient's of-ficial care plan. Other agencies require a sepa-rate care plan, whereas still others see the two plans as redundant and time-consuming. If a pa-tient is receiving more than one service, such as physical or occupational therapy, agencies use an interdisciplinary care plan. (See *Interdisciplinary care plan,* page 232.)

Legally speaking, a care plan is the most di-rect evidence of your nursing judgment. If you outline a care plan and then deviate from it, a court may decide that you strayed from a reason-able standard of care. Be sure to update your care plan and make sure that it fits the patient's individualized needs.

To document most effectively on your care plan, follow these suggestions:
▶ Keep a copy of the care plan in the patient's home for easy reference by him and his family.
▶ Make sure that the plan is comprehensive by including more than the patient's physiologic problems. Also chart the home environment, the resources needed, and the attitudes of the patient, family, and caregiver.
▶ Document physical changes that need to be made in the patient's home for him to re-ceive proper care. Help the family find the resources to implement them.
▶ Describe the primary caregiver, including whether he lives with the patient, their rela-tionship, his age and physical ability, and his willingness to help the patient. The patient's well-being may depend on this person's abili-ties.

(Text continues on page 231.)

ChartWizard

Using the OASIS-B1 form

The OASIS-B1 form includes more than 80 topics, such as socioeconomic, physiologic, and functional data; service utilization information; and mental, behavioral, and emotional data.

OUTCOME AND ASSESSMENT INFORMATION SET (OASIS-B1)

START OF CARE Assessment (also used for Resumption of Care Following Inpatient Stay)	Client's Name: _Rojer Rabino_ Client Record No. _723641_

The Outcome and Assessment Information Set (OASIS) is the intellectual property of The Center for Health Services and Policy Research. Copyright ©2000 Used with Permission.

DEMOGRAPHIC/GENERAL INFORMATION

1. **(M0010)** Agency Medicare Provider Number:

2. **(M0012)** Agency Medicaid Provider Number:

Branch Identification *(Optional, for Agency Use)*
3. **(M0014)** Branch State: _____
4. **(M0016)** Branch ID Number:

   Agency-assigned

5. **(M0020)** Patient ID Number:
   QCB/811757

6. **(M0030)** Start of Care Date: _02_ / _02_ / _2007_
   month day year

7. **(M0032)** Resumption of Care Date:
   ____ / ____ / ____   ☒ NA - Not Applicable
   month day year

8. **(M0040)** Patient Name:
   Terry   _S_
   First   MI
   Elliot   _Mr._
   Last   Suffix

   Patient Address:
   11 Second Street
   Street, Route, Apt. Number
   Hometown
   City

   (M0050) Patient State of Residence: _PA_
   (M0060) Patient Zip Code: _____ 10981_ - _1234_
   Phone: (_881_) _555_ - _2937_

9. **(M0063)** Medicare Number:
   _134765482 A_
                        including suffix
   ☐ NA - No Medicare

10. **(M0064)** Social Security Number:
    _111_ - _22_ - _3333_
    ☐ UK - Unknown or Not Available

11. **(M0065)** Medicaid Number:

    ☒ NA - No Medicaid

12. **(M0066)** Birth Date: _07_ / _08_ / _1932_
    month day year

13. **(M0069)** Gender:
    ☒ 1 - Male   ☐ 2 - Female

14. **(M0072)** Primary Referring Physician ID:
    _222222_   (UPIN#)
    ☐ UK - Unknown or Not Available
    Name _Dr. Kyle Stevens_
    Address _10 State St._
    Hometown, PA 10981
    Phone: (_881_) _555_ - _6900_
    FAX: (_881_) _555_ - _6974_

15. **(M0080)** Discipline of Person Completing Assessment:
    ☒ 1-RN   ☐ 2-PT   ☐ 3-SLP/ST   ☐ 4-OT

16. **(M0090)** Date Assessment Completed:
    _02_ / _02_ / _2007_
    month day year

Using the OASIS-B1 form *(continued)*

17. (M0100) This Assessment is Currently Being Completed for the Following Reason:

Start/Resumption of Care
- ☒ 1 - Start of care — further visits planned
- ☐ 3 - Resumption of care (after inpatient stay)

Follow-Up
- ☐ 4 - Recertification (follow-up) reassessment [Go to *M0150*]
- ☐ 5 - Other follow-up [Go to *M0150*]

Transfer to an Inpatient Facility
- ☐ 6 - Transferred to an inpatient facility — patient not discharged from agency [Go to *M0150*]
- ☐ 7 - Transferred to an inpatient facility — patient discharged from agency [Go to *M0150*]

Discharge from Agency — Not to an Inpatient Facility
- ☐ 8 - Death at home [Go to *M0150*]
- ☐ 9 - Discharge from agency [Go to *M0150*]

18. Marital status:
- ☐ Not Married   ☒ Married   ☐ Widowed
- ☐ Divorced   ☐ Separated   ☐ Unknown

19. (M0140) Race/Ethnicity (as identified by patient): (Mark all that apply.)
- ☐ 1 - American Indian or Alaska Native
- ☐ 2 - Asian
- ☐ 3 - Black or African-American
- ☐ 4 - Hispanic or Latino
- ☐ 5 - Native Hawaiian or Pacific Islander
- ☒ 6 - White
- ☐ UK - Unknown

20. Emergency contact:

Name *Susan Elliot*

Address *11 Second St.*

Hometown, PA 10981

Phone: (*881*) *555* - *2937*

21. (M0150) Current Payment Sources for Home Care: (Mark all that apply.)
- ☐ 0 - None; no charge for current services
- ☒ 1 - Medicare (traditional fee-for-service)
- ☐ 2 - Medicare (HMO/managed care)
- ☐ 3 - Medicaid (traditional fee-for-service)
- ☐ 4 - Medicaid (HMO/managed care)
- ☐ 5 - Workers' compensation
- ☐ 6 - Title programs (e.g., Title III, V, or XX)
- ☐ 7 - Other government (e.g., CHAMPUS, VA, etc.)
- ☐ 8 - Private insurance
- ☐ 9 - Private HMO/managed care
- ☐ 10 - Self-pay
- ☐ 11 - Other (specify) _____
- ☐ UK - Unknown

PATIENT HISTORY

22. (M0175) From which of the following **Inpatient Facilities** was the patient discharged *during the past 14 days*? (Mark all that apply.)
- ☐ 1 - Hospital
- ☐ 2 - Rehabilitation facility
- ☐ 3 - Skilled nursing facility
- ☐ 4 - Other nursing home
- ☐ 5 - Other (specify) _____
- ☒ NA - Patient was not discharged from an inpatient facility [If NA, go to *M0200*]

23. (M0180) Inpatient Discharge Date (most recent):

_____ / _____ / _____
month   day   year
- ☐ UK - Unknown

(continued)

Using the OASIS-B1 form (continued)

24. **(M0190)** **Inpatient Diagnoses** and ICD code categories (three digits required; five digits optional) *for only those conditions treated during an inpatient facility stay within the last 14 days* (no surgical or V-codes):

Inpatient Facility Diagnosis	ICD
a. _____	(_____ . _____)
b. _____	(_____ . _____)

25. **(M0200)** **Medical or Treatment Regimen Change Within Past 14 Days:** Has this patient experienced a change in medical or treatment regimen (e.g., medication, treatment, or service change due to new or additional diagnosis, etc.) within the last 14 days?

  ☐ 0 - No   [If No, go to *M0220*]
  ☒ 1 - Yes

26. **(M0210)** List the patient's **Medical Diagnoses** and ICD code categories (three digits required; five digits optional) or those conditions requiring changed medical or treatment regimen (no surgical or V-codes):

Changed Medical Regimen Diagnosis	ICD
a. *open wound Ⓛ ankle*	(*891* . *00*)
b. _____	(_____ . _____)
c. _____	(_____ . _____)
d. _____	(_____ . _____)

27. **(M0220)** **Conditions Prior to Medical or Treatment Regimen Change or Inpatient Stay Within Past 14 Days:** If this patient experienced an inpatient facility discharge or change in medical or treatment regimen within the past 14 days, indicate any conditions which existed *prior* to the inpatient stay or change in medical or treatment regimen. **(Mark all that apply.)**

  ☐ 1 - Urinary incontinence
  ☐ 2 - Indwelling/suprapubic catheter
  ☐ 3 - Intractable pain
  ☐ 4 - Impaired decision making
  ☐ 5 - Disruptive or socially inappropriate behavior
  ☐ 6 - Memory loss to the extent that supervision required
  ☒ 7 - None of the above
  ☐ NA - No inpatient facility discharge *and* no change in medical or treatment regimen in past 14 days
  ☐ UK - Unknown

28. **(M0230/M0240)** **Diagnoses and Severity Index:** List each medical diagnosis or problem for which the patient is receiving home care and ICD code category (three digits required; five digits optional — no surgical or V-codes) and rate them using the following severity index. (Choose one value that represents the most severe rating appropriate for each diagnosis.)

  0 - Asymptomatic, no treatment needed at this time
  1 - Symptoms well controlled with current therapy
  2 - Symptoms controlled with difficulty, affecting daily functioning; patient needs ongoing monitoring
  3 - Symptoms poorly controlled, patient needs frequent adjustment in treatment and dose monitoring
  4 - Symptoms poorly controlled, history of rehospitalizations

(M0230) Primary Diagnosis · ICD

a. *open wound Ⓛ ankle* (*891* . *00*)

Severity Rating ☐ 0 ☐ 1 ☒ 2 ☐ 3 ☐ 4

(M0240) Other Diagnoses · ICD

b. *Type 2 diabetes* (*250* . *72*)

Severity Rating ☐ 0 ☐ 1 ☒ 2 ☐ 3 ☐ 4

c. *PVD* (*443* . *89*)

Severity Rating ☐ 0 ☐ 1 ☐ 2 ☒ 3 ☐ 4

d. _____ (_____ . _____)

Severity Rating ☐ 0 ☐ 1 ☐ 2 ☐ 3 ☐ 4

e. _____ (_____ . _____)

Severity Rating ☐ 0 ☐ 1 ☐ 2 ☐ 3 ☐ 4

f. _____ (_____ . _____)

Severity Rating ☐ 0 ☐ 1 ☐ 2 ☐ 3 ☐ 4

29. **Patient/family knowledge and coping level regarding present illness:**

Patient *Knowledgeable about disease process*

Family *Anxious to assist in care*

30. **Significant past health history:** _____

  PVD
  Type 2 diabetes
  Ⓡ BKA

Using the OASIS-B1 form *(continued)*

Effective 10/1/03

31. (M0245) Payment Diagnosis (optional): If a V-code was reported in M0230 in place of a case mix diagnosis, list the primary diagnosis and ICD-9-CM code, determined in accordance with OASIS requirements in effect before October 1, 2003 – no V-codes, E-codes, or surgical codes allowed. ICD-9-CM sequencing requirements must be followed. Complete both lines (a) and (b) if the case mix diagnosis is a manifestation code or in other situations where multiple coding is indicated for the primary diagnosis: otherwise, complete line (a) only.

(M0245) Primary Diagnosis   ICD-9-CM

a. _____   (_____ • _____)

(M0245) Primary Diagnosis   ICD-9-CM

b. _____   (_____ • _____)

32. (M0250) **Therapies** the patient receives *at home*:
(Mark all that apply.)

☐ 1 - Intravenous or infusion therapy (excludes TPN)

☐ 2 - Parenteral nutrition (TPN or lipids)

☐ 3 - Enteral nutrition (nasogastric, gastrostomy, jejunostomy, or any other artificial entry into the alimentary canal)

☒ 4 - None of the above

33. (M0260) **Overall Prognosis:** BEST description of patient's prognosis for *recovery from this episode of illness*.

☐ 0 - Poor: little or no recovery is expected and/or further decline is imminent

☒ 1 - Good/Fair: partial to full recovery is expected

☐ UK - Unknown

34. (M0270) **Rehabilitative Prognosis:** BEST description of patient's prognosis for *functional status*.

☒ 0 - Guarded: minimal improvement in functional status is expected; decline is possible

☐ 1 - Good: marked improvement in functional status is expected

☐ UK - Unknown

35. (M0280) **Life Expectancy:** (Physician documentation is not required.)

☐ 0 - Life expectancy is greater than 6 months

☒ 1 - Life expectancy is 6 months or fewer

36. Immunization/screening tests:

Immunizations:

Flu   ☒ Yes ☐ No   Date   10/05

Tetanus   ☒ Yes ☐ No   Date   3/02

Pneumonia   ☒ Yes ☐ No   Date   10/05

Other _____ Date _____

Screening:

Cholesterol level   ☒ Yes ☐ No   Date   11/06

Mammogram   ☐ Yes ☒ No   Date _____

Colon cancer
screen   ☒ Yes ☐ No   Date   11/06

Prostate cancer
screen   ☒ Yes ☐ No   Date   11/06

Self-exam frequency:

Breast self-exam frequency _____

Testicular self-exam frequency _____

37. Allergies: NKA _____

38. (M0290) **High Risk Factors** characterizing this patient:
(Mark all that apply.)

☒ 1 - Heavy smoking

☐ 2 - Obesity

☐ 3 - Alcohol dependency

☐ 4 - Drug dependency

☐ 5 - None of the above

☐ UK - Unknown

LIVING ARRANGEMENTS

39. (M0300) **Current Residence:**

☒ 1 - Patient's owned or rented residence (house, apartment, or mobile home owned or rented by patient/couple/significant other)

☐ 2 - Family member's residence

☐ 3 - Boarding home or rented room

☐ 4 - Board and care or assisted living facility

☐ 5 - Other (specify) _____

(continued)

Using the OASIS-B1 form *(continued)*

40. (M0340) Patient Lives With: (Mark all that apply.)

- [ ] 1 - Lives alone
- [X] 2 - With spouse or significant other
- [ ] 3 - With other family member
- [ ] 4 - With a friend
- [ ] 5 - With paid help (other than home care agency staff)
- [ ] 6 - With other than above

Comments: ....

41. Others living in household: ....

Name *Susan*   Age *74*   Sex *F*
Relationship *wife*   Able/willing to assist [X] Yes [ ] No
Name .... Age........ Sex ....
Relationship .... Able/willing to assist [ ] Yes [ ] No
Name .... Age........ Sex ....
Relationship .... Able/willing to assist [ ] Yes [ ] No
Name .... Age........ Sex ....
Relationship .... Able/willing to assist [ ] Yes [ ] No
Name .... Age........ Sex ....
Relationship .... Able/willing to assist [ ] Yes [ ] No
Name .... Age........ Sex ....
Relationship .... Able/willing to assist [ ] Yes [ ] No

SUPPORTIVE ASSISTANCE

42. Persons/Organizations providing assistance: ....

43. (M0350) Assisting Person(s) Other than Home Care Agency Staff: (Mark all that apply.)

- [ ] 1 - Relatives, friends, or neighbors living outside the home
- [X] 2 - Person residing in the home (EXCLUDING paid help)
- [ ] 3 - Paid help
- [ ] 4 - None of the above
  [If None of the above, go to *Review of Systems*]
- [ ] UK - Unknown [If Unknown, go to *Review of Systems*]

44. (M0360) Primary Caregiver taking *lead* responsibility for providing or managing the patient's care, providing the most frequent assistance, etc. (other than home care agency staff):

- [ ] 0 - No one person [If No one person, go to *M0390*]
- [X] 1 - Spouse or significant other
- [ ] 2 - Daughter or son
- [ ] 3 - Other family member
- [ ] 4 - Friend or neighbor or community or church member
- [ ] 5 - Paid help
- [ ] UK - Unknown [If Unknown, go to *M0390*]

45. (M0370) How Often does the patient receive assistance from the primary caregiver?

- [X] 1 - Several times during day and night
- [ ] 2 - Several times during day
- [ ] 3 - Once daily
- [ ] 4 - Three or more times per week
- [ ] 5 - One to two times per week
- [ ] 6 - Less often than weekly
- [ ] UK - Unknown

Using the OASIS-B1 form *(continued)*

46. (M0380) Type of Primary Caregiver Assistance:

(Mark all that apply.)

☒ 1 - ADL assistance (e.g., bathing, dressing, toileting, bowel/bladder, eating/feeding)

☒ 2 - IADL assistance (e.g., meds, meals, housekeeping, laundry, telephone, shopping, finances)

☐ 3 - Environmental support (housing, home maintenance)

☒ 4 - Psychosocial support (socialization, companionship, recreation)

☒ 5 - Advocates or facilitates patient's participation in appropriate medical care

☐ 6 - Financial agent, power of attorney, or conservator of finance

☐ 7 - Health care agent, conservator of person, or medical power of attorney

☐ UK - Unknown

Comments: _____

REVIEW OF SYSTEMS

SENSORY STATUS

(Mark S for subjective, O for objectively assessed problem. If no problem present or if not assessed, mark NA.)

Head *NA* Dizziness

NA Headache (describe location, duration) _____

Eyes *O* Glasses *NA* Cataracts *NA* Blurred/double vision

O PERRL _____ Other (specify) _____

47. (M0390) Vision with corrective lenses if the patient usually wears them:

☒ 0 - Normal vision: sees adequately in most situations; can see medication labels, newsprint.

☐ 1 - Partially impaired: cannot see medication labels or newsprint, but *can* see obstacles in path, and the surrounding layout; can count fingers at arm's length.

☐ 2 - Severely impaired: cannot locate objects without hearing or touching them *or* patient nonresponsive.

Ears *NA* Hearing aid *NA* Tinnitus

_____ Other (specify) _____

48. (M0400) Hearing and Ability to Understand Spoken Language in patient's own language (with hearing aids if the patient usually uses them):

☒ 0 - No observable impairment. Able to hear and understand complex or detailed instructions and extended or abstract conversation.

☐ 1 - With minimal difficulty, able to hear and understand most multi-step instructions and ordinary conversation. May need occasional repetition, extra time, or louder voice.

☐ 2 - Has moderate difficulty hearing and understanding simple, one-step instructions and brief conversation; needs frequent prompting or assistance.

☐ 3 - Has severe difficulty hearing and understanding simple greetings and short comments. Requires multiple repetitions, restatements, demonstrations, additional time.

☐ 4 - *Unable* to hear and understand familiar words or common expressions consistently, *or* patient nonresponsive.

Oral _____ Gum problems _____ Chewing problems

_____ Dentures _____ Other (specify) _____

49. (M0410) Speech and Oral (Verbal) Expression of Language (in patient's own language):

☒ 0 - Expresses complex ideas, feelings, and needs clearly, completely, and easily in all situations with no observable impairment.

☐ 1 - Minimal difficulty in expressing ideas and needs (may take extra time; makes occasional errors in word choice, grammar or speech intelligibility; needs minimal prompting or assistance).

☐ 2 - Expresses simple ideas or needs with moderate difficulty (needs prompting or assistance, errors in word choice, organization, or speech intelligibility). Speaks in phrases or short sentences.

☐ 3 - Has severe difficulty expressing basic ideas or needs and requires maximal assistance or guessing by listener. Speech limited to single words or short phrases.

☐ 4 - *Unable* to express basic needs even with maximal prompting or assistance but is not comatose or unresponsive (e.g., speech is nonsensical or unintelligible).

☐ 5 - Patient nonresponsive or unable to speak.

Nose and sinus

NA Epistaxis _____ Other (specify) _____

Neck and throat

NA Hoarseness *NA* Difficulty swallowing

_____ Other (specify) _____

(continued)

Using the OASIS-B1 form (continued)

Musculoskeletal, Neurological

N/A Hx arthritis   *N/A* Joint pain   *N/A* Syncope

N/A Gout   *N/A* Weakness   *N/A* Seizure

N/A Stiffness   *S* Leg cramps   *N/A* Tenderness

N/A Swollen joints   *S* Numbness   *N/A* Deformities

N/A Unequal grasp   *O* Temp changes   *N/A* Comatose

N/A Tremor   *N/A* Aphasia/inarticulate speech

N/A Paralysis (describe) _____

N/A Amputation (location) _____

N/A Other (specify) _____

Coordination, gait, balance (describe) *Gait steady*

_____

_____

Comments (Prosthesis, appliances) *Uses a walker*

_____

_____

Patient's perceived pain level: *4*   (Scale 1-10)

50. (M0420) Frequency of Pain interfering with patient's activity or movement:

- [ ] 0 - Patient has no pain or pain does not interfere with activity or movement
- [ ] 1 - Less often than daily
- [X] 2 - Daily, but not constantly
- [ ] 3 - All of the time

51. (M0430) Intractable Pain: Is the patient experiencing pain that is *not easily relieved*, occurs at least daily, and affects the patient's sleep, appetite, physical or emotional energy, concentration, personal relationships, emotions, or ability or desire to perform physical activity?

- [X] 0 - No
- [ ] 1 - Yes

Comments (pain management) _____

_____

_____

_____

INTEGUMENTARY STATUS

O Hair changes (where)   *Balding* _____

N/A Pruritus   Other (specify) _____

Skin condition (Record type # on body area. Indicate size to right of numbered category.)

#5

Type	Size
1. Lesions	
2. Bruises	
3. Masses	
4. Scars	
5. Stasis Ulcers	*1/2" round*
6. Pressure Ulcers	
7. Incisions	
8. Other (specify)	

52. (M0440) Does this patient have a **Skin Lesion** or an **Open Wound**? This excludes "OSTOMIES."

- [ ] 0 - No [If No, go to *Cardio/respiratory status*]
- [X] 1 - Yes

53. (M0445) Does this patient have a **Pressure Ulcer**?

- [X] 0 - No [If No, go to *M0468*]
- [ ] 1 - Yes

Using the OASIS-B1 form (continued)

54. **(M0450)** Current Number of Pressure Ulcers at Each Stage: (Circle one response for each stage.)

Pressure Ulcer Stages	Number of Pressure Ulcers
a) Stage 1: Nonblanchable erythema of intact skin; the heralding of skin ulceration. In darker-pigmented skin, warmth, edema, hardness, or discolored skin may be indicators.	0 1 2 3 4 or more
b) Stage 2: Partial thickness skin loss involving epidermis and/or dermis. The ulcer is superficial and presents clinically as an abrasion, blister, or shallow crater.	0 1 2 3 4 or more
c) Stage 3: Full-thickness skin loss involving damage or necrosis of subcutaneous tissue which may extend down to, but not through, underlying fascia. The ulcer presents clinically as a deep crater with or without undermining of adjacent tissue.	0 1 2 3 4 or more
d) Stage 4: Full-thickness skin loss with extensive destruction, tissue necrosis, or damage to muscle, bone, or supporting structures (e.g., tendon, joint capsule, etc.)	0 1 2 3 4 or more

e) In addition to the above, is there at least one pressure ulcer that cannot be observed due to the presence of eschar or a nonremovable dressing, including casts?

- ☐ 0 - No
- ☐ 1 - Yes

55. **(M0460)** Stage of Most Problematic (Observable) Pressure Ulcer:

- ☐ 1 - Stage 1
- ☐ 2 - Stage 2
- ☐ 3 - Stage 3
- ☐ 4 - Stage 4
- ☐ NA - No observable pressure ulcer

56. **(M0464)** Status of Most Problematic (Observable) Pressure Ulcer:

- ☐ 1 - Fully granulating
- ☐ 2 - Early/partial granulation
- ☐ 3 - Not healing
- ☐ NA - No observable pressure ulcer

57. **(M0468)** Does this patient have a **Stasis Ulcer**?

- ☐ 0 - No [If No, go to *M0482*]
- ☒ 1 - Yes

58. **(M0470)** Current Number of Observable Stasis Ulcer(s):

- ☐ 0 - Zero
- ☒ 1 - One
- ☐ 2 - Two
- ☐ 3 - Three
- ☐ 4 - Four or more

59. **(M0474)** Does this patient have at least one Stasis Ulcer that **Cannot be Observed** due to the presence of a nonremovable dressing?

- ☒ 0 - No
- ☐ 1 - Yes

60. **(M0476)** Status of Most Problematic (Observable) Stasis Ulcer:

- ☐ 1 - Fully granulating
- ☒ 2 - Early/partial granulation
- ☐ 3 - Not healing
- ☐ NA - No observable stasis ulcer

61. **(M0482)** Does this patient have a **Surgical Wound**?

- ☒ 0 - No [If No, go to *Cardio/Respiratory Status*]
- ☐ 1 - Yes

62. **(M0484)** Current Number of (Observable) Surgical Wounds: (If a wound is partially closed but has *more* than one opening, consider each opening as a separate wound.)

- ☐ 0 - Zero
- ☐ 1 - One
- ☐ 2 - Two
- ☐ 3 - Three
- ☐ 4 - Four or more

63. **(M0486)** Does this patient have at least one **Surgical Wound that Cannot be Observed** due to the presence of a nonremovable dressing?

- ☐ 0 - No
- ☐ 1 - Yes

64. **(M0488)** Status of Most Problematic (Observable) Surgical Wound:

- ☐ 1 - Fully granulating
- ☐ 2 - Early/partial granulation
- ☐ 3 - Not healing
- ☐ NA - No observable surgical wound

(continued)

Using the OASIS-B1 form *(continued)*

CARDIO/RESPIRATORY STATUS

Temperature _99°_   Respirations _18_

Blood pressure
   Lying _132/80_ Sitting _130/78_ Standing _130/76_

Pulse
   Apical rate _72_   Radial rate _72_
   Rhythm _Regular_   Quality _____

Cardiovascular
   _NA_ Palpitations   _NA_ Chest pains
   _S_ Claudication   _NA_ Murmurs
   _S_ Fatigues easily   _O_ Edema
   _NA_ BP problems   _NA_ Cyanosis
   _NA_ Dyspnea on exertion _NA_ Varicosities
   _NA_ Paroxysmal nocturnal dyspnea
   _NA_ Orthopnea (# of pillows)
   _NA_ Cardiac problems (specify)_____
   _NA_ Pacemaker _____
                (Date of last battery change)
   Other (specify) _____
   Comments _____

Respiratory
   History of
   _NA_ Asthma   _NA_ Pleurisy
   _NA_ TB   _NA_ Pneumonia
   _S_ Bronchitis   _NA_ Emphysema
   Other (specify) _____
   Present condition
   _S_ Cough (describe) _Dry_
   _O_ Breath sounds (describe) _Clear_
   _NA_ Sputum (character and amount) _____
   Other (specify) _____

65. (M0490) When is the patient dyspneic or noticeably **Short of Breath**?
   ☒ 0 - Never, patient is not short of breath
   ☐ 1 - When walking more than 20 feet, climbing stairs
   ☐ 2 - With moderate exertion (e.g., while dressing, using commode or bedpan, walking distances less than 20 feet)
   ☐ 3 - With minimal exertion (e.g., while eating, talking, or performing other ADLs) or with agitation
   ☐ 4 - At rest (during day or night)

66. (M0500) **Respiratory Treatments** utilized at home:
   (Mark all that apply.)
   ☐ 1 - Oxygen (intermittent or continuous)
   ☐ 2 - Ventilator (continually or at night)
   ☐ 3 - Continuous positive airway pressure
   ☐ 4 - None of the above
   Comments _____

ELIMINATION STATUS

Genitourinary Tract
   _NA_ Frequency   _NA_ Prostate disorder
   _NA_ Pain   _NA_ Dysmenorrhea
   _NA_ Hematuria   _NA_ Lesions
   _NA_ Vaginal discharge/bleeding _NA_ Hx hysterectomy
   _S_ Nocturia   _NA_ Gravida/Para
   _NA_ Urgency   _NA_ Contraception
   _NA_ Date last PAP _____
   Other (specify) _____

67. (M0510) Has this patient been treated for a **Urinary Tract Infection** in the past 14 days?
   ☒ 0 - No
   ☐ 1 - Yes
   ☐ NA - Patient on prophylactic treatment
   ☐ UK - Unknown

68. (M0520) **Urinary Incontinence or Urinary Catheter Presence:**
   ☒ 0 - No incontinence or catheter (includes anuria or ostomy for urinary drainage) [If No, go to *M0540*]
   ☐ 1 - Patient is incontinent
   ☐ 2 - Patient requires a urinary catheter (i.e., external, indwelling, intermittent, suprapubic) [Go to *M0540*]

Using the OASIS-B1 form *(continued)*

69. (M0530) When does **Urinary Incontinence** occur?

☐ 0 - Timed-voiding defers incontinence

☐ 1 - During the night only

☐ 2 - During the day and night

Comments (e.g., appliances and care, bladder programs, catheter type, frequency of irrigation and change) ....

....

....

....

....

....

Gastrointestinal Tract

N/A Indigestion   *N/A* Rectal bleeding

N/A Nausea/vomiting   *N/A* Hemorrhoids

N/A Ulcers   *N/A* Gallbladder problems

N/A Pain   *N/A* Jaundice

N/A Diarrhea/constipation   *N/A* Tenderness

N/A Hernias (where) ....

Other (specify) ....

70. (M0540) Bowel Incontinence Frequency:

☒ 0 - Very rarely or never has bowel incontinence

☐ 1 - Less than once weekly

☐ 2 - One to three times weekly

☐ 3 - Four to six times weekly

☐ 4 - On a daily basis

☐ 5 - More often than once daily

☐ NA - Patient has ostomy for bowel elimination

☐ UK - Unknown

71. (M0550) Ostomy for Bowel Elimination: Does this patient have an ostomy for bowel elimination that (within the last 14 days):

a) was related to an inpatient facility stay, *or*

b) necessitated a change in medical or treatment regimen?

☒ 0 - Patient does *not* have an ostomy for bowel elimination.

☐ 1 - Patient's ostomy was *not* related to an inpatient stay and did *not* necessitate change in medical or treatment regimen.

☐ 2 - The ostomy *was* related to an inpatient stay or *did* necessitate change in medical or treatment regimen.

Comments (bowel function, stool color, bowel program, GI series, abd. girth) ....

....

Nutritional status

N/A Weight loss/gain last 3 mos. (Give amount _____)

N/A Over/under weight   *N/A* Change in appetite

Diet   *20% protein 30% fat*

Other (specify) ....

Meals prepared by   *Wife*

Comments ....

....

....

....

....

Breasts (For both male and female)

N/A Lumps   *N/A* Tenderness

N/A Discharge   *N/A* Pain

Other (specify) ....

Comments ....

....

....

....

NEURO/EMOTIONAL/BEHAVIORAL STATUS

N/A Hx of previous psych. illness

Other (specify) ....

72. (M0560) Cognitive Functioning: (Patient's current level of alertness, orientation, comprehension, concentration, and immediate memory for simple commands.)

☐ 0 - Alert/oriented, able to focus and shift attention, comprehends and recalls task directions independently.

☒ 1 - Requires prompting (cueing, repetition, reminders) only under stressful or unfamiliar conditions.

☐ 2 - Requires assistance and some direction in specific situations (e.g., on all tasks involving shifting of attention), or consistently requires low stimulus environment due to distractibility.

☐ 3 - Requires considerable assistance in routine situations. Is not alert and oriented or is unable to shift attention and recall directions more than half the time.

☐ 4 - Totally dependent due to disturbances such as constant disorientation, coma, persistent vegetative state, or delirium.

(continued)

Using the OASIS-B1 form *(continued)*

73. **(M0570)** When Confused (Reported or Observed):

☒ 0 - Never

☐ 1 - In new or complex situations only

☐ 2 - On awakening or at night only

☐ 3 - During the day and evening, but not constantly

☐ 4 - Constantly

☐ NA - Patient nonresponsive

74. **(M0580)** When Anxious (Reported or Observed):

☐ 0 - None of the time

☐ 1 - Less often than daily

☒ 2 - Daily, but not constantly

☐ 3 - All of the time

☐ NA - Patient nonresponsive

75. **(M0590)** Depressive Feelings Reported or Observed in Patient: (Mark all that apply.)

☐ 1 - Depressed mood (e.g., feeling sad, tearful)

☐ 2 - Sense of failure or self-reproach

☒ 3 - Hopelessness

☐ 4 - Recurrent thoughts of death

☐ 5 - Thoughts of suicide

☐ 6 - None of the above feelings observed or reported

76. **(M0610)** Behaviors Demonstrated *at Least Once a Week* (Reported or Observed): (Mark all that apply.)

☐ 1 - Memory deficit: failure to recognize familiar persons/places, inability to recall events of past 24 hours, significant memory loss so that supervision is required

☐ 2 - Impaired decision making: failure to perform usual ADLs or IADLs, inability to appropriately stop activities, jeopardizes safety through actions

☐ 3 - Verbal disruption: yelling, threatening, excessive profanity, sexual references, etc.

☐ 4 - Physical aggression: aggressive or combative to self and others (e.g., hits self, throws objects, punches, dangerous maneuvers with wheelchair or other objects)

☐ 5 - Disruptive, infantile, or socially inappropriate behavior (**excludes** verbal actions)

☐ 6 - Delusional, hallucinatory, or paranoid behavior

☒ 7 - None of the above behaviors demonstrated

77. **(M0620)** Frequency of Behavior Problems (Reported or Observed) (e.g., wandering episodes, self-abuse, verbal disruption, physical aggression, etc.):

☒ 0 - Never

☐ 1 - Less than once a month

☐ 2 - Once a month

☐ 3 - Several times each month

☐ 4 - Several times a week

☐ 5 - At least daily

78. **(M0630)** Is this patient receiving **Psychiatric Nursing Services** at home provided by a qualified psychiatric nurse?

☒ 0 - No

☐ 1 - Yes

Comments _____

_____

_____

Endocrine and hematopoietic

_S_ Diabetes   _NA_ Polydipsia

_NA_ Polyuria   _NA_ Thyroid problem

_NA_ Excessive bleeding or bruising

_S_ Intolerance to heat and cold

Fractionals

Usual results _____

Frequency checked _____

Other (specify) _____

Comments _____

_____

Using the OASIS-B1 form *(continued)*

ADL/IADLs

For M0640-M0800, complete the "Current" column for all patients. For these same items, complete the "Prior" column only at start of care and at resumption of care; mark the level that corresponds to the patient's condition 14 days prior to start of care date (M0030) or resumption of care date (M0032). In all cases, record what the patient is *able to do.*

79. (M0640) Grooming: Ability to tend to personal hygiene needs (i.e., washing face and hands, hair care, shaving or makeup, teeth or denture care, fingernail care).

Prior Current

☒ ☐ 0 - Able to groom self unaided, with or without the use of assistive devices or adapted methods.

☐ ☒ 1 - Grooming utensils must be placed within reach before able to complete grooming activities.

☐ ☐ 2 - Someone must assist the patient to groom self.

☐ ☐ 3 - Patient depends entirely upon someone else for grooming needs.

☐ UK - Unknown

80. (M0650) Ability to Dress *Upper* Body (with or without dressing aids) including undergarments, pullovers, front-opening shirts and blouses, managing zippers, buttons, and snaps:

Prior Current

☒ ☐ 0 - Able to get clothes out of closets and drawers, put them on and remove them from the upper body without assistance.

☐ ☒ 1 - Able to dress upper body without assistance if clothing is laid out or handed to the patient.

☐ ☐ 2 - Someone must help the patient put on upper body clothing.

☐ ☐ 3 - Patient depends entirely upon another person to dress the upper body.

☐ UK - Unknown

81. (M0660) Ability to Dress *Lower* Body (with or without dressing aids) including undergarments, slacks, socks or nylons, shoes:

Prior Current

☒ ☐ 0 - Able to obtain, put on, and remove clothing and shoes without assistance.

☐ ☐ 1 - Able to dress lower body without assistance if clothing and shoes are laid out or handed to the patient.

☐ ☒ 2 - Someone must help the patient put on undergarments, slacks, socks or nylons, and shoes.

☐ ☐ 3 - Patient depends entirely upon another person to dress lower body.

☐ UK - Unknown

82. (M0670) Bathing: Ability to wash entire body. *Excludes* grooming (washing face and hands only).

Prior Current

☐ ☐ 0 - Able to bathe self in *shower or tub* independently

☒ ☐ 1 - With the use of devices, is able to bathe self in shower or tub independently.

☐ ☐ 2 - Able to bathe in shower or tub with the assistance of another person:
(a) for intermittent supervision or encouragement or reminders, *OR*
(b) to get in and out of the shower or tub, *OR*
(c) for washing difficult-to-reach areas.

☐ ☒ 3 - Participates in bathing self in shower or tub, *but* requires presence of another person throughout the bath for assistance or supervision.

☐ ☐ 4 - *Unable* to use the shower or tub and is bathed in *bed or bedside chair.*

☐ ☐ 5 - Unable to effectively participate in bathing and is totally bathed by another person.

☐ UK - Unknown

83. (M0680) Toileting: Ability to get to and from the toilet or bedside commode.

Prior Current

☒ ☒ 0 - Able to get to and from the toilet independently with or without a device.

☐ ☐ 1 - When reminded, assisted, or supervised by another person, able to get to and from the toilet.

☐ ☐ 2 - *Unable* to get to and from the toilet but is able to use a bedside commode (with or without assistance).

☐ ☐ 3 - *Unable* to get to and from the toilet or bedside commode but is able to use a bedpan/urinal independently.

☐ ☐ 4 - Is totally dependent in toileting.

☐ UK - Unknown

(continued)

Using the OASIS-B1 form *(continued)*

84.(M0690) Transferring: Ability to move from bed to chair, on and off toilet or commode, into and out of tub or shower, and ability to turn and position self in bed if patient is bedfast.

Prior Current

☐ ☐ 0 - Able to independently transfer.

☒ ☒ 1 - Transfers with minimal human assistance or with use of an assistive device.

☐ ☐ 2 - *Unable* to transfer self but is able to bear weight and pivot during the transfer process.

☐ ☐ 3 - Unable to transfer self and is *unable* to bear weight or pivot when transferred by another person.

☐ ☐ 4 - Bedfast, unable to transfer but is able to turn and position self in bed.

☐ ☐ 5 - Bedfast, unable to transfer and is *unable* to turn and position self.

☐   UK - Unknown

85.(M0700) Ambulation/Locomotion: Ability to *SAFELY* walk, once in a standing position, or use a wheelchair, once in a seated position, on a variety of surfaces.

Prior Current

☒ ☐ 0 - Able to independently walk on even and uneven surfaces and climb stairs with or without railings (i.e., needs no human assistance or assistive device).

☐ ☒ 1 - Requires use of a device (e.g., cane, walker) to walk alone or requires human supervision or assistance to negotiate stairs or steps or uneven surfaces.

☐ ☐ 2 - Able to walk only with the supervision or assistance of another person at all times.

☐ ☐ 3 - Chairfast, *unable* to ambulate but is able to wheel self independently.

☐ ☐ 4 - Chairfast, unable to ambulate and is *unable* to wheel self.

☐ ☐ 5 - Bedfast, unable to ambulate or be up in a chair.

☐   UK - Unknown

86.(M0710) Feeding or Eating: Ability to feed self meals and snacks. **Note: This refers only to the process of** *eating, chewing,* **and** *swallowing, not preparing* **the food to be eaten.**

Prior Current

☒ ☒ 0 - Able to independently feed self.

☐ ☐ 1 - Able to feed self independently but requires:
(a) meal set-up; *OR*
(b) intermittent assistance or supervision from another person; *OR*
(c) a liquid, pureed or ground meat diet.

☐ ☐ 2 - *Unable* to feed self and must be assisted or supervised throughout the meal/snack.

☐ ☐ 3 - Able to take in nutrients orally *and* receives supplemental nutrients through a nasogastric tube or gastrostomy.

☐ ☐ 4 - *Unable* to take in nutrients orally and is fed nutrients through a nasogastric tube or gastrostomy.

☐ ☐ 5 - Unable to take in nutrients orally or by tube feeding.

☐   UK - Unknown

87.(M0720) Planning and Preparing Light Meals (e.g., cereal, sandwich) or reheat delivered meals:

Prior Current

☒ ☐ 0 - (a) Able to independently plan and prepare all light meals for self or reheat delivered meals; OR
(b) Is physically, cognitively, and mentally able to prepare light meals on a regular basis but has not routinely performed light meal preparation in the past (i.e., prior to this home care admission).

☐ ☒ 1 - *Unable* to prepare light meals on a regular basis due to physical, cognitive, or mental limitations.

☐ ☐ 2 - Unable to prepare any light meals or reheat any delivered meals.

☐   UK - Unknown

88.(M0730) Transportation: Physical and mental ability to *safely* use a car, taxi, or public transportation (bus, train, subway).

Prior Current

☐ ☐ 0 - Able to independently drive a regular or adapted car; OR uses a regular or handicap-accessible public bus.

☒ ☒ 1 - Able to ride in a car only when driven by another person; OR able to use a bus or handicap van only when assisted or accompanied by another person.

☐ ☐ 2 - Unable to ride in a car, taxi, bus, or van, and requires transportation by ambulance.

☐   UK - Unknown

Using the OASIS-B1 form *(continued)*

89.(M0740) Laundry: Ability to do own laundry — to carry laundry to and from washing machine, to use washer and dryer, to wash small items by hand.

Prior   Current

☐   ☐   0 - (a) Able to independently take care of all laundry tasks; *OR*
(b) Physically, cognitively, and mentally able to do laundry and access facilities, but has not routinely performed laundry tasks in the past (i.e., prior to this home care admission).

☒   ☐   1 - Able to do only light laundry, such as minor hand wash or light washer loads. Due to physical, cognitive, or mental limitations, needs assistance with heavy laundry such as carrying large loads of laundry.

☐   ☒   2 - *Unable* to do any laundry due to physical limitation or needs continual supervision and assistance due to cognitive or mental limitation.

☐   UK - Unknown

90.(M0750) Housekeeping: Ability to safely and effectively perform light housekeeping and heavier cleaning tasks.

Prior   Current

☐   ☐   0 - (a) Able to independently perform all housekeeping tasks; *OR*
(b) Physically, cognitively, and mentally able to perform *all* housekeeping tasks but has not routinely participated in housekeeping tasks in the past (i.e., prior to this home care admission).

☐   ☐   1 - Able to perform only *light* housekeeping (e.g., dusting, wiping kitchen counters) tasks independently.

☐   ☐   2 - Able to perform housekeeping tasks with intermittent assistance or supervision from another person.

☐   ☐   3 - *Unable* to consistently perform any housekeeping tasks unless assisted by another person throughout the process.

☒   ☒   4 - Unable to effectively participate in any housekeeping tasks.

☐   UK - Unknown

91.(M0760) Shopping: Ability to plan for, select, and purchase items in a store and to carry them home or arrange delivery.

Prior   Current

☐   ☐   0 - (a) Able to plan for shopping needs and independently perform shopping tasks, including carrying packages; *OR*
(b) Physically, cognitively, and mentally able to take care of shopping, but has not done shopping in the past (i.e., prior to this home care admission).

☐   ☐   1 - Able to go shopping, but needs some assistance:
(a) By self is able to do only light shopping and carry small packages, but needs someone to do occasional major shopping; *OR*
(b) *Unable* to go shopping alone, but can go with someone to assist.

☒   ☒   2 - *Unable* to go shopping, but is able to identify items needed, place orders, and arrange home delivery.

☐   ☐   3 - Needs someone to do all shopping and errands.

☐   UK - Unknown

92.(M0770) Ability to Use Telephone: Ability to answer the phone, dial numbers, and *effectively* use the telephone to communicate.

Prior   Current

☒   ☒   0 - Able to dial numbers and answer calls appropriately and as desired.

☐   ☐   1 - Able to use a specially adapted telephone (i.e., large numbers on the dial, teletype phone for the deaf) and call essential numbers.

☐   ☐   2 - Able to answer the telephone and carry on a normal conversation but has difficulty with placing calls.

☐   ☐   3 - Able to answer the telephone only some of the time or is able to carry on only a limited conversation.

☐   ☐   4 - *Unable* to answer the telephone at all but can listen if assisted with equipment.

☐   ☐   5 - Totally unable to use the telephone.

☐   ☐   NA - Patient does not have a telephone.

☐   UK - Unknown

MEDICATIONS

93.(M0780) Management of Oral Medications: *Patient's ability* to prepare and take all prescribed oral medications reliably and safely, including administration of the correct dosage at the appropriate times/intervals. *Excludes* injectable and I.V. medications. (NOTE: This refers to ability, not compliance or willingness.)

Prior   Current

☒   ☒   0 - Able to independently take the correct oral medication(s) and proper dosage(s) at the correct times.

☐   ☐   1 - Able to take medication(s) at the correct times if:
(a) individual dosages are prepared in advance by another person; *OR*
(b) given daily reminders; *OR*
(c) someone develops a drug diary or chart.

☐   ☐   2 - *Unable* to take medication unless administered by someone else.

☐   ☐   NA - No oral medications prescribed.

☐   UK - Unknown

(continued)

Using the OASIS-B1 form *(continued)*

94.(M0790) **Management of Inhalant/Mist Medications:**
Patient's ability to prepare and take all prescribed inhalant/mist medications (nebulizers, metered dose devices) reliably and safely, including administration of the correct dosage at the appropriate times/intervals. *Excludes* all other forms of medication (oral tablets, injectable and I.V. medications).

Prior Current

☐ ☐ 0 - Able to independently take the correct medication and proper dosage at the correct times.

☐ ☐ 1 - Able to take medication at the correct times if:
(a) individual dosages are prepared in advance by another person, OR
(b) given daily reminders.

☐ ☐ 2 - *Unable* to take medication unless administered by someone else.

☒ ☒ NA - No inhalant/mist medications prescribed.

☐ UK - Unknown

95.(M0800) **Management of Injectable Medications:** *Patient's ability* to prepare and take all prescribed injectable medications reliably and safely, including administration of correct dosage at the appropriate times/intervals. *Excludes* I.V. medications.

Prior Current

☒ ☒ 0 - Able to independently take the correct medication and proper dosage at the correct times.

☐ ☐ 1 - Able to take injectable medication at correct times if:
(a) individual syringes are prepared in advance by another person, OR
(b) given daily reminders.

☐ ☐ 2 - Unable to take injectable medications unless administered by someone else.

☐ ☐ NA - No injectable medications prescribed.

☐ UK - Unknown

EQUIPMENT MANAGEMENT

96.(M0810) **Patient Management of Equipment (includes *ONLY* oxygen, I.V./infusion therapy, enteral/parenteral nutrition equipment or supplies):** *Patient's ability* to set up, monitor and change equipment reliably, and safely add appropriate fluids or medication, clean/store/dispose of equipment or supplies using proper technique. **(NOTE: This refers to ability, not compliance or willingness.)**

☐ 0 - Patient manages all tasks related to equipment completely independently.

☐ 1 - If someone else sets up equipment (i.e., fills portable oxygen tank, provides patient with prepared solutions), patient is able to manage all other aspects of equipment.

☐ 2 - Patient requires considerable assistance from another person to manage equipment, but independently completes portions of the task.

☐ 3 - Patient is only able to monitor equipment (e.g., liter flow, fluid in bag) and must call someone else to manage the equipment.

☐ 4 - Patient is completely dependent on someone else to manage all equipment.

☒ NA - No equipment of this type used in care [If NA, go to *M0825*]

97.(M0820) **Caregiver Management of Equipment (includes *ONLY* oxygen, I.V./infusion equipment, enteral/parenteral nutrition, ventilator therapy equipment or supplies):** *Caregiver's ability* to set up, monitor, and change equipment reliably and safely, add appropriate fluids or medication, clean/store/dispose of equipment or supplies using proper technique. **(NOTE: This refers to ability, not compliance or willingness.)**

☐ 0 - Caregiver manages all tasks related to equipment completely independently.

☐ 1 - If someone else sets up equipment, caregiver is able to manage all other aspects.

☐ 2 - Caregiver requires considerable assistance from another person to manage equipment, but independently completes significant portions of task.

☐ 3 - Caregiver is only able to complete small portions of task (e.g., administer nebulizer treatment, clean/store/dispose of equipment or supplies).

☐ 4 - Caregiver is completely dependent on someone else to manage all equipment.

☐ NA - No caregiver

☐ UK - Unknown

THERAPY NEED

98.(M0825) **Therapy Need:** Does the care plan of the Medicare payment period for which this assessment will define a case mix group indicate a need for therapy (physical, occupational, or speech therapy) that meets the threshold for a Medicare high-therapy case mix group?

☒ 0 - No

☐ 1 - Yes

☐ NA - Not applicable

Using the OASIS-B1 form *(continued)*

EQUIPMENT AND SUPPLIES

Equipment needs (check appropriate box)

Has	Needs	
☐	☐	Oxygen/Respiratory Equip.
☐	☐	Wheelchair
☐	☐	Hospital Bed
☒	☐	Other (specify) *Walker*

Supplies needed and comments regarding equipment needs

Financial problems/needs

SAFETY

Safety measures recommended to protect patient from injury
NA

Emergency plans
Wife will call 911 for emergency care if needed

CONCLUSIONS

Conclusions/impressions and skilled interventions performed this visit
Wound care performed per care plan. Initiated teaching regarding wound care signs & symptoms of wound infection and emergency measures. Patient tolerated wound care well with pain rated less than 1 on a scale of 0 to 5, and verbalized understanding of instructions.

Date of assessment *2/2/07*

Signature of Assessor *Holly Dougherty, RN, BSN*

▶ Show in your documentation how you made the most of the patient's strengths and resources. Strengths include support systems, good health habits and coping behaviors, a safe and healthful environment, and financial security. Resources include the practitioner, pharmacy, and medical equipment supplier.

Progress notes

Each time you visit a patient, you must write a progress note that documents:

▶ changes in the patient's condition
▶ skilled nursing interventions performed that are related to the care plan
▶ the patient's responses to the services provided
▶ event or incident in the home that would affect the treatment plan
▶ vital signs and systemic assessment

▶ patient and home caregiver education (includes written instructional materials and brochures as well as the patient's response to the instruction and any return demonstrations)
▶ communication with other team members or support staff during your visit or since the previous visit
▶ discharge plans
▶ the time you arrived at the home and the time you left the home.

The following guidelines will help you chart safely and efficiently on progress notes:

▶ Chart all events in chronological order.
▶ Avoid addendums.
▶ Provide a heading for each entry, such as "Nursing progress note," because many members of the health care team use the progress notes.

ChartWizard

Interdisciplinary care plan

The care plan is individualized for each patient. An example of this form is shown below.

Patient name:	_Mary Long_	Init. cert. period: _____
		Recert. period _____
Primary nurse:	_N. Smith, RN_	Init. cert. period: _____

PROBLEM	GOAL	APPROACH	INITIAL CERT	RECERT #1	RECERT #2
Atrial fibrillation (12/1/06)	Maintain optimal cardiac output	1. Meds as ordered 2. Monitor vs. inc. apical rhythm and rate 3. observe for chest pain, dyspnea, palpitations, anxiety, etc.	GOAL MET? Y N INIT:_____	GOAL MET? Y N INIT:_____	GOAL MET? Y N INIT:_____
Heart Failure (2/1/01)	1. Maintain fluid and electrolyte balance 2. Promote optimal gas exchange.	1. Meds as ordered 2. Nebulizer as ordered 3. Draw labs as ordered 4. I and O daily 5. Monitor edema 6. ✔ for SOB, dyspnea, congestion (lung sounds) 7. amb. as tol 8. semi Fowler's when sitting	GOAL MET? Y N INIT:_____	GOAL MET? Y N INIT:_____	GOAL MET? Y N INIT:_____
Gastrostomy tube insertion (2/3/01)	1. Maintain optimal nutritional status 2. Prevent skin break-down	1. Magnacal 80 ml/hr 2. Follow G-tube protocol, including site care and oral hygiene 3. Weekly weights 4. I and O daily 5. ✔ for N/V, diarrhea	GOAL MET? Y N INIT:_____	GOAL MET? Y N INIT:_____	GOAL MET? Y N INIT:_____

Intervention Codes

(please circle all that apply)

- A1. Skilled observation
- A2. Foley insertion
- A3. Bladder installation
- A4. Irrigation care (wd. dsg.)
- A5. Irrigation decub. care - meds.
- A6. Venipuncture
- A7. Restorative nursing
- A8. Postcataract care
- A9. Bowel/Bladder training

- A10. Chest physical (incl. postural drainage)
- A11. Administer vit. B_{12}
- A12. Prepare/Administer insulin
- A13. Administer other
- A14. Administer I.V.
- A15. Teach ostomy care
- A16. Teach nasogastric feeding
- A17. Reposition nasogastric feeding tube
- A18. Teach gastrostomy
- A19. Teach parenteral nutrition

- A20. Teach care of trach
- A21. Administer care of trach
- A22. Teach inhalation Rx
- A23. Administer inhalation Rx
- A24. Teach administration of injections
- A25. Teach diabetic care
- A26. Disimpaction/enema
- A27. Other
    Foot care (diabetic)
    Teach diet
    Teach disease process

- Teach use of O_2
    Instruct re: Medication child
- A28. Wound care/dsg - closed
- A29. Decubitus care - simple
- A30. Teach care of indwelling catheter
- A31. Management and evaluation of patient care plan
- A32. Teaching and training (other)

Nursing summaries

As a home health care nurse, you must compile a summary of the patient's progress (and discharge from home health care, when appropriate). You must also submit a patient progress report to the attending practitioner and to the reimburser to confirm the need for continuing services.

When writing these summaries, include the following information:

▶ current problems, treatments, interventions, and instructions
▶ home health care provided by other health care professionals, such as physical therapists, speech pathologists, occupational therapists, social workers, and home health care aides
▶ reason for any change in services
▶ patient outcomes and responses—both physical and emotional—to services provided.

Patient or caregiver teaching

Correct documentation will help justify to your agency and to third-party payers that your visits to teach the patient or caregiver were necessary. Learn about the patient's and family's needs, resources, and support systems. This will help you outline a basic plan for teaching.

Remember that teaching is usually an ongoing process requiring more than one visit. Until the patient becomes independent, your documentation will help other nurses continue the teaching and identify additional areas where teaching is needed. (See *Certification of instruction,* page 234.)

Keep a list of teaching and reference materials you've supplied to the patient or caregiver. Also document modifications made to accommodate the patient's or caregiver's literacy skills and native language.

If the patient isn't physically or mentally able to perform the skills himself and no caregiver is available, report this in your documentation. Never leave a patient alone to perform a procedure until he can express understanding of it and perform it competently.

Be careful to call equipment by the same names used on the packages and in teaching literature. Consider providing a glossary of terms and labeling machines to match your instructions. Make sure that the patient can identify devices when speaking on the telephone. Document all teaching materials given to the patient, and keep copies in your records. You may want to videotape your instructions and leave the tape in the home if more than one caregiver will be providing care.

Most agencies require patients to sign a teaching documentation record indicating that they accept responsibility for learning self-care activities. This is a critical piece of documentation for the home health care chart.

Recertification

To ensure continued home health care services for patients who need them, you'll have to prove that the patient still requires and qualifies for home health care. Medicare and many managed care plans certify an initial 60-day period during which your agency can receive reimbursement for the patient's home health care. When that period is over, the insurer may certify an additional 60 days. This period is called the recertification period.

Naturally, your documentation requesting recertification must clearly support the patient's need for continued care within the insurer's guidelines. A clinical summary of care must be compiled and sent to the patient's practitioner and then to the insurer. For Medicare, you'll

ChartWizard

Certification of instruction

The model patient-teaching form below shows what was taught to a home-care patient with an I.V. This type of form will help you document your teaching sessions clearly and completely.

CONTENT (check all that apply; fill in blanks as indicated)

1. ☐ Reason for therapy

2. Drug/Solution
- ☐ Dose
- ☐ Schedule
- ☐ Label accuracy
- ☐ Storage
- ☐ Container integrity

3. Aseptic technique
- ☐ Handwashing
- ☐ Prepping caps/connections
- ☐ Tubing/cap/needs
- ☐ Needleless adaptor changes

4. Access device maintenance
Type/Name: _____
- ☒ Device / Site Inspection
- ☐ Site care/Dsg. changes
- ☐ Catheter clamping
- ☒ Maintaining patency
  - ☒ Saline flushing
  - ☐ Heparin locking
  - ☐ Fdg. Tube /declogging
  - ☐ Self insertion of device

5. Drug preparation
- ☒ Premixed containers
- ☐ Compounding
- ☐ Piggyback lipids
- ☐ Client additives

6. Method of administration
- ☐ Gravity
- ☒ Pump (name): _IVAC-pump_
- ☐ Continuous   ☒ Intermittent
- ☐ Cycle/Taper:

7. Administration technique
- ☒ Pump rate/calibration
- ☐ Priming tubing   ☐ Filter
- ☐ Filling syringe
- ☐ Loading pump
- ☒ Access device hookup/disconnect

8. Potential complications/Adverse effects
- ☐ Patient drug information sheet reviewed
- ☒ Pump alarms/troubleshooting
- ☒ Phlebitis/infiltration
- ☐ Clotting/dislodgment
- ☒ Infection ☐ Air embolus
- ☐ Breakage/cracking
- ☐ Electrolyte imbalance
- ☐ Fluid balance
- ☐ Glucose intolerance
- ☐ Aspiration
- ☐ N / V / D / Cramping
- ☐ Other: _____

9. Self monitoring:
- ☐ Weight ☒ Temperature   ☐ P   ☐ PB
- ☐ Urine S & A   ☐ Fingersticks
- ☐ Other: _____

10. Supply handling/disposal
- ☒ Disposal of sharps/supplies ☐ Narcotics
- ☐ Cleaning pump
- ☒ Changing batteries
- ☐ Blood/fluid precautions
- ☐ Chemo/spill precautions

11. Information given to client re:
- ☐ Pharmacy counseling
- ☐ Advance directives
- ☐ Inventory checks _____
- ☐ Deliveries _____
- ☒ 24-hour on-call staff _____
- ☒ Reimbursement _____
- ☐ Service complaints _____

12. Safety/Disaster plan
- ☐ Back up pump batteries _____
- ☒ Emergency room use _____
- ☐ Electrical _____
- ☒ Disaster _____
- ☐ Other: _____
_____

13. Written instructions
- ☒ Yes ☐ No   If no, why _____
_____
_____
_____

☐ Client or caregiver demonstrates or verbalizes competency to perform home infusion therapy.

COMMENTS: _Wife incorrectly changed pump battery. Procedure reviewed. Wife then demonstrated correct procedure. Wife also concerned about frequency of dressing changes. Access site nonreddened and not edematous. Protocol reviewed and patient states he is satisfied to wait until scheduled dressing change tomorrow._

Theory/Skill reviewed/Return demonstration completed:

Chris Banner, RN   _1-21-01_
Signature of RN Educator   Date

CERTIFICATION OF INSTRUCTION

I agree that I have been instructed as described above and understand that the above functions will be performed in the home by myself and caregiver, outside a hospital or medically supervised environment.

Robert Burns   _1-21-01_
Client/caregiver signature   Date

need to submit a new care plan on Form 485 as well as a medical update on Form 486. Make sure that this form includes data as amended by verbal order since the start of care.

Finally, when you record the primary diagnosis, make sure that it is a valid medical diagnosis and reflects the patient's current needs, not the original reason for the home health care.

Discharge summary

You'll prepare a discharge summary to obtain the practitioner's approval to discharge a patient, for notifying reimbursers that services have been terminated, and for officially closing the case. When preparing this document, summarize:

▶ the time frame covered
▶ the services provided and the names and titles of assigned staff
▶ the third-party payer and whether the patient is eligible for future payment (he may have exhausted his annual benefits)
▶ the clinical and psychosocial conditions of the patient at discharge
▶ recommendations for further care
▶ caregiver involvement in care
▶ interruptions in home care, such as readmission to the hospital
▶ referral to community agencies
▶ OASIS discharge information
▶ the patient's response to and comprehension of patient-teaching efforts
▶ the patient's current medication list
▶ outcomes attained.

Community referrals

If you work in a home health care setting, you'll want to think about local community resources that can help maintain and promote your patients' health and well-being. Such resources may consist of a free mobile health care unit or services to provide emotional support. Whenever you make a referral for community services, be sure to document your actions and the reasons for the referral. Your agency's medical social worker is often a useful resource in educating the patient about community referrals and in obtaining them.

▶

Documentation guidelines

Update the record with any changes in the patient's condition or care plan and document that you reported these changes to the practitioner. Keep in mind that Medicare and Medicaid won't reimburse for skilled services implemented but not reported to the practitioner. Make sure that all of your documentation is accurate. Accuracy ensures proper reimbursement and prevents the appearance of fraud.

Be certain to state in your documentation that the patient is homebound and provide the reason for this. An example of a valid reason for being homebound is dyspnea on minimal activity; an invalid reason would be not having a car. Again, keep in mind that Medicare requires that a patient receiving skilled care in the home must be homebound (although some commercial insurers don't require this).

If an emergency arises in the home during your presence, accompany the patient to the hospital or emergency department and stay with him until another professional caregiver takes over. Document all assessments and interventions performed for the patient until you're relieved. Note the date and time of transfer and the name of the caregiver who assumes responsibility for the patient.

Make sure that the documentation reflects consistent adherence to the care plan by all caregivers involved.

Whenever possible, use flow sheets and checklists to record vital signs, intake and output measurements, and nutritional data. Encourage the patient or home caregiver to complete these forms when appropriate. Doing so involves the patient and his family in the patient's progress and increases their feeling of control.

At least once a week, remove completed documentation materials that have been left in the patient's home. This keeps volumes of paper from piling up or becoming misplaced. It also makes the records available for review by the agency supervisor.

Selected references

Brown, E.L., et al. "Transition to Home Care: Quality of Mental Health, Pharmacy, and Medical History Information," *International Journal of Psychiatry in Medicine* 36(3):339-49, 2006.

Caffrey, R.A. "Community Care Gerontological Nursing: The Independent Nurse's Role," *Journal of Gerontological Nursing* 31(7):18-25, July 2005.

Clarke, J.N. "Mother's Home Healthcare: Emotion Work When a Child has Cancer," *Cancer Nursing* 29(1):58-65, January-February 2006.

Eaton, M.K. "Nurse and Client Perceptions of Home Health Wound Care Effectiveness after a Change in Medicare Reimbursement," *Policy, Politics & Nursing Practice* 6(4):285-95, November 2005.

Jones, M.J. "How to Navigate and Sail the Waters Around OASIS M0440," *Home Healthcare Nurse* 23(5):279-82, May 2005.

Lowder, J.L., et al. "The Caregiver Balancing Act: Giving Too Much or Not Enough," *Care Management Journals* 6(3):159-65, Fall 2005.

Owen, K. "Documentation in Nursing Practice," *Nursing Standard* 19(32):48-49, April 2005.

Stadt, J., and Molare, E. "Best Practices: That Improved Patient Outcomes and Agency Operational Performance," *Home Healthcare Nurse* 23(9):587-93, September 2005.

Teenier, P. "The Clinician's Role in Medicare Prospective Payment: Part 4—Medicare Adjustments," *Home Healthcare Nurse* 23(5):331-34, May 2005.

Tice, M.A. "Nurse Specialists in Home Health Nursing: The Certified Hospice and Palliative Care Nurse," *Home Healthcare Nurse* 24(3):145-47, March 2006.

Zeisset, A. "ICD-9-CM Coding Changes for Home Care: Effective October 1, 2004," *Home Healthcare Nurse* 22(9):624-32, September 2004.

DOCUMENTATION IN AMBULATORY CARE

9

Ambulatory care has evolved greatly over the past 30 years. Many aspects of health care that were once unique to hospital inpatient settings, such as the performance of invasive procedures and emergency services, are now commonplace in ambulatory, outpatient, and community health care centers, which makes the necessity for accurate, complete documentation even more important. Whether your ambulatory care facility is small or large and part of an integrated health care system or an independent, superior documentation remains a core component of effective and efficient patient care.

Functions of documentation in ambulatory care

The three major functions of nursing documentation in ambulatory care are communication, regulation, and litigation. *Communication* is the recording and exchange of information to facilitate and manage patient care. *Regulation* involves fulfilling the mandates of various accrediting bodies, governmental controls, and programmatic guidelines that allow ambulatory care facilities to operate and receive payment for their services. *Litigation* addresses the need for nurses and other health care providers to support their practices against possible legal challenges. In this section, you'll learn how each of these functions affects your documentation responsibilities.

Communication

The first function of nursing documentation in ambulatory care, as in other professional practice settings, is to communicate about patient care. Accurate, complete, timely, and accessible documentation provides the most important link between understanding a patient's previous health care encounters and planning his current care. The need to coordinate patient care increases dramatically as health care systems spread out geographically and add services.

One goal of The Joint Commission 2007 National Patient Safety Goals is to improve the effectiveness of communication among caregivers. The specific requirements The Joint Commission expects organizations to implement in order to accomplish this goal are covered throughout this chapter. Also covered are two additional safety goals that affect ambulatory care: reconciling medications and improving the safety of their use.

In the "good old days," when many patients received most of their primary care in small, independent physician practices, there was likely to be only one medical record for each patient, which was stored in one office and accessed whenever the need arose. The current trend in health care, in which many practitioners and other health care providers are involved in each patient's care, creates new challenges to health care communication and coordination. The expansion of non-physician, non-nurse personnel in the staffing of ambulatory care facilities has also increased the complexity of the communication function. Because of these changes in the health care system, your role in designing, monitoring, and instructing others in the use of forms and systems that work for the whole ambulatory care team is more critical than ever.

When considering changes to a documentation system, look to the nursing process to provide a consistent framework. A systematic, problem-solving method that's well understood by professional nurses, the nursing process has the following advantages:

▶ compatible with the scientific method applied in medicine
▶ easily taught to unlicensed assistive personnel and other types of health care providers
▶ helps to organize record keeping
▶ most adaptable to local requirements
▶ most easily understood framework.

The nursing process aspects of documentation adapted to ambulatory care include assessment, planning, documentation of services provided, education of the patient and his family, evaluation, and directions for follow-up care. (See *The nursing process in ambulatory care.*)

Regulation

The second function of documentation is to meet regulatory requirements. Health care facilities need reimbursement to survive financially. Most ambulatory care facilities, like the vast majority of other health care organizations, rely heavily on payments from federal, state, and local governments; "third party" insurance companies; and various capitated or managed health plans, such as health maintenance organizations and preferred provider organizations.

MEDICARE AND MEDICAID
The federal Medicare program reimburses for many of the services offered in ambulatory care facilities. To obtain Medicare reimbursement, an ambulatory care facility must obtain a Medicare Provider Number and operate within established guidelines. There are specific screens that must be satisfied through specific documentation in patient records. A *screen* is a criterion, or element, that must be met for a record to be in compliance with the regulations. For example, one Medicare screen is that all entries must be fully dated and signed. Record audits may be performed at any time. When records are audit-

The nursing process in ambulatory care

The nursing process can serve as a framework for documentation in ambulatory care. Documentation should include the areas below.

ASSESSMENT

Assessment is dependent on the type of patient and the nature of the health care encounter. When the encounter involves nursing assessment, you need to complete a targeted assessment relevant to the age, culture, and presenting concerns of the patient. If necessary, you may also need to direct data collection by unlicensed assistive personnel.

One of your roles in ambulatory care is the application of critical thinking to rapidly adapt the history and physical assessment based on patient needs. Every patient presenting for care doesn't necessarily need or want a comprehensive head-to-toe nursing assessment, so decisions about how to do a rapid focused assessment (what to ask, how to ask it, and how to interpret the findings) are central.

PLANNING

Planning is also dependent on the type of patient and nature of the health care encounter. Because practitioners are commonly in the position to direct medical care, they're responsible for much of the planning. It's your job to carry out the prescribed medical regimen.

However, developing a nursing plan is part of your independent nursing practice and should be based on your professional assessment, adapted for the patient's age and cultural needs, and negotiated with the patient and his family.

For example, when there's an identified need for referral to a specific community resource to assist a patient or family, you make plans with the family and document the details of the referral, including the rationale (Why?), the contact information (Who's making contact? With whom?), the method of contact (How? By mail, phone, e-mail, walk-in?), and when the contact can be made.

INTERVENTIONS

Documenting interventions is the next step. Nursing interventions may be in response to the ordered medical plan for treatment or within the scope of professional nursing practice. Document everything done to, for, or with the patient, family, or significant others. Include clear information about exactly what was done, when, and by whom. In most circumstances, the person actually providing the care is responsible for documenting the care.

Education of patients, family members, and other caregivers is the most frequently used nursing intervention in ambulatory care. It's vital for patients and their caregivers to understand their condition and the responsibilities that go with care and treatment. You need to evaluate each patient's developmental level, ability to learn, and potential barriers to learning. You must specifically record what's taught (content), how material was presented (video, brochure, discussion, demonstration) and the level of patient understanding. If family members or others are included in teaching, record who was involved as well as their level of understanding.

EVALUATION

An element that's commonly overlooked in documentation is the description of the patient's response to intervention. Whenever care is provided, there needs to be documentation in the medical record stating the patient's response to care. The ambulatory care setting isn't exempt from this rule no matter how brief the patient's visit is.

The amount of documentation required is based on the level of care delivered, the condition of the patient, and the anticipated outcomes. The classic phrase, "Patient tolerated well," is inadequate to meet increasing regulatory and legal requirements. In the record, you must clearly in-

(continued)

The nursing process in ambulatory care *(continued)*

clude a postintervention assessment of the patient's condition with regard to relevant parameters. For example, is there redness or irritation after an injection? Is the patient complaining of pain? Is there any indication of an adverse reaction?

The specific areas of assessment and description will be determined by the nature of the intervention and the status of the specific patient. When the primary intervention is health teaching, be sure to record the patient's response. Specify "level of understanding," as with tolerance for other interventions, in greater detail than "patient understood." Describe what the patient or family said or did during the teaching intervention to facilitate understanding. Can the patient return a demonstration of the skill being taught? Can the patient or family member correctly summarize what they have learned? What further teaching might be indicated? Based on postintervention evaluation, further intervention may be required and the nursing process continues.

DIRECTIONS FOR FOLLOW-UP CARE

Directions for follow-up care are a universal intervention in ambulatory care nursing. When patients leave an ambulatory care facility, they often return for additional interventions, testing, or monitoring. There's no time limit: Follow-up care may be within a couple days or it may not be for several months. When follow-up care is required, a written description of the follow-up recommendations should be noted. A simple framework for documenting follow-up recommendations is the formula used in journalism: who, what, when, where, why. *Who* is to do the follow-up (patient, family)? *What* is recommended or required (tests, laboratory work, nursing visit)? *When* does the care need to be done or when should the appointments be made? *Where* should the patient go for follow-up care? *Why* is the follow-up required (diagnosis, monitoring, importance to life and health)? Be sure to document the patient's and family's response to follow-up care instructions.

If a practitioner is handing off complete patient responsibility by transferring that responsibility to another practitioner (that is, follow-up will occur with a different practitioner), he must follow the organization's hand-off communication procedures according to The Joint Commission's 2007 National Patient Safety Goals. These procedures must include passing specified information on to the receiving practitioner, such as: current information about the patient's care, treatment, condition, recent or anticipated changes, as well as a complete and accurate list of the patient's current medications. The receiving practitioner must then have an opportunity to verify the information received, a chance to ask any questions, and an opportunity to review relevant historical data for that patient.

ed, the auditor is looking for information that's easy to find, complete, and signed by the appropriate person. Medicare has the option to refuse payment if care isn't documented according to the published requirements. The consequences for failure to meet Medicare documentation requirements range from nonpayment of specific accounts to withdrawal of the Medicare Provider Number, which, in essence, strips the facility of its ability to bill for services.

Although not all facilities provide services to Medicare recipients, many other payers use compliance with federal Medicare requirements as an indicator of eligibility for reimbursement from other sources. The Medicaid program requirements at the state level, for example, commonly follow the federal regulations for deciding reimbursement eligibility.

Due to the significant influence of federal Medicare guidelines, many ambulatory care facilities perform regular internal audits to make sure that Medicare requirements are being appropriately and consistently met. Although the Medicare and Medicaid requirements are numerous, they're clearly published and updated and can be used to develop a comprehensive self-evaluation tool for internal audits. The participation of all levels and disciplines of health care providers in internal audits serves to educate staff about requirements for documentation content and style, anticipate and correct deficits before external reviews, and generally raise the level of quality documentation.

Centers for Medicare and Medicaid Services

The Centers for Medicare and Medicaid Services (CMS), formerly known as the Health Care Financing Administration, is the regulatory body that has the authority to grant Medicare and Medicaid Provider Numbers. CMS has the option to directly survey (visit or audit) a health care organization or to accept the organization's accreditation by another group CMS recognizes. The Joint Commission, the American Osteopathic Association, and the International Quality Systems Directory are examples of accrediting organizations currently recognized by CMS.

OTHER REGULATORS

Managed care plans and "third-party" payers often have specific additional medical record provisions. Review all payment contracts and identify what type of medical record documentation will be required for reimbursement. Due to the potentially large number of separate payers in the ambulatory care setting, each with distinctive requirements, you may also want to consult with a medical records professional to be certain that the documentation practices and forms of your facility are in compliance.

Litigation

The third function of documentation in ambulatory care nursing is to provide legal proof of the nature and quality of care the patient received. Much of the documentation that's done in ambulatory care, as in other health care settings, revolves around avoidance of litigation and defense against litigation. Of course, there's no such thing as a "suit-proof" medical record, but there are steps that you can take to protect yourself and your facility from legal action. Consider your facility's past legal problems in the design, implementation, and evaluation of recording systems to prevent recurrence. Also consider issues surrounding access to recorded information and documentation maintenance.

Documentation of ambulatory care services

As indicated at the beginning of this chapter, there are multiple types of ambulatory care visits. Each type of visit requires specific documentation. In this section, you're given recommendations for the documentation of clinic and office, procedure and surgical, emergency, and chemotherapy visits; short stay and clinical decision unit assessments; and telephone encounters.

Clinic and office visits

In a clinic or professional office, each patient visit is typically documented with a narrative note from the practitioner or nurse who provides the care. The note should reflect the current condition of the patient, reason for the visit (history, chief concern, or presenting complaint), current condition (assessment), the care plan (planning), what was discussed or done with the patient (interventions), a description of the patient's response to the intervention (evaluation), and recommendations for follow-up.

Make sure that routine information is available, including a history, allergies, medications currently being taken, medication history, vital signs, immunization records, current laboratory and other tests, and any specific patient monitoring information such as diabetic management. If the patient has a designated "patient advocate" or specified person holding a Medical Power of Attorney for Health Care, make it clear in the clinical history; add any missing information.

Document all of your patient teaching, including what was taught, learning deficits that you observed (and what you did to accommodate them), and the patient's response or level of understanding. Your documentation should also reflect when family members or others are included in the health teaching.

If the ambulatory care facility is surveyed by The Joint Commission, you must include a summary list in the patient's record by his third clinic visit. This is a list of the types of encounters the patient has had at the facility, such as a well visit, sick visit, visit for immunizations, or otherwise. This list summarizes significant diagnoses, procedures, drug allergies, and medications and should be readily accessible to practitioners. The purpose of a summary list is to facilitate continuity of care and to support safe and high-quality patient care.

Procedure and surgical visits

When a patient undergoes a procedure in an ambulatory care facility, the health care provider who performs the procedure documents patient consent, the procedure description, and recommended follow-up. Your nursing documentation should include a preprocedure assessment (in-

cluding vital signs and surgical site verification), all nursing care provided before, during, and after the procedure, a postprocedure assessment (including vital signs), and the patient's postprocedure instructions for follow-up. As with other types of visits, make sure that you record all patient and family teaching.

SURGICAL SITE VERIFICATION

For operative procedures in the ambulatory setting, it's essential that all requirements of The Joint Commission's Universal Protocol for Preventing Wrong Site, Wrong Procedure, Wrong Person Surgery are followed and documented appropriately. The first step is to conduct a preoperative verification process to make sure that all relevant documents and studies are collected and reviewed, and that all discrepancies, inconsistencies, or missing data are addressed. This must occur before the start of the procedure, along with verification of the intended patient, procedure, and site. The second step is identifying and unambiguously marking the operative site for procedures that involve right or left distinction, multiple levels (for example, spinal procedures), or multiple structures (for example, fingers or toes). Finally, a "time-out" step must occur immediately before the procedure starts for final confirmation of the correct patient, procedure, site, and special equipment, if applicable. These operative procedures should be documented according to your facility's policy. (See *Steps for surgical site verification.*)

Another one of The Joint Commission's 2007 National Patient Safety Goals for ambulatory care is to reduce the risk of surgical fires. Facilities are required to establish guidelines regarding oxygen concentration under surgical drapes and to educate surgical staff members on how to control heat sources.

ChartWizard

Steps for surgical site verification

This is an example of a form for verifying the correct patient, procedure, and site before surgery.

Preoperative patient identification
Surgical site verification

Date: _2/13/07_

STEP 1
BEFORE ENTERING THE PROCEDURE ROOM
A. Identify the patient using two patient identifiers:
   1. Ask the patient to state his full name.
   2. Ask the patient to state his date of birth.
   Patient's name: _Carol Parker_
B. Ask the patient to state the side, site, and procedure to be performed and have him point to the actual surgical site.
C. Be sure that patient consent, relevant data in the medical record, and surgical schedule are consistent with the patient's responses.
D. Mark the surgical site over or adjacent to the incision site.
   Site: _Right knee_ ☐ N/A

Enter time completed and your signature:
Time: _0700_
Signature: _Elizabeth Ladd, RN_

STEP 2
IN THE PROCEDURE ROOM
A. Confirm the patient's identity, consent obtained, patient's position, operative procedure, laterality, site mark, correct implants, and any special equipment.
B. Review the medical record for consistency in identifying the correct surgical site.
C. Be sure that the operating physician hangs correct imaging studies.

Enter time completed and your signature:
Time: _0745_
Signature: _Elizabeth Ladd, RN_

STEP 3
IMMEDIATELY BEFORE THE PROCEDURE
A. Conduct a "time out" immediately before the procedure for final team verification of the correct patient, correct site, correct procedure, X-rays displayed on correct patient, and that correct implants are available.
Document team members present for "time out":
   David Aims   Anesthesia
   Kelley Banfield   Technician
   Julie Cho, RN   Other
   Maggie Krum, RN   Other

Enter time completed and signatures:
Time: _0810_
Signature: _Elizabeth Ladd, RN_   Physician
Time: _0810_
Signature: _Elizabeth Ladd, RN_   R.N.

LIST ANY DISCREPANCIES:
None

Physician notified: _____
Date: _____ Time: _____
Notes: _____

VISITS FOR PROCEDURES WITH MODERATE SEDATION

Some procedures, such as cardiac catheterization and endoscopy, require the patient to receive moderate sedation. *Moderate sedation* minimally lowers the patient's level of consciousness (LOC) and provides pain control while retaining the patient's protective reflexes, a patent airway, and continuous vital signs. When a patient is scheduled to receive moderate sedation, complete and document a nursing assessment before the procedure. In the assessment, make sure you include:

▶ patient identification
▶ verification of documented consent
▶ chief complaint
▶ diagnosis
▶ planned procedure
▶ ambulation status
▶ emotional status
▶ neurological status
▶ fasting status
▶ pain status
▶ color
▶ drug allergies
▶ medications
▶ review of laboratory or other testing completed before the procedure
▶ condition of procedure site
▶ level of anesthesia to be provided.

Before beginning the moderate sedation, document all care provided, including vital signs checked, I.V. lines started, medications administered, patient instruction given, and abnormal test results noted; and confirm that a "time out" was taken immediately before starting the procedure. You'll work closely with the health care provider performing each procedure to ensure consideration of assessment findings (especially those that lie outside of the normal range). Be certain that these communications are fully documented.

As part of the National Patient Safety Goals to improve medication safety, it's required that medication containers or other solutions be labeled on and off the sterile field. Include the drug name, strength, amount, expiration date, and expiration time on the medication label. Only one medication or solution may be labeled at a time, and labeling occurs when the substance is transferred from the original container to a different container. If the person preparing the medication won't be giving it, the labels are verified verbally and visually by two qualified people. At the end of the procedure, the labeled containers must be discarded. Document these procedures according to your facility's policy.

During the operative phase—when moderate sedation is given—you're responsible for documenting vital signs (including pulse oximetry, the monitoring of which is critical during moderate sedation), medications administered, patient positioning, and all other nursing interventions. Also document your ongoing assessment and the patient's response to interventions. (See *Outpatient procedure record*.)

After the procedure, perform an assessment of the patient when he arrives in the recovery area. In this assessment, you'll document the patient's LOC, cardiovascular status, respiratory rate, skin condition and color, and range of motion of extremities. You'll also perform a complete pain assessment and note drains and dressings that are present, drug allergies or adverse responses, and fluid intake and output. As always, fully document your nursing care, being sure to include all communications with the health care provider who performed the procedure and the patient's responses to your interventions.

ChartWizard

Outpatient procedure record

This is an example of an outpatient procedure record. Note how the preoperative, intraoperative, and discharge assessment all go on the same form.

Clinical Ambulatory Services
Outpatient Procedure Record

Date: _2/19/07_
Medical record number: _021839_
Name: _Cynthia Sanders_

Pre-operative assessment: Nurse: _Julie Haas, RN_ Physician: _Dr. Pat McTigue_
Condition on arrival: _"Anxious to have the procedure completed."_
Consent signed: ☐ NA ☒ Yes NPO since: _2/18/07 2200_
                                                        Date/time
Allergies: _Sulfa drugs_

Pregnant: ☐ NA ☒ No ☐ Yes Trimester: _____ Dentures removed: ☒ NA ☐ No ☐ Yes
Disposition of dentures: _____
Pre-op procedure prep completed by patient: ☐ NA ☐ No ☒ Yes
Patient belongings: ☒ With patient ☐ Given to family
BP: _120/68_ Temp: _98.7°F_ P: _68_ R: _18_ Skin warmth, color, dryness: _Warm, pink, dry_
Pre-op medications: _None_ Time: _____ Route: _____
_____ Time: _____ Route: _____
_____ Time: _____ Route: _____
Anesthesia used: _Midazolam 1.5 mg_ Time: _1045_ Route: _I.V._
Morphine 5 mg Time: _1045_ Route: _I.V._
I.V. access: Solution: _NSS_ Needle type: _20G_ Site: _® AC_ Time: _1040_ Rate: _10 ml/hr_
          Solution: _____ Needle type: _____ Site: _____ Time: _____ Rate: _____

Intra-operative assessment: Procedure performed: _Upper endoscopy_
If intra and postoperative vital signs are not applicable, check here ☐

	TIME	TEMP	BP	P	R	O₂ SAT	O₂ RATE	LEVEL OF CONSCIOUSNESS	SKIN	MEDICATIONS TREATMENTS	NURSE'S SIGNATURE
Intra-operative	1047	98.3°	118/70	67	18	98	2 L/min	Sleeping	Warm		J. Haas RN
	1050		122/72	70	20	97	2 L/min	Sleeping	Warm	Biopsy taken	J. Haas RN
	1052		120/68	70	22	98	2 L/min	Sleeping	Warm	Procedure completed	J. Haas RN
Post-operative	1055	98.6°	124/66	68	20	99	2 L/min	Easily aroused	Warm		J. Haas RN
	1100		126/74	70	22	99	O₂ discontinued	Awake	Warm	IV discontinued	J. Haas RN
	1110		128/74	72	20	99		Awake	Warm		J. Haas RN
	1125		126/72	70	20	99		Awake	Warm	PO liquids tolerated	J. Haas RN

Nursing notes/
interventions/
monitoring
equipment

Patient attached to C/R monitor, blood pressure monitor, and pulse ox. VSS. Anesth. Dr. Klein inserted 20G IV in R AC, without complications. NSS hung and infusing at 10 ml/hr. Morphine and midazolam administered via IV. pt. sleeping but easily aroused. Upper endoscopy performed by Dr. McTigue. VSS throughout procedure. Pt. easily aroused after procedure. O₂ and IV discontinued and discharge instructions reviewed and written for patient and husband. Pt. verbalized understanding. Pt. discharged to home with husband.————— J. Haas, RN

Specimens: ☐ NA X ☐ Yes _Gastric biopsy_ Solution _Buffered formalin_ Disposition: _Outside lab_

Discharge assessment: Condition at discharge: _Alert, VSS_
Discharged to: ☒ Home ☐ IPD room: _____ ☐ Emergency room ☐ Other: _____
Discharged per: ☒ Ambulatory ☐ Wheelchair ☐ Stretcher
Accompanied by: ☐ Self ☒ Family member ☐ Other: _____
Nurse's signature/title _Julie Haas, RN_

Form used courtesy of the Henry Ford Health System, West Bloomfield, Michigan.

Use a discharge summary checklist to document the patient's readiness for discharge. This checklist should include information on the patient's physical and mental status, follow-up care, and response to instructions. Include the following patient information:

Physical and mental status

When recording a patient's physical status, note his vital signs (including their stability), level of motor control, absence or control of nausea, voiding status, comfort level, and the condition of dressings or appliances. When recording a patient's mental status, note the patient's alertness and ability to understand directions.

Follow-up care

Make sure that when a patient who receives moderate sedation is discharged home, he's given adequate information for obtaining emergent or needed care. Because sedation temporarily impairs memory and cognition, give follow-up instructions to a responsible adult who'll be escorting the patient home so that he can instruct the patient after the sedation wears off; also provide these instructions in writing with your facility's phone number so the patient or family can call with questions. Before discharge, document your review of all prescriptions, the evaluation by the health care provider of the procedure, the disposition and return of all personal patient property (such as clothing), and the patient's response to all instructions.

Your facility may also require that you place and document a follow-up phone call to the patient 72 hours after the moderate sedation. During this phone call, you'll collect important information, including level of pain, presence of nausea and vomiting, oral intake, sleep comfort or disturbances, bleeding or discharges, voiding, and activity patterns. Also be sure to address and document patient and family questions at this time. If the patient was referred to another health care provider at the time of discharge, assess and document the patient's referral status as well as The Joint Commission-required hand-off procedures.

If the patient or a family member can't be reached after a predetermined number of attempts, a message should be left for the patient and the failure to reach the patient should be noted. Many patients who have procedures or ambulatory surgery are back to work or out of the home by the day after surgery. All calls and call attempts must be documented fully. When voice-mail or message-recording devices are used to facilitate patient contact, due caution must be used so that the message doesn't violate the patient's confidentiality in any way.

Emergency visits

For patients receiving emergency services in an ambulatory care facility, documentation requirements are the same as they would be for an emergency department visit at an inpatient facility. See chapter 11, Documentation of Selected Clinical Specialties, for more information on documentation in the emergency department.

Chemotherapy visits

Many ambulatory care facilities now perform chemotherapy, and a growing number of patients are taking advantage of this new role. It's your job to document their care effectively. At every visit, note the patient's weight, infection symptoms and, if present, new lesions, and document your assessment findings. Include information on the patient's hydration and antiemetic regimen, the specific chemotherapeutic and dose given, up-to-date laboratory results, and other significant comments. Fully describe changes in treatment and teaching. If the patient is in a research study or on a clinical trial protocol, make sure that you're including documentation that's specific to the study. When a patient is new to chemotherapy, teach him about self-care measures and when to call for assistance. Also provide written instructions for home care and written information about the specific chemotherapeutic drug that has been prescribed. (See *Oncology flow sheet,* page 248.)

Short-stay, observation, and clinical decision units

Short-stay units offer the opportunity for patients to receive care or be observed for up to 23 hours in an ambulatory care facility. As with inpatient settings, assess every patient upon admission. (See *Short-stay nurses' admission assessment form,* page 249.) Also note the reason for the patient's admission, which could be for surgery, infusion therapy, medical monitoring, or some other reason. Ambulatory care facilities commonly develop patient care protocols for each patient type to help direct and support the care delivered.

On discharge, you should give the patient written discharge instructions and have the patient or caregiver sign them. Per The Joint Commission, you must also provide the patient with a complete and accurate medication list.

Telephone encounters

Telephone encounters, common in ambulatory care, may request an initial visit, ask advice from you or another health care provider, or initiate a prescription renewal or a follow-up visit—each requiring documentation. To prevent confusion, your facility should develop a format for documenting these encounters. This documentation helps to prevent the omission of significant information and provides a way to accurately organize the information you obtain.

Useful information includes the date and time of the phone call; who called (the patient or his caregiver); the patient's name and primary health care provider; and the patient's chief complaint, reported temperature, pregnancy status (if applicable), allergies, chronic diseases, and current medications. At the end of the phone call, be sure to document your assessment of the situation and the advice you gave.

If a patient calls asking for a prescription to be refilled, document the medication's name, strength, dosage, quantity, and refill amount as well as the name of the patient's pharmacy and the telephone number.

Keep the telephone encounter form in the patient's record. (See *Telephone encounter form,* page 250.) All paper, including informal "scratch" notes made during phone encounters, should be secured to ensure patient confidentiality. Notes that in any way identify a patient by name, address, telephone number, or clinical condition must be either filed as part of the official record or securely destroyed by shredding.

(*Text continues on page 251.*)

ChartWizard

Oncology flow sheet

Oncology flow sheets, such as the example below, can be used for chemotherapy administration in the ambulatory care setting.

ONCOLOGY FLOW SHEET

Date _1/28/07_
Medical record number _01863_
Name _Andrea Martin_

DATE			1/28/07				
DAY ON STUDY							
TREATMENT	1	Anzemet I.V. ‡	100 mg				
	2	Decadron I.V. ‡	10 mg				
	3	Adriamycin I.V. ‡	100 mg				
	4	Cytoxan I.V. ‡	1000 mg				
	5	Antibiotics (✓)					
	6	Transfusions amt.					
	7						
	8	X R T ( )					
MARROW	9	Cellularity (N-I-D)					
	10	Tumor cells %					
	11						
	12						
LAB	13	Hgb gm	12.5				
	14	Hct Vol %					
	15	Retics %					
	16	Platelets mm^3 (10^3)	350,000				
	17	WBC mm^3 (10^3)	4.5				
	18	Neutrophils %	60 %				
	19	Lymphocytes %					
	20	Monocytes %					
	21	Eosinophils %					
	22	ANC	2.7				
	23	BUN mg%					
	24						
	25						
	26						
	27						
	28						
	29						
	30						
	31						
	32						
PHYSICAL	33	Temp					
	34	Weight (kg) (lb)	150 lb				
	35	Hemorrhage •					
	36	Infection •					
	37						
	38						
	39						
MEASURABLE LESIONS	40						
	41						
	42						
	43						
	44						
	45						
	46	New lesions (✓)					
SYMPTOMS	47	Performance status					
	48	•					
	49	•					
	50	•					
	51	•					
TOXICITY	52	•					
	53	•					
	54	•					
	55	•					
	56	•					
RESP	57	Objective †					
	58	Subjective †					

Pt. No. _____ Reg. Date _____
Study _____ Rx. No. _____
Disease Category _____

Progress notes and remarks:
(Signature/Title/Date each)

_1/28/07 at 1330_
Pt. and family viewed video "So Many Questions." Reviewed medication names, side effects, and management with pt. and family. All questions answered. Weight 150 lb, Height 65", BSA 2.0 ——— I.V. started with 22G angiocatheter, ⊕ blood return. 500cc NSS hung and infusing. I.V. patent. Pt. premedicated with Anzemet and Decadron, followed by Adriamycin and Cytoxan — each infused via I.V. without incident. I.V. discontinued. Patient will see doctor prior to next treatment, to have weekly CBC, and will call with any questions or problems. — Ana Cumming, RN

‡ Record amount of drug administered in manner specified in protocol
• Describe under remarks and rate severity: 0 = none; 1 = mild; 2 = moderate; 3 = severe; 4 = fatal
† Rate response as: C (Complete), P (Partial), M (Mixed), N (No change), or I (Increasing disease)

Form used courtesy of the Henry Ford Health System, West Bloomfield, Michigan.

ChartWizard

Short-stay nurses' admission assessment form

Short-stay, observation, or clinical decision units have their own admission assessment forms for nurses. See the example below.

Short Stay/CDU
Nurses' Admission Assessment Form

Date: _2/25/07_

Name: _Susanna Jackson_

Medical record number: _018263_

Patient type: ☐ DEM ☐ MED ☒ SURG ☐ OTHER _____

Arrival time: _1130_ Arrived: ☐ Walking ☒ Wheelchair ☐ Other _____

Patient identified: ☒ Name ☒ Bracelet Age: _41_ Height: _5' 6"_ Weight: _135 lb_

Emotional status: ☒ Calm ☐ Apprehensive ☐ Combative ☐ Crying

Neurological: ☒ Oriented ☒ Awake ☐ Easily aroused ☐ Confused ☐ Lethargic ☐ Asleep ☐ Unresponsive

Color: ☒ Pink ☐ Pale ☐ Cyanotic ☐ Jaundiced Skin: ☒ Warm ☐ Cool ☒ Dry ☐ Moist

---

Diagnosis: _Cholecystitis, S/P laparoscopic cholecystectomy_

Consents correct and signed: ☒ Yes ☐ No Explain: _____

Nursing care considerations: _Monitor vital signs, wound checks for bleeding, pain management, nausea management._

Personal items:

Dentures/Partials	Glasses/Contacts	Hearing aids
☐ Retained	☐ Retained	☐ Retained
☐ Removed	☐ Removed	☐ Removed
☒ None	☒ None	☒ None

Drug allergies/sensitivities: _Penicillin: rash_ ☐ NKDA

Current medications: _Prochlorperazine 5 mg IV Q4° prn nausea and vomiting; morphine 5 mg IV Q4° prn pain._

Pertinent medical history:

☐ Diabetes ☐ Pulmonary disease ☐ Arthritis ☐ Cardiovascular disease

☒ Hypertension ☐ Psychiatric disease ☐ Seizure disorder ☐ Stroke

☐ Kidney disease ☐ Substance abuse ☐ Migraine headache ☐ No significant history

☐ Other _____

Initial vital signs: BP _138/80_ P _76_ R _20_ T _98.4°F_ Spo$_2$ _98_ % ☐ RA ☒ O$_2$ _2_ L/min

Signature/Title: _Karen Sands, RN_ Date: _2/25/07_ Time: _1200_

Form used courtesy of the Henry Ford Health System, West Bloomfield, Michigan.

ChartWizard

Telephone encounter form

Some ambulatory care facilities have developed forms to be used for telephone encounters, which become part of the medical record. The bottom section of the sample form below can be used for patients requiring prescription refills.

Telephone Encounter Form

MRN: _0193802_
Patient's name: _Joseph DiLorenzo_
DOB: _4/18/1939_

Date of call: 2/14/07	Time of call: 1045	Site: Twin City Health Clinic		
Caller: Emily DiLorenzo, patient's wife		Telephone number: (843)555-3547	Provider: Dr. McManus	Insurance: Medicare

Chief complaint:
States her husband has been complaining of muscle weakness, and he has been nauseous since yesterday, has vomited twice today.

Temperature: 98.9°F orally	Pregnant: ☒N ☐Y	Allergies: ☐N ☒Y penicillin

Chronic diseases:
Hypertension, heart failure

Current medications:
Digoxin 0.5 mg PO daily
Enalapril 2.5 mg PO b.i.d.
Furosemide 40 mg PO b.i.d.

Assessment/Advice:
Pt's wife stated that her husband's symptoms started yesterday. He took Maalox yesterday for nausea but received no relief. Stated he had cardiology appointment on 2/11/07 and that the doses of his "heart" medicines were increased. Reports no signs or symptoms of infection. Advised to bring him to clinic today for evaluation and digoxin level.

Lauren Wilson, RN		_2/14/07_
Signature	Title	Date

Pharmacy name: _____   Telephone number: _____

Medications:	Strength:	Dosage:	Quantity:	Refill:

Provider's signature: _____
      Signature   Title   Date

Called by: _____
      Signature   Title   Date

Form used courtesy of the Henry Ford Health System, West Bloomfield, Michigan.

Selected references

Alavy, B., et al. "Emergency Department as the Main Source of Asthma Care," *Journal of Asthma* 43(7):527-32, September 2006.

Brixner, D.I., et al. "Documentation of Chemotherapy Infusion Preparation Costs in Academic- and Community-based Oncology Practices," *Journal of National Comprehensive Cancer Network* 4(3):99-101, April-June 2006.

Gladfelter, J. "Managing the Ever Expanding Plastic Surgery Office: Part 3," *Plastic Surgical Nursing* 26(2):99-101, April-June 2006.

Guglielmo, W. "Your Guide to OSHA Regulations," *RN* 67(7):28on2-4, July 2004.

Lake, F.R., and Vickery, A.W. "Teaching on the Run Tips 14: Teaching in Ambulatory Care," *Medical Journal of Australia* 185(3):166-67, August 2006.

Macnee, C.L., et al. "Evaluation of NOC Standardized Outcome of 'Health Seeking Behavior' in Nurse-managed Clinics," *Journal of Nursing Care Quality* 21(3):242-47, July-September 2006.

McCaiq, L.F., and Nawar, E.W. "National Hospital Ambulatory Medical Care Survey: 2004 Emergency Department Summary," *Advance Data* (372):1-29, June 2006.

Schauberger, C. W., and Larson, P. "Implementing Patient Safety Practices in Small Ambulatory Settings," *Joint Commission Journal on Quality and Patient Safety* 32(9):419-25, August 2006.

Summers, L., and McCartney, M. "Liability Concerns: A View from the American College of Nurse-Midwives," *Journal of Midwifery & Women's Health* 50(6):531-35, November-December 2005.

Tenrreiro, K.N. "Time-efficient Strategies to Ensure Vaccine Risk/Benefit Communication," *Journal of Pediatric Nursing* 20(6):469-76, December 2005.

Williams, D. "Setting Up a Cardiovascular Clinic in Primary Care," *Nursing Standard* 20(43):45-50, July 2006.

DOCUMENTATION IN ACTION

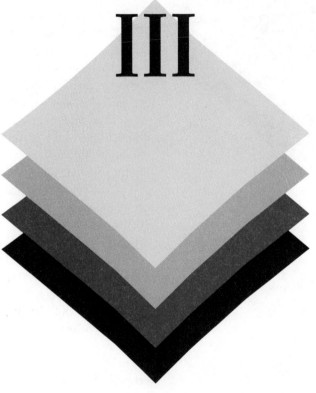

III

DOCUMENTATION OF EVERYDAY EVENTS

10

Your patient's medical record communicates important information about his condition and course of treatment to other nurses and members of the health care team. Without this record, neither you nor other caregivers can do the job effectively. That's why incomplete or improper charting has enormous implications.

Poor charting poses a threat to your patient's health and to your career. To avoid serious problems, take the time in both routine and exceptional situations to document legibly, accurately, objectively, and thoroughly, as well as consistently and in a timely manner.

In this chapter, you'll read about specific situations that you may encounter in your practice. Each situation is followed by a documentation example. Among the situations discussed are routine nursing procedures, common charting flaws, patient noncompliance, interdisciplinary communication, practitioners' orders, and incidents.

Routine nursing procedures

Your notes about routine nursing procedures should appear in the patient's chart. Include information about the procedure, who performed it, how it was performed, how the patient tolerated it (if applicable), and subsequent adverse effects (if applicable). Also include any patient teaching that was provided before and after the procedure.

Typically, your documentation will include drug administration, I.V. therapy, supportive care, assistive procedures, infection control, diagnostic tests, pain control, codes, change in the patient's condition, intake and output monitoring, skin and wound care, the patient's personal property, shift reports, and patient teaching. Some facilities use flow sheets to document repetitive procedures, such as wound care and I.V. therapy.

Drug administration

Your employer probably includes a medication administration record (MAR) in your documentation system. Commonly included in a card file (a medication Kardex) or on a separate medication administration sheet, the MAR serves as the central record of medication orders and their execution. Some documentation systems have the MAR included in an electronic format or as part of a clinical information system. It's part of the patient's permanent record.

When using the MAR, follow these guidelines:

▶ Know and follow your facility's policies and procedures for recording drug orders and charting drug administration.

▶ Make sure that all drug orders include the patient's full name, the date, the drug's name, dose, administration route or method, and frequency. When appropriate, include the specific number of doses given or the stop date. When administering a drug dose immediately—or stat—be sure to record the time. Also be sure to include drug allergy information.

▶ Write legibly.

▶ Use only standard abbreviations approved by your facility. When doubtful about an abbreviation, write out the word or phrase.

▶ Before administering medications, be sure to confirm the patient's identity using two patient identifiers, according to facility policy, and record that you've done so.

▶ After giving the first dose, sign your full name, licensure status, and initials in the appropriate space on the MAR.

▶ When transcribing a one-time order to be given on another shift, be sure to communicate information to the next shift during report, or use a medication alert sticker to flag the order.

▶ Record drugs immediately after administration so that another nurse doesn't give the drug again. (See *The medication Kardex,* pages 256 and 257.)

If you document medication administration by computer, chart your information for each drug right after you give it. This is particularly important if you don't use printouts as a backup. By keying in information immediately, you ensure that all health care team members have access to the latest drug administration data for the patient.

If you can't administer a prescribed drug as scheduled, document the reason (for example, the patient is having a test, which requires him not to take the drug). Many nurses omit this critical information.

Occasionally, you may suspect a connection between a patient's medication and an adverse event, such as illness, injury, or even death. In such a case, follow your facility's policy on reporting adverse drug events. This information should be reported to the U.S. Food and Drug Administration (FDA) on a MedWatch form issued by the FDA. (See *Reporting adverse events and product problems to the FDA,* pages 258 and 259.)

DRUGS GIVEN "AS NEEDED"

Chart all drugs administered "as needed." For eye, ear, or nose drops, chart the number of drops and where they were inserted. For suppositories, chart the type of suppository (rectal, vaginal, or urethral) and how the patient tolerated it. For topical drugs, chart the size and location of

(*Text continues on page 260.*)

ChartWizard

The medication Kardex

One type of Kardex is the medication Kardex. It contains a permanent record of the patient's medications. The medication Kardex may also include the patient's diagnosis and information about allergies and diet. A sample form is shown below.

Oettel, Robert
765432

NURSE'S FULL SIGNATURE, STATUS AND INITIALS						
Ray Charles, RN	INIT. RC		INIT.			INIT.
Theresa Hopkins, RN	TH					

DIAGNOSIS: Heart failure, Atrial flutter

ALLERGIES: ASA   DIET: Cardiac

ROUTINE/DAILY ORDERS/FINGERSTICKS/ INSULIN COVERAGE			DATE: 1/24/07	DATE: 1/25/07	DATE: 1/26/07	DATE:	DATE:	DATE:	DATE:	DATE:	DATE:	DATE:

ORDER DATE	MEDICATIONS DOSE, ROUTE, FREQUENCY	TIME	SITE	INT.	SITE	INT.	SITE	INT.	SITE	INT.	SITE	INT.	SITE	INT.	SITE	INT.	SITE	INT.	SITE	INT.	SITE	INT.
1/24/07	digoxin 0.125 mg	0900	®s.c.	RC																		
RC	I.V. daily	HR	68																			
1/24/07	furosemide 40 mg	0900	®s.c.	RC																		
RC	I.V. q12h	2100	®s.c.	TH																		
1/24/07	enalapril 1.25 mg	0500	®s.c.	TH																		
RC	I.V. q6h	1100	®s.c.	RC																		
		1700	®s.c.	RC																		
		2300	®s.c.	TH																		

The medication Kardex *(continued)*

Oettel, Robert
765432

PRN MEDICATION

ALLERGIES:

INITIAL	SIGNATURE & STATUS	INITIAL	SIGNATURE & STATUS	INITIAL	SIGNATURE & STATUS	INITIAL	SIGNATURE & STATUS
RC	Roy Charles, RN						
TH	Theresa Hopkins, RN						

YEAR 2007   P.R.N. MEDICATIONS

ORDER DATE: 1/24/07 RENEWAL DATE: / DISCONTINUED DATE: /	DATE	1/24/07			
MEDICATION: acetaminophen	DOSE 650 mg	TIME GIVEN 0930			
DIRECTION: p.r.n. mild pain	ROUTE: P.O.	SITE P.O.			
		INIT. RC			
ORDER DATE: 1/24/07 RENEWAL DATE: / DISCONTINUED DATE: /	DATE	1/24/07			
MEDICATION: morphine sulfate	DOSE 2 mg	TIME GIVEN 0930			
DIRECTION: 15 minutes prior to changing ® heel dressing	ROUTE: I.V.	SITE ® s.c.			
		INIT. RC			
ORDER DATE: 1/24/07 RENEWAL DATE: / DISCONTINUED DATE: /	DATE	1/24/07			
MEDICATION: Milk of Magnesia	DOSE 30ml	TIME GIVEN 2115			
DIRECTION: q6h p.r.n.	ROUTE: P.O.	SITE P.O.			
		INIT. TH			
ORDER DATE: 1/25/07 RENEWAL DATE: / DISCONTINUED DATE: 1/25/07	DATE	1/25/07	1/25/07		
MEDICATION: prochlorperazine	DOSE 5 mg	TIME GIVEN 1100	2230		
DIRECTION: q8h p.r.n.	ROUTE: I.M.	SITE ®glut.	©glut.		
prn nausea and vomiting		INIT. RC	TH		
ORDER DATE: / RENEWAL DATE: / DISCONTINUED DATE: /	DATE				
MEDICATION:	DOSE	TIME GIVEN			
DIRECTION:	ROUTE:	SITE			
		INIT.			
ORDER DATE: / RENEWAL DATE: / DISCONTINUED DATE: /	DATE				
MEDICATION:	DOSE	TIME GIVEN			
DIRECTION:	ROUTE:	SITE			
		INIT.			
ORDER DATE: / RENEWAL DATE: / DISCONTINUED DATE: /	DATE				
MEDICATION:	DOSE	TIME GIVEN			
DIRECTION:	ROUTE:	SITE			
		INIT.			

ChartWizard

Reporting adverse events and product problems to the FDA

Even large, well-designed clinical trials can't guarantee that adverse reactions will never arise after a drug or medical device is approved for use. An adverse reaction that occurs in only 1 in 5,000 patients could easily be missed in clinical trials. The drug could also interact with other drugs in ways unrevealed during clinical trials.

As a nurse, you play a key role in reporting adverse events and product problems. Reporting such problems helps ensure the safety of products that the Food and Drug Administration (FDA) regulates. The FDA's Medical Products Reporting Program supplies health care professionals with MedWatch forms on which they can report adverse events and product problems.

WHAT TO REPORT

Complete a MedWatch form when you suspect that a drug, medical device, special nutritional product, or other products regulated by the FDA are responsible for:
► congenital anomaly
► death
► disability
► initial or prolonged hospitalization
► life-threatening illness
► the need for any medical or surgical intervention to prevent a permanent impairment or an injury.

Also, promptly inform the FDA of product quality problems, such as:
► defective devices
► inaccurate or unreadable product labels
► intrinsic or extrinsic contamination or stability problems
► packaging or product mix-ups
► particulates in injectable drugs
► product damage.

YOUR RESPONSIBILITY IN REPORTING

When filing a MedWatch form, keep in mind that you're not expected to establish a connection between the product and the problem. You don't have to include a lot of details; you only have to report the adverse event or the problem with the drug or the product.

Additionally, you don't even have to wait until the evidence seems compelling. FDA regulations protect your identity and the identities of your patient and employer.

FURTHER GUIDELINES

The MedWatch form merges the individual forms used in the past to report adverse drug reactions, drug quality product problems, device quality product problems, and adverse reactions to medical devices. Send completed forms to the FDA by using the fax number or mailing address on the form.

File a separate MedWatch form for each patient, and attach additional pages if needed. If appropriate, report product problems to the manufacturer as well as to the FDA. Also, remember to comply with your health care facility's protocols for reporting adverse events associated with drugs and medical devices.

Product lot numbers are used in product identification, tracking, and product recall; therefore, the lot number should be retained and a copy of the report should be kept on file by your supervisor.

FDA RESPONSE

The FDA will report back to you on the actions it takes and will continue to work to instruct health care professionals about adverse events.

U.S. Department of Health and Human Services

MEDWATCH
The FDA Safety Information and Adverse Event Reporting Program

For **VOLUNTARY** reporting
of adverse events
and product problems

Page _1_ of _1_

Form Approved: OMB No. 0910-0291 Expires: 10/31/08
See OMB statement on reverse

FDA Use Only

Triage unit
sequence #

A. Patient information

1. Patient identifier	2. Age at time of event:		3. Sex	4. Weight
23674 _In confidence_	or ___ Date of birth: 11/14/60		☑ female ☐ male	___ lbs or 59 kgs

B. Adverse event or product problem

1. ☐ **Adverse event** and/or ☐ **Product problem** (e.g., defects/malfunctions)

2. Outcomes attributed to adverse event (check all that apply)
- ☐ death ___ (mo/day/yr)
- ☐ life-threatening
- ☐ hospitalization -- initial or prolonged
- ☐ disability
- ☐ congenital anomaly
- ☐ required intervention to prevent permanent impairment/damage
- ☐ other: ___

3. Date of event (mo/day/yr) 2/8/07	4. Date of this report (mo/day/yr) 2/8/07

5. Describe event or problem

After reconstituting 100 mg vial with
10 ml of bacteriostatic water, the drug
crystallized and turned yellow.

Drug was not given.

6. Relevant tests/laboratory data, including dates

7. Other relevant history, including preexisting medical conditions (e.g., allergies, race, pregnancy, smoking and alcohol use, hepatic/renal dysfunction, etc.)

PLEASE TYPE OR USE BLACK INK

C. Suspect medication(s)

1. Name (give labeled strength & mfr/labeler, if known)

#1 Leucovorin Calcium for injection — 100 mg vial

#2

2. Dose, frequency & route used	3. Therapy dates (if unknown, give duration) from/to (or best estimate)
#1 100 mg IV X 1	#1 2/8/07
#2	#2

4. Diagnosis for use (indication)

#1 Megaloblastic Anemia

#2

5. Event abated after use stopped or dose reduced
- #1 ☐ yes ☐ no ☑ doesn't apply
- #2 ☐ yes ☐ no ☐ doesn't apply

6. Lot # (if known)	7. Exp. date (if known)
#1 #891	#1
#2	#2

8. Event reappeared after reintroduction
- #1 ☐ yes ☐ no ☐ doesn't apply
- #2 ☐ yes ☐ no ☐ doesn't apply

9. NDC # (for product problems only)
- ___ — ___ — ___

10. Concomitant medical products and therapy dates (exclude treatment of event)

D. Suspect medical device

1. Brand name

2. Type of device

3. Manufacturer name & address

4. Operator of device
- ☐ health professional
- ☐ lay user/patient
- ☐ other: ___

5. Expiration date (mo/day/yr)

6.
model # ___
catalog # ___
serial # ___
lot # ___
other # ___

7. If implanted, give date (mo/day/yr)

8. If explanted, give date (mo/day/yr)

9. Device available for evaluation? (Do not send to FDA)
- ☐ yes ☐ no ☐ returned to manufacturer on ___ (mo/day/yr)

10. Concomitant medical products and therapy dates (exclude treatment of event)

E. Reporter (see confidentiality section on back)

1. Name & address | phone #

Patricia Cohen
987 Elm Ave
Cincinatti, Ohio

2. Health professional?	3. Occupation	4. Also reported to
☑ yes ☐ no	RN	☐ manufacturer ☑ user facility ☑ distributor

5. If you do NOT want your identity disclosed to the manufacturer, place an "X" in this box. ☐

FDA

Mail to: **MEDWATCH**
5600 Fishers Lane
Rockville, MD 20852-9787

or FAX to:
1-800-FDA-0178

FDA Form 3500 (1/96)   Submission of a report does not constitute an admission that medical personnel or the product caused or contributed to the event.

the area to which you applied the drug, and describe the condition of the skin or wound. For skin patches, chart the location of the patch.

If you administer all drugs according to the accepted standards, you don't need to include more specific information in the chart. However, if the MAR doesn't include space to document exceptional data (such as the patient's response to drugs given "as needed" or deviations from the drug order such as patient refusal), document the information as narrative in the chart, including any interventions required on your part.

2/8/07	0900	Pt. refused KCL elixir, stating
		that it makes her feel nause-
		ated and that she can't stand
		the taste. Dr. Miller notified.
		K-Dur tabs ordered and given.
		Pt. tolerated K-Dur well and
		denies nausea.——Betty Griffin, RN

SINGLE-DOSE MEDICATIONS

Single-dose medications, which can include a supplemental dose or a stat dose, should be documented both in the MAR and in the progress notes. Your documentation should include who gave the order, why the order was given, and the patient's response to the medication. For example, if you gave a one-time dose of I.V. Lasix, you would write:

2/3/07	0900	Lasix 40 mg I.V. given as per
		Dr. Singh's order. Pt. with SOB,
		crackles bilaterally, and O_2
		saturation decreased to 93%
		on room air. —— Ann Barrow, RN
2/3/07	1000	Pt. responded with urine out-
		put of 1500 ml, decreased SOB,
		and O_2 saturation increased to
		97% on room air. ———
		——— Ann Barrow, RN

OPIOIDS

When you administer an opioid, you must give the drug and document its administration according to federal, state, and institutional regulations. These regulations require opioids to be counted after each nursing shift to ensure an accurate drug count. Before administering an opioid, verify the amount of the drug in the container, and sign out the medication on the appropriate form.

Many facilities now use an automated storage system for opioids that eliminates the need for counting them at the end of the shift. This system allows the nurse easy access (via an I.D. and password) to medications (including other drugs and floor stocks for nursing units). Nurses may remove one or more medications by selecting the patient, medication, and amount needed on the keypad. The nurse must then count the amount of the drug remaining in the system and enter that number. Each transaction is recorded, and copies are sent to the pharmacy and billing department.

Many facilities still require that a second nurse document your activity and observe you if part or all of a dose of an opioid must be wasted.

If you discover a discrepancy in the opioid count, follow your facility's policy for reporting this and file an incident report. An investigation will follow. (See *Opioid control sheet.*)

I.V. therapy

Currently, more than 80% of hospitalized patients receive some form of I.V. therapy. Whether providing fluid or electrolyte replacement, total parenteral nutrition (TPN), drugs, or blood products, you'll need to carefully document all facets of I.V. therapy—including the administration and any subsequent complications of the therapy.

ChartWizard

Opioid control sheet

The sample opioid control sheet demonstrates proper documentation of opioids and an end-of-shift opioid count.

CITY HOSPITAL

Unit __45__   Date __1/5/07__

24-HOUR RECORD CONTROLLED SUBSTANCES

7 a.m. INVENTORY	CODEINE 30 MG TAB	PERCOCET TAB	TYLENOL #3 TAB	VALIUM 2 MG TAB	VALIUM 5 MG TAB	TEMAZEPAM 15 MG TAB	DEMEROL 50 MG INJ	DEMEROL 75 MG INJ	DEMEROL 100 MG INJ	DILAUDID 2 MG INJ	MORPHINE 2 MG INJ	MORPHINE 2 MG INJ	MIDAZOLAM 10 MG INJ	MIDAZOLAM 2 ML INJ	DOSE	AMOUNT WASTED	Signature	Witness
	25	20	18	15	16	10		10	8	5	10	15	13	3				

Time	Patient name	Patient number																	Signature	Witness
0915	Orr, Carl	555112													12		5mg	5mg	M. Stevens, RN	D. Buzon, RN
1000	Davis, Donna	555161			16												ii		M. Koller, RN	
1115	McGowen, John	555111					15										i		K. Collins, RN	

Keep in mind that an accurate description of your care provides a clear record of the treatments and drugs received by your patient. This record provides legal protection for you and your employer and furnishes health care insurers with the data they need to approve and provide reimbursement for equipment and supplies.

Depending on your facility's policy, you'll document I.V. therapy on a special I.V. therapy sheet, nursing flow sheet, or in another format. (See *Using a flow sheet to document I.V. therapy.*)

If a venipuncture requires more than one attempt, document the number of attempts made and the type of assistance required. Be sure to follow your facility's policy regarding this.

When you establish an I.V. route, remember to document the date, time, and venipuncture site together with the equipment used, such as the type and gauge of catheter or needle. You'll need to update your records each time you change the insertion site or the I.V. tubing. Also document any reason for changing the I.V. site, such as extravasation, phlebitis, occlusion, patient removal, or a routine change according to facility policy.

1/16/07	0200	Pt. complained of pain in Ⓛ
		hand at I.V. site. Hand red-
		dened from I.V. insertion site
		to 2" above site, tender and
		warm to touch. Slight swelling
		noted. I.V. discontinued and a
		warm, moist towel applied to
		left hand. I.V. started in right
		forearm. ————————————
		———————— Kathy Costello, RN

On each shift, be sure to document the type, amount, and flow rate of I.V. fluid, along with the condition of the I.V. site. Document each time that you flush the I.V. line and identify the type and amount of fluid used, including any medication.

Take the time to document any complication precisely. For example, if extravasation occurs, stop the I.V. Then assess the amount of fluid infiltrated, provide appropriate nursing intervention, and notify the practitioner. Be sure to document all pertinent information.

If a chemotherapeutic drug extravasates, follow the procedure specified by your facility. In the chart, document the appearance of the I.V. site, the type of treatment given (especially any drug used as an antidote), the kind of dressing applied to the site, and that the practitioner was notified. Also be sure to record every time that you flush this kind of I.V. line and the type and amount of fluid used.

If an allergic reaction occurs while the patient is receiving I.V. therapy, notify the practitioner immediately and complete an adverse reaction form. Document all pertinent information about the reaction, such as the type of reaction, when the reaction was identified, the extent of the reaction, and that it was reported to the practitioner. In addition, you must document treatments and the patient's response to them.

Record any patient teaching that you perform with the patient and his family, such as explaining the purpose of I.V. therapy, describing the procedure itself, and discussing any possible complications.

TPN

TPN is the administration of a solution of dextrose, proteins, electrolytes, vitamins, and trace elements in amounts that exceed the patient's energy expenditure and thereby achieve anabolism. Because this solution has about six times the solute concentration of blood, it requires dilution by delivery into a high-flow central vein to avoid injury to the peripheral vasculature. Typically, the solution is delivered to the superior vena cava through an indwelling subclavian vein catheter. Generally, TPN is prescribed for any

ChartWizard

Using a flow sheet to document I.V. therapy

This sample shows the typical features of an I.V. therapy flow sheet.

I.V. THERAPY FLOW SHEET

Patient: Jeanne Gallagher
Diagnosis: ℞ mastectomy
Venipuncture limitations: ℄ arm only
Permanent access: None

Date and time	1/14/07 1400	1/15/07 0800						
Patient visit	2	1						
Site status	1	1						
Procedure	R	C						
Gauge I.V. device	20	√						
Catheter type	PIV	PIV						
Location	LPF	LPF						
Date of insertion	1/14	1/14						
Routine site rotation	—	—						
Phlebitis	1 +	1						
Infiltration	1 +	0 +						
Other	1	—						
No. of failed attempts	0	—						
Lock status	—	—						
Flush	—	—						
Tubing: Macrodrip	√	√						
Minidrip								
Valleylab								
Filter								
Extension	√	√						
Dressing change	√	—						
Blood sample drawn	—	—						
Subcutaneous access port	—	—						
Patient response	1	1						
Patient teaching	1	1						
Nurse's initials	BG	KC						

Initials	Signature		Initials	Signature
BG	Betty Griffin, RN			
KC	Kathy Collins, RN			

(continued)

Using a flow sheet to document I.V. therapy *(continued)*

Date	Time	Patient care notes
1/14/07	1400	I.V. D5-1/2 NSS c̄ 40 mEq KCL infusing at 125 ml/hr. —————— Patricia Quinn, LPN

KEY

Patient visit
1   Routine rounds
2   Unit request
3   Patient not available for rounds

Site status
1   Within normal limits
2   Dressing intact

Procedure
S   Start
R   Restart
C   Check
D   Discontinue
CD   Cutdown

Catheter type
GR   Groshong catheter
PIV   Peripheral intravenous catheter
PICC Peripherally inserted central catheter
TL   Triple-lumen catheter
HI   Hickman catheter
SC   Subclavian catheter
SG   Swan-Ganz catheter
TE   Tenckhoff catheter
BR   Broviac catheter

Location
RH   Right hand
RW   Right wrist
RA   Right arm
RPF   Right posterior forearm
RC   Right cubital
RU   Right upper arm

LH   Left hand
LW   Left wrist
LA   Left arm
LPF   Left posterior forearm
LC   Left cubital
LU   Left upper arm
RF   Right foot
LF   Left foot
RJ   Right jugular
LJ   Left jugular
AB   Abdomen

Phlebitis
1   No pain to slight pain at site; erythema and no edema; no streak; no palpable cord
1+   Pain at site; erythema and/or edema; no streak, no palpable cord
2+   Pain at site; erythema and/or edema; streak formation; nonpalpable cord
3+   Pain at site; erythema and/or edema; streak formation; palpable cord

Infiltration
0+   Slight edema — no infiltration
1+   Slight puffiness at site
2+   Swelling above or below site
3+   Skin cool and pale; large area of swelling above or below site

Other
1   Leaking
2   Occluded
3   Patient removed catheter
4   Other (see patient care notes)

Lock status
1   Site locked
2   Site unlocked
3   Caps changed

Flush
1   Heparin
2   Saline

Patient response
1   Patient tolerated
2   Unresponsive
3   Patient agitated/combative
4   Other (see patient care notes)

Patient teaching
1   Patient/family member indicates understanding procedure
2   Instructed to call nurse for signs of redness, swelling, leaking, pain, or problem
3   Patient unable to comprehend

patient who can't absorb nutrients through the GI tract for more than 10 days.

Because TPN solution supports bacterial growth and the central venous (CV) line gives systemic access, contamination and sepsis are always a risk. Strict surgical asepsis is required during solution, dressing, tubing, and filter changes. Site care and dressing changes should be performed according to your facility's policy, every 48 hours for gauze dressings that prevent site visualization (once per week for transparent dressings) and whenever the dressing becomes wet, soiled, or nonocclusive. Tubing and filter changes should be performed every 72 hours; tubing used for lipids should be changed every 24 hours, according to your facility's policy.

If a patient is receiving TPN, document the type and location of the central line, the condition of the insertion site, and the volume and rate of the solution infused. Monitor any patient receiving TPN for adverse reactions and document your observations and interventions.

When you discontinue a central or peripheral I.V. line for TPN, record the date, time, and type of dressing applied. Also describe the appearance of the administration site.

1/31/07	2020	2-L bag of TPN hung at 2000.
		Infusing at 65 ml/hr via infusion
		pump through ℞ subclavian CV
		line. Transparent dressing intact,
		and site is without redness,
		drainage, swelling, or tenderness.
		Told pt. to call nurse if dressing
		becomes loose or soiled, site
		becomes tender or painful, or
		tubing or catheter becomes
		dislodged. Reviewed reasons for
		TPN and answered pt.'s questions
		about its purpose. ————
		———————— Meg Callahan, RN

BLOOD TRANSFUSIONS

Whenever you administer blood or blood components, such as packed cells, plasma, platelets, or cryoprecipitate, you must use proper identification and crossmatching procedures to ensure that the patient receives the correct blood product for transfusion. Verify the patient's identity using two patient identifiers according to facility policy. Then match the patient's name, medical record number, blood group (or type) and Rh factor (both the patient's and the donor's), the crossmatch data, and the blood bank identification number with the label on the blood bag, and clearly document that you did so. The blood or blood component must be identified and documented properly by two health care professionals, so you'll need to have a colleague assist you.

After you've determined that all the information is correct and matches, the consent form has been signed, and the patient's vital signs are within acceptable parameters per your facility's policy, you may administer the transfusion. On the transfusion record, document the date and time the transfusion was started and completed, the name of the health care professional who verified the information, the type and gauge of the catheter, and the total amount of the transfusion. Record the patient's vital signs before, during, and after the transfusion, as well as any blood-warming unit or infusion device used and the infusion flow rate.

For autologous blood transfusions, document the amount of blood retrieved and reinfused in the intake and output records. Monitor and document laboratory data during and after the autotransfusion as well as the patient's vital signs before and after the transfusion.

Pay particular attention to the patient's coagulation profile, hematocrit, and hemoglobin, arterial blood gas (ABG), and calcium levels.

Transfusion reaction

During a blood transfusion, the patient is at risk for developing a transfusion reaction. If he develops signs of a reaction, stop the transfusion immediately, remove the blood tubing, and hang new tubing with normal saline solution running to maintain vein patency. Notify the practitioner and the laboratory.

2/13/07	1400	Pt. reports nausea and chills.
		Cyanosis of the lips noted at
		1350 hours, with PRBCs trans-
		fusing. Infusion stopped,
		approximately 100 ml infused.
		Tubing changed. I.V. of
		1,000 ml D₅NSS infusing at
		30 ml/hour in Ⓡ arm. Notified
		Dr. Cahill. BP, 168/88; P, 104; R,
		25; T, 97.6° R. Blood sample
		taken from PRBCs. Two red-
		top tubes of blood drawn from
		pt. and sent to the laboratory.
		Urine specimen obtained from
		catheter. Urine specimen sent
		to lab for UA. Gave pt.
		diphenhydramine 50 mg I.M.
		Two blankets placed on pt.———
		———— Maryann Belinsky, RN
2/13/07	1415	Pt. reports he's getting warmer
		and less nauseated. BP 148/80;
		P, 96; R, 20; T, 98.2° R.———
		———— Maryann Belinsky, RN
2/13/07	1430	Pt. no longer complaining of
		nausea or chills. I.V. of 1,000 ml
		D₅NSS infusing at 125 ml/hr in
		Ⓡ arm. BP, 138/76; P, 80; R, 18;
		T, 98.4° R.———
		———— Maryann Belinsky, RN

Be sure to document the time and date of the reaction, the type and amount of infused blood or blood products, the time you started the transfusion, and the time you stopped it. Also record the signs of the reaction in order of occurrence, the patient's vital signs, a urine specimen or blood sample sent to the laboratory for analysis, treatment given, and the patient's response to the treatment.

Some health care facilities require the completion of a transfusion reaction report that must be sent to the blood bank. (See *Transfusion reaction report.*)

Supportive care procedures

Your daily nursing interventions constitute supportive care measures. Many of these can be documented on graphic forms and flowcharts; others must be described in progress notes or other forms. Among the most commonly documented nursing interventions are those that are provided before and after a surgical procedure (for example, pacemaker insertion, peritoneal dialysis, peritoneal lavage, suture removal, or thoracic drainage) and those provided to support the patient throughout treatment (for example, cardiac monitoring, chest physiotherapy, mechanical ventilation, nasogastric [NG] tube insertion and removal, seizure management, tube feedings, and withdrawing arterial blood for analysis).

PREOPERATIVE DOCUMENTATION

Effective nursing documentation during the preoperative period focuses on two primary elements—the baseline preoperative assessment and patient teaching. Documenting both of these elements encourages accurate communication among caregivers. Most facilities use a preoperative checklist to verify that required data have been collected, that preoperative teaching has occurred, and that prescribed procedures and safety precautions have been executed. (See *Preoperative checklist and surgical identification form,* page 269.) In addition, be sure to follow The Joint Commission's Universal

(*Text continues on page 270.*)

ChartWizard

Transfusion reaction report

If your facility requires a transfusion reaction report, you'll include the following types of information.

TRANSFUSION REACTION REPORT

Nursing report

1. Stop transfusion immediately. Keep I.V. line open with saline infusion.
2. Notify responsible physician.
3. Check all identifying names and numbers on the patient's wristband, unit, and paperwork for discrepancies.
4. Record patient's post-transfusion vital signs.
5. Draw posttransfusion blood samples (clotted and anti-coagulated) avoiding mechanical hemolysis.
6. Collect posttransfusion urine specimen from patient.
7. Record information as indicated below.
8. Send discontinued bag of blood, administration set, attached I.V. solutions, and all related forms and labels to the blood bank with this form completed.

Clerical errors
- ☑ None detected
- ☐ Detected

Vital signs

	Pre-TXN	Post-TXN
Temp.	98.4°F	98°F
B.P.	120/60	134/80
Pulse	88	80

Signs and Symptoms

- ☑ Urticaria
- ☐ Fever
- ☐ Chills
- ☐ Chest pain
- ☐ Hypotension
- ☐ Nausea
- ☑ Flushing
- ☐ Dyspnea
- ☐ Headache
- ☐ Perspiration
- ☐ Shock
- ☐ Oozing
- ☐ Back pain
- ☐ Infusion site pain
- ☐ Hemoglobin-uria
- ☐ Oliguria or anuria

Reaction occurred

During administration? _yes_
After administration? _____
How long? _____
Medications added? _____
Previous I.V. fluids? _1 unit FFP_
Blood warmed? _No_

Specimen collection

Blood: Difficulty collecting? _____
Urine: Voided _Yes – Sent lab_   Catheterized _____

Comments:

Signature _Jacqueline Brown, RN_   Date _2/10/07_

BLOOD BANK REPORT

Unit #
22FM80507

Component Returned
Yes

Volume Returned
185 ml

1. Clerical errors
- ☑ None detected
- ☐ Detected

Comments:

2. Hemolysis:

Note: If hemolysis is present in the posttransfusion sample, a posttransfusion urine sample must be tested for free hemoglobin immediately.

	None	Slight	Moderate	Marked
Patient pre-TXN sample	☑	☐	☐	☐
Patient post-TXN sample	☑	☐	☐	☐
Blood Bag	☑	☐	☐	☐
Urine HGB (centrifuged)	☐	☐	☑	☐

(continued)

Transfusion reaction report *(continued)*

BLOOD BANK REPORT *(continued)*

3. Direct antiglobulin test

Pretransfusion _____   Posttransfusion _____

If No. 2 and No. 3 are negative, steps 4 through 6 are not required. Report results to the blood bank physician. Steps 7 and 8 or further testing will be done as ordered by blood bank physician.

4. ABO and Rh Groups

Repeat testing	Cell reaction with								Serum reaction with		ABO/Rh
	Anti-A	Anti-B	Anti-A,B	Anti-D	Cont.	Du	Cont.	CCC	A₁ cells	B cells	
Pretransfusion											
Posttransfusion											
Unit #											
Unit #											

5. Red cell antibody screen

Pretransfusion	Cell	Saline/AB				INT
		RT	37°C	AHG	CCC	
Date of sample	I					
	II					
By:	Auto					

Posttransfusion	Cell	Saline/AB				INT
		RT	37°C	AHG	CCC	
Date of sample	I					
	II					
By:	Auto					

Specificity of antibody detected: _____

6. Crossmatch compatibility testing

Use patient pre- and post-TXN serum and the suspected unit red cells obtained from inside the container or from a segment still attached to bag. Observe appearance of blood in bag and administration tubing.

Pretransfusion	Albumin				INT
	RT	37°C	AHG	CCC	
Unit #					
Unit #					

Posttransfusion	Albumin				INT
	RT	37°C	AHG	CCC	
Unit #					
Unit #					

All units on hold for future transfusion must be recrossmatched with the posttransfusion sample.

7. Bacteriologic testing

Pretransfusion _____   Posttransfusion _____

8. Other testing results

Total bilirubin	Coagulation studies	Urine output studies
Patient pre-TXN _____ mg/dl		
Patient 6 hrs. post-TXN ___ mg/dl		

Pathologist's conclusions:

Signature _____   Date _____

ChartWizard

Preoperative checklist and surgical identification form

To document preoperative procedures, data collection, and teaching, most facilities use a checklist like the one below.

Woodview
Hospital

Patient ID

Mangin, Thomas
236489

**Pre-Operative Checklist
and Surgical Identification Form**

*Instructions: All items checked "No" requires follow up. Follow up is to be documented.
In "Additional Information / Comment" section until resolved.*

Pre-Op Checklist	Yes	No	Resolved	Initials
ID Band On	✔			NRC
Allergies Noted / Bracelet	✔			NRC
History & Physical (Present & Reviewed)	✔			NRC
Surgical Informed Consent Signed	✔			NRC
Anesthesia Informed Consent	✔			NRC
Pre-Op Teaching	✔			NRC
Prep. as Ordered	N/A			
NPO After Midnight	✔			NRC
Dentures, Capped Teeth, Cosmetics, Glasses, Contact Lenses, Wig Removed	N/A			
Voided/Catheter Inserted	✔			NRC
Medical Clearance/Physician's Name	✔			NRC
TEDS, as Ordered	N/A			
SCD, as Ordered	N/A			
PCA Teaching, as Ordered	✔			NRC
Type & Cross/Screen Drawn (If Ordered Must Have Blood Informed Consent Signed)	N/A			
**Blood Informed Consent Signed				
*Lab Results on Chart	✔			NRC
*EKG on Chart	✔			NRC
*Chest X-ray on Chart	✔			NRC

*Abnormal Results Results Reported To H&H   Dr. Schoblitz
Time & Date 2/28/07   0800
Reported By NRC

Temp. 98.6   Pulse 84   Resp. 18   B/P 132/82

Valuables
Destination: ☐ To Safe   ☐ To Family, Name _____

✗ Norma R. Clay, RN   NRC
Signature of Nurse   Initials

_____

✗ _____
Signature of Transferring RN   Date   Time

Additional Information /Comments

Surgical Patient Identification Form

Nursing Floor RN Patient Identification

☑ Patient I.D. Bracelet Personally Observed
☑ Patient Questioned Verbally Regarding I.D., Procedure & Site
☑ Patient's Chart Reviewed to Verify I.D., Procedure & Site

✗ Norma R. Clay, RN   2/28/07   0800
R.N.'s Signature   Date   Time

Pre-Op Anesthesia Patient Identification

☐ Patient's I.D. Bracelet Personally Observed
☐ Patient Questioned Verbally Regarding I.D., Procedure & Site
☐ Patient's Chart Reviewed to Verify I.D., Procedure & Site

✗ _____
Anesthesiologist/Anesthetist's Signature   Date   Time

Operating Room and Anesthesia Personnel Patient Identification

Operative Procedure & Site: _____

ANES	CIRC Nurse	
☐	☐	Patient I.D. Bracelet Personally Observed
☐	☐	Patient Questioned Verbally Regarding I.D., Procedure & Site
☐	☐	Patient's Chart Reviewed to Verify I.D., Procedure & Site
☐	☐	Surgical Site Confirmed

✗ _____
Anesthesiologist/Anesthetist's Signature   Time

✗ _____
CIRC Nurse's Signature   Time

Surgeon's Patient Identification Statement

☐ Patient I.D. Bracelet Personally Observed
☐ Patient Questioned Verbally Regarding I.D., Procedure & Site
☐ Surgical Site Marked

✗ _____
Surgeon's Signature   Time

Protocol for Preventing Wrong Site, Wrong Procedure, Wrong Person Surgery and complete the appropriate documentation. (See chapter 9, Documentation in Ambulatory Care.)

Be sure to document the name of the person you notified of any abnormalities or discrepancies that could affect the patient's response to the surgical procedure or any deviations from facility standards. For example, if you find there isn't a completed history or physical, your note might read as follows:

2/14/07	0800	No completed history and phy-
		sical found in pt's medical
		record. O.R. charge nurse,
		Margaret Little, notified. Also
		called Dr. Steven Adler's an-
		swering service. Message given
		to Operator 34.
		————Susan Altman, RN

SURGICAL INCISION CARE

In addition to documenting vital signs and level of consciousness (LOC) when the patient returns from surgery, pay particular attention to maintaining records pertaining to the surgical incision and drains and the care you provide.

Also read the records that travel with the patient from the postanesthesia care unit. (See *Documenting postsurgical status.*) Look for a practitioner's order directing whether you or the practitioner will perform the first dressing change. The following features of documenting surgical wound care are important:

▶ the date, time, and type of wound care performed

▶ the wound's appearance (size, condition of margins, necrotic tissue, if any), odor (if any), location of any drains, and drainage characteristics (type, color, consistency, and amount)

▶ dressing information, such as the type and amount of new dressing or pouch applied

▶ additional wound care procedures provided, such as drain management, irrigation, packing, or application of a topical medication

▶ the patient's tolerance of the procedure.

Record special or detailed wound care instructions and pain management measures on the nursing care plan. Document the color and amount of measurable drainage on the intake and output form.

2/10/07	0830	Dressing removed from mid-
		line abd. incision; no drainage
		noted on dressing. Incision
		well approximated and intact
		with staples. Margins ecchymo-
		tic; dime-sized area of sero-
		sanguineous drainage noted
		from distal portion of wound.
		Dry 4" x 4" sterile gauze pad
		applied. JP in LLQ draining
		serosanguineous fluid. Emptied
		40 ml. JP drain intact. Inser-
		tion site without redness or
		drainage. Split 4" x 4" gauze
		applied to site and taped se-
		curely.
		———— Grace Fedor, RN

If the patient will need wound care after discharge, provide and document appropriate instruction. The record should show that you explained aseptic technique, described how to examine the wound for signs of infection and other complications, demonstrated how to change the dressing, and provided written instructions for home care.

PACEMAKER CARE

Record the type and model of the pacemaker used, the date and time of pacemaker placement, the physician who inserted it, the reason for placement, the pacemaker settings, and the patient's response.

Smarter charting

Documenting postsurgical status

When your patient recovers sufficiently from the effects of anesthesia, he can be transferred from the operating room–postanesthesia care unit (OR–PACU) to his assigned unit for ongoing recovery and care. As the nurse on this service, you're responsible for the four-part documentation that travels with the patient. Here are some tips for making sure that all parts of the patient's record are present and complete.

PART 1: HISTORY
Make sure that this section of the OR–PACU report includes the patient's pertinent medical and surgical history (information that might affect the patient's response to anesthesia and his postoperative course).

Include drug allergies, medication history, chronic illnesses (coronary artery disease or chronic obstructive pulmonary disease, for example), significant surgical history and hospitalizations, and smoking history.

PART 2: OPERATION
Check that the following information is recorded in this section of the report, describing the surgery itself:
▶ the surgical site verification
▶ the procedure performed
▶ the type and dosage of anesthetics administered
▶ the length of time the patient was anesthetized
▶ the patient's vital signs throughout surgery
▶ the volume of fluid lost and replaced
▶ drugs administered
▶ surgical complications
▶ tourniquet time
▶ any drains, tubes, implants, or dressings used in surgery and removed or still in place.

PART 3: POSTANESTHESIA PERIOD
Make sure that this part of the record includes information about:

▶ pain medications and pain control devices that the patient received and how he responded to them
▶ the patient's postanesthesia recovery scores on arrival and discharge in these areas: activity level, respiration, circulation, level of consciousness (LOC), and color (all recorded on a flow sheet)
▶ unusual events or complications that occurred on the PACU—for instance, nausea or vomiting, shivering, hypothermia, arrhythmias, central anticholinergic syndrome, sore throat, back or neck pain, corneal abrasion, tooth loss during intubation, swollen lips or tongue, pharyngeal or laryngeal abrasion, and postspinal headache
▶ interventions that should continue on the unit. (For example, if the patient underwent leg surgery and had a tourniquet on for a long time, he'll need more frequent circulatory, motor, and neurologic checks. Additionally, if the anesthesiologist inserted an epidural catheter, the record should note any practitioner's orders regarding medication administration or special care procedures.)

PART 4: CURRENT STATUS
Expect this section to describe the patient's status at the time of transfer. Information should include the patient's vital signs, LOC, and sensorium.

Document the patient's LOC and vital signs, noting which arm you used to obtain the blood pressure reading. Also note any complications (such as infection, chest pain, pacemaker malfunction, or arrhythmias) and interventions performed (such as X-ray studies to verify correct electrode placement).

Document the information obtained from a 12-lead electrocardiogram (ECG). Obtain and include rhythm strips in the medical record at these times: before, during, and after pacemaker placement; any time pacemaker settings change; and any time the patient receives treatment resulting from a pacemaker complication.

1/9/07	0920	Pt. c̄ temporary transvenous
		pacemaker in Ⓛ subclavian vein.
		Rate 70, mA2, mV full demand.
		100% ventricular paced rhythm
		noted on monitor. ECG obtained.
		Pacer sensing & capturing
		correctly. Site w/o redness or
		swelling. Dressing D & I.———
		——————— John Mora, RN

As ECG monitoring continues, note capture, sensing rate, intrinsic beats, and competition of paced and intrinsic rhythms.

If the patient has a transcutaneous pacemaker, document the reason for this kind of pacing, the time pacing started, and the locations of the electrodes.

PERITONEAL DIALYSIS

Peritoneal dialysis is indicated for patients with chronic renal failure who have cardiovascular instability, vascular access problems that prevent hemodialysis, fluid overload, or electrolyte imbalances. In this procedure, dialysate—the solution instilled into the peritoneal cavity by a catheter—draws waste products, excess fluid, and electrolytes from the blood across the semipermeable peritoneal membrane. After a prescribed period, the dialysate is drained from the peritoneal cavity, removing impurities with it. The dialysis procedure is then repeated, using a new dialysate each time until waste removal is complete and fluid, electrolyte, and acid-base

balances have been restored. Peritoneal dialysis may be performed manually or by using an automatic or semiautomatic cycle machine.

During and after dialysis, monitor and document the patient's response to treatment. Record his vital signs every 10 to 15 minutes for the first 1 to 2 hours of exchanges, then every 2 to 4 hours or as often as necessary. If you detect any abrupt changes in the patient's condition, document them, notify the practitioner, and document your notification.

Document the amount of dialysate infused and drained and any medications added. Be sure to complete a peritoneal dialysis flowchart every 24 hours. Keep a record of the effluent's characteristics and the assessed negative or positive fluid balance at the end of each infusion-dwell-drain cycle. Also record each time you notify the practitioner of an abnormality.

Chart the patient's daily weight (immediately after the drain phase) and abdominal girth. Note the time of day and any variations in the weighing-measuring technique. Also document physical assessment findings and fluid status daily.

1/15/07	0700	Pt. receiving exchanges q2hr of
		1500 ml 4.25 dialysate with 500
		units heparin and 2 mEq KCL.
		Dialysate infused over 15 min. Dwell
		time 75 min. Drain time 30 min.
		Drainage clear, pale-yellow fluid.
		Weight 135 lb, abdominal girth 40°.
		Lungs clear, normal heart sounds,
		mucous membranes moist, good skin
		turgor. VSS (See flow sheets for
		fluid balance and frequent VS
		assessments.) Pt. tolerating
		procedure. No c/o cramping or
		discomfort. Skin warm, dry at RLQ
		catheter site, no redness or
		drainage. Dry split 4° X 4° dressing
		applied after site cleaned per
		protocol. ——— Liz Schaeffer, RN

Keep a record of equipment problems, such as kinked tubing or mechanical malfunction, and your interventions. Also note the condition of the patient's skin at the dialysis catheter site, the patient's reports of unusual discomfort or pain, and your interventions.

PERITONEAL LAVAGE

Used as a diagnostic procedure in a patient with blunt abdominal trauma, peritoneal lavage helps detect bleeding in the peritoneal cavity. The test may proceed through several steps. Initially, the practitioner inserts a catheter through the abdominal wall into the peritoneal cavity and aspirates the peritoneal fluid with a syringe. If he can't see blood in the aspirated fluid, he then infuses a balanced saline solution and siphons the fluid from the cavity. He inspects the siphoned fluid for blood and also sends fluid samples to the laboratory for microscopic examination.

Frequently monitor and document the patient's vital signs and any signs or symptoms of shock—for example, tachycardia, decreased blood pressure, diaphoresis, dyspnea, or vertigo.

Keep a record of the incision site's condition and document the type and size of peritoneal dialysis catheter used, the type and amount of solution instilled and withdrawn from the peritoneal cavity, and the amount and color of fluid returned. Note whether the fluid flowed freely into and out of the abdomen. Record which specimens were obtained and sent to the laboratory.

Also note any complications that occurred and the nursing actions you took to manage them.

SUTURE REMOVAL

Although suture removal is primarily a practitioner's responsibility, this procedure may be delegated to a skilled nurse with a written medical order. When documenting this procedure, note the appearance of the suture line, the date and time the sutures were removed, and whether the wound site contained purulent drainage. If you suspect infection at the site, notify the practitioner, collect a specimen, and send it to the laboratory for analysis.

1/2/07	1500	NG tube inserted via Ⓡ nostril
		and connected to low continuous
		suction, draining small amount of
		greenish colored fluid, hematest
		negative #16 Fr. Foley catheter
		inserted to straight drainage.
		Drained 200 ml clear amber
		urine, negative for blood. Dr.
		Fisher inserted #15 peritoneal
		dialysis catheter below umbilicus
		via trocar. Clear fluid withdrawn.
		700 ml warm NSS instilled as
		ordered and clamped. Pt. turned
		from side to side. NSS dwell
		time of 10 min. NSS drained
		freely from abdomen. Fluid
		samples sent to lab, as ordered.
		Peritoneal catheter removed
		and incision closed by Dr. Fisher.
		4" X 4" gauze pad with povidone-
		iodine ointment applied to site.
		Pt. tolerated procedure well.
		Preprocedure P 92, BP 110/64,
		RR 24. Postprocedure P 88, BP
		116/66, RR 18. ————————
		———— Angela Novack, RN

2/14/07	1030	Order obtained from MD to
		remove sutures from index
		finger. Suture line well approx-
		imated and healed. No drainage
		present upon assessment. Site
		clean and dry. No redness.
		Patient complaining of "a numb
		feeling" when the finger is
		touched. All three sutures
		removed without difficulty. Dry
		Bandaid applied to the finger.
		———— Pauline Primas, RN

THORACIC DRAINAGE

Record the date and time thoracic drainage began, the type of system used, the amount of suction applied to the system, and the initial presence or absence of bubbling or fluctuation in the water-seal chamber. (Bubbling in the water-seal chamber may indicate an air leak.) Also record the initial amount and type of drainage and the patient's respiratory status.

Document how frequently you inspected the drainage system. Again, note the presence or absence of bubbling or fluctuation in the water-seal chamber, and enter the patient's respiratory status.

2/11/07	0900	℞ anterior CT intact to Pleur-
		evac suction system to 20 cm of
		suction. All connections intact.
		50 ml bright red bloody drain-
		age noted since 0800. No air
		leak noted + water chamber
		fluctuation. CT site dressing
		D&I, no crepitus palpated. Lungs
		clear bilaterally. Chest expansion
		equal bilaterally. No SOB noted.
		RR 18-20 nonlabored. O₂ at 2
		L/min via NC. ————
		———— Andrew Ortiz, RN

Also record the condition of the chest dressings; the name, amount, and route of any pain medication you gave; complications that developed; and any subsequent interventions that you performed.

When documenting ongoing drainage characteristics, describe the color, consistency, and amount of thoracic drainage in the collection chamber. Be sure to include the time and date of each instance that you make such observations.

Keep a record of patient-teaching sessions and subsequent activities that the patient will perform, such as coughing and deep-breathing exercises, sitting upright, and splinting the insertion site to minimize pain.

Record the results of your respiratory assessments, including the rate and quality of the patient's respirations and auscultation findings. Also document the time and date when you notify the practitioner of serious patient conditions, such as cyanosis, rapid or shallow breathing, subcutaneous emphysema, chest pain, or excessive bleeding.

Be sure to document each chest tube dressing change and findings related to the patient's skin condition at the chest tube site.

CARDIAC MONITORING

In your notes, document the date and time that monitoring began and the monitoring leads used. Commit all rhythm strip readings to the record. Be sure to label the rhythm strip with the patient's name, his room number, and the date and time. Also document any changes in the patient's condition, and be sure to include a rhythm strip in the patient's chart that was printed during the condition change.

1/8/07	0720	Pt. on 5-lead electrode system.
		ECG strip shows NSR at a rate
		of 80 ĉ occasional PACs PR .16,
		QRS .08; 6-sec. episode of PAT
		– rate 160 noted at 0710 hr.
		Dr. Durkin notified. Pt. asympto-
		matic. Peripheral pulses normal;
		no edema noted. Heart ĉ RRR.
		No murmurs, gallops or rubs.
		Pt. denies chest pain/discom-
		fort, SOB and palpitations.
		———— Diane Goldman, RN

If cardiac monitoring will continue after the patient's discharge, document which caregivers can interpret dangerous rhythms and perform cardiopulmonary resuscitation. Also teach troubleshooting techniques to use if the monitor malfunctions, and document your teaching efforts or referrals (for example, to equipment suppliers).

CHEST PHYSIOTHERAPY

Whenever you perform chest physiotherapy, document the date and time of your interventions, the patient's positions for secretion drainage and length of time the patient remains in each position, the chest segments percussed or vibrated, and the characteristics of the secretion expelled (including color, amount, odor, viscosity, and the presence of blood). Also record indications of complications, the nursing actions taken, and the patient's tolerance of the treatment.

2/20/07	1415	Pt. placed on ℚ side c̄ foot of
		bed elevated. Chest PT and
		postural drainage performed for
		10 min. from lower to middle
		then upper lobes, as ordered.
		Pt. had productive cough and
		expelled approximately 5 ml of
		thick yellow sputum. Lungs clear
		p̄ chest PT. Procedure tolerated
		w/o difficulty. ————————
		———————— Jane Goddard, RN

MECHANICAL VENTILATION

Document the date and time that mechanical ventilation began. Note the type of ventilator used for the patient and its settings. Describe the patient's subjective and objective responses to mechanical ventilation (including vital signs, breath sounds, use of accessory muscles, comfort level, and physical appearance).

Throughout mechanical ventilation, list any complications and subsequent interventions. Record all pertinent laboratory data, including results of any ABG analyses and oxygen saturation findings.

2/16/07	1015	Pt. on Servo ventilator set at
		TV 750; FIO_2, 45%; 5 cm PEEP;
		AC of 12. RR 20 nonlabored. #8
		ETT in ℝ corner of mouth,
		taped securely at 22-cm mark.
		Suctioned via ETT for large
		amt. of thick white secretions.
		Pulse oximeter reading 98%. ℚ
		lung clear. ℝ lung with basilar
		crackles and expiratory wheezes.
		No SOB noted. ————————
		———————— Janice Del Vecchio, RN

If the patient is receiving pressure support ventilation or using a T-piece or tracheostomy collar, note the duration of spontaneous breathing and the patient's ability to maintain the weaning schedule. If the patient is receiving intermittent mandatory ventilation, with or without pressure-support ventilation, record the control breath rate, the time of each breath reduction, and the rate of spontaneous respirations.

Record any adjustments made in ventilator settings as a result of ABG levels, and document any adjustments of ventilator components, such as draining condensate into a collection trap and changing, cleaning, or discarding the tubing.

Note interventions implemented to promote mobility, to protect skin integrity, or to enhance ventilation. For example, record when and how you perform active or passive range-of-motion exercises, turn the patient, or position him upright for lung expansion. Also record any tracheal suctioning done and the character of secretions.

Document assessment findings related to peripheral circulation, urine output, decreased cardiac output, fluid volume excess, or dehydration. When possible, document sleep and wake periods, noting significant trends as appropriate.

Record any teaching efforts (involving the patient and appropriate caregivers) that you carried out in preparation for the patient's discharge. Take special care to record teaching associated with ventilator care and settings, artificial airway care, communication, nutrition, and therapeutic exercise.

Also indicate teaching discussions and demonstrations related to signs and symptoms of infection and equipment functioning. List any referrals you made to equipment vendors, home health agencies, and other community resources.

NG TUBE INSERTION AND REMOVAL

Record the type and size of the NG tube inserted; the date, time, and route of insertion; the reason for the insertion; and confirmation of proper placement. Describe the type and amount of suction (if used); drainage characteristics, such as amount, color, consistency, and odor; and the patient's tolerance of the insertion procedure. Record when the NG tube was irrigated and the amount of solution used.

Include in your notes any signs and symptoms signaling complications, such as nausea, vomiting, and abdominal distention. Document any subsequent irrigation procedures and continuing problems after irrigation.

1/15/07	1605	# 12 Fr. NG tube placed in Ⓛ nostril. Placement verified and attached to low intermittent suction as ordered. Drainage pale green; heme negative. Irrigated with 30 ml NSS q 2 hr. Pt. tolerated procedure. Hypoactive B.S. in all 4 quadrants.————————— Vijay Rao, RN

Record the date and time of NG tube clamping or removal, the patient's tolerance of the procedure, and any unusual events accompanying NG tube removal, such as nausea, vomiting, abdominal distention, and food intolerance.

SEIZURE MANAGEMENT

Note in the medical record that the patient requires seizure precautions, and record all precautions taken. Record the date and time that a seizure began, as well as its duration and any precipitating factors. Identify any sensation that may be considered an aura. Describe any involuntary behavior occurring at onset, such as lip smacking, chewing movements, or hand and eye movements. Record any incontinence occurring during the seizure.

1/19/07	1712	At 1615 Pt. observed with generalized seizure activity lasting 2 ½ min. Pt. sleeping at time of onset. Urinary incontinence during seizure. Seizure pads in place on bed before seizure. Pt. placed on Ⓛ side, airway patent, no N/V. Dr. Gordon notified of seizure. Diazepam 10 mg given I.V. as ordered. VS taken q 15 min. and p.r.n. (see flow sheet). Pt. currently obtunded (see neurologic flow sheet). No further seizure activity noted.————— Gale Hartman, RN

Document the patient's response to the seizure, the medications given, any complications resulting from the medications or the seizure, and any interventions performed. Finally, record your assessment of the patient's postictal mental and physical status.

TUBE FEEDINGS

In addition to frequently assessing and documenting the patient's tolerance of the procedure and the feeding formula, keep careful records of the kind of tube feeding the patient is receiving (for example, duodenal or jejunal feedings or continuous drip or bolus) as well as the amount, rate, route, and method of feeding.

If you need to dilute a feeding formula, note the dilution strength for the record (for example, half- or three-quarters strength).

When you flush the feeding tube to maintain patency, be sure to document the time and the flushing solution (such as water or cranberry juice) as intake amounts. If you must replace the feeding tube, document this activity as well.

Regularly assess and document the patient's gastric function and note any prescribed medications or treatments to relieve constipation or diarrhea.

When administering continuous feedings, check and document the infusion rate regularly. When administering bolus feedings, document the residual contents and amount as well as placement and patency of the tube before feeding.

Regularly record such laboratory test findings as the patient's urine and serum glucose, serum electrolyte, and blood urea nitrogen levels as well as serum osmolality. Be sure to document any feeding complications, such as hyperglycemia, glycosuria, and diarrhea.

If the patient will continue receiving tube feedings after discharge, document any instructions you give to the patient and appropriate caregivers and any referrals you make to suppliers or support agencies.

WITHDRAWAL OF ARTERIAL BLOOD

When you must obtain blood for ABG analysis, keep careful records of the patient's vital signs and temperature, the arterial puncture site, and the results of Allen's test. Also document any indications of circulatory impairment, such as bleeding at the puncture site and swelling, discoloration, pain, numbness, or tingling in the bandaged arm or leg.

Document the time that the blood sample was drawn, the length of time pressure was applied to the site to control bleeding and, if appropriate, the type and amount of oxygen therapy that the patient was receiving.

| 2/25/07 | 0700 | Full-strength Pulmocare infusing via Flexiflow pump thru Dobhoff tube in Ⓡ nostril at 50 ml/hr. Tube placement checked and pt. maintained with HOB raised about 45°. 5 ml residual obtained. Pt. denies any N/V. Normal active bowel sounds auscultated x 4 quad. Diphenoxylate elixir 2.5 mg given via F.T. for continuous diarrhea. Tube flushed with 30 ml H₂O this shift as ordered. Pt. instructed to tell nurse of discomfort. ————————————————————— Sandra Mann, RN |

| 2/12/07 | 1010 | Blood drawn from Ⓡ radial artery p̄ positive Allen's test c̄ brisk capillary refill. Pressure applied to site for 5 min. and pressure drsg. applied. No bleeding, hematoma, or swelling noted. Hand pink, warm c̄ 2-sec. capillary refill. Dr. Smith notified of ABG results. O2 increased to 40% nonbreather mask at 0845. Pt. in no resp. distress. ————————————————————— Pat Toricelli, RN |

When filling out a laboratory request for ABG analysis, be sure to include the following information for laboratory records: the patient's current temperature and respiratory rate, his most recent hemoglobin level and, if he's receiving mechanical ventilation, the fraction of inspired oxygen, tidal volume, and control rate. In many facilities, this information is entered as a computerized order.

Assistive procedures

When you assist a practitioner in such procedures as bone marrow aspiration, esophageal tube insertion, insertion or removal of arterial or central venous lines, lumbar puncture, paracentesis, or thoracentesis, your role also involves patient support, patient teaching, and evaluation of the patient's response.

Careful charting of these procedures is your responsibility. Document the name of the practitioner performing the procedure, the equipment used, the patient's response to the procedure, the patient teaching provided, and any other pertinent information.

BONE MARROW ASPIRATION

When assisting the practitioner with a bone marrow aspiration, document the date and time and the name of the practitioner performing the procedure. Also describe the appearance of the specimen aspirated, the patient's response to the procedure, and the appearance of the aspiration

1/30/07	1000	Assisted Dr. Shelbourne while
		he performed a bone marrow
		aspiration at 0915 hr. The
		procedure was performed on
		the ® anterior iliac crest. Pt.
		tolerated the procedure well
		with little discomfort. Speci-
		mens sent to lab, as ordered.
		No bleeding at site. VS: BP,
		142/82; P, 88; R, 22. Pt.
		afebrile. Bed rest being main-
		tained.————— Margaret Little, RN

site. Monitor the patient's vital signs after the procedure, and observe the aspiration site for bleeding. Document any pertinent information about the specimen sent to the laboratory.

ESOPHAGEAL TUBE INSERTION AND REMOVAL

Make sure your documentation includes the date and time that you assisted with insertion and removal of the esophageal tube and the name of the practitioner who performed the procedure.

As applicable, record the type of sedation administered, the intragastric balloon pressure, the amount of air injected into the gastric balloon port, the amount of fluid used for gastric irrigation, and the color, consistency, and amount of gastric return both before and after lavage.

Because intraesophageal balloon pressure varies with respirations and esophageal contractions, be sure to record the baseline pressure, which is the most important pressure.

Document the patient's tolerance of both the insertion and removal procedures.

2/11/07	1210	Sengstaken-Blakemore tube
		placed w/o difficulty by Dr.
		Fisher via ® nostril. 50 ml air
		injected into gastric balloon.
		Abdominal X-ray obtained to
		confirm placement. Gastric
		balloon inflated c̄ 500 ml air.
		Tube secured to football hel-
		met traction. Large amt. bright
		red bloody drainage noted.
		Tube irrigated c̄ 1,800 ml of
		iced NSS until clear. NG tube
		placed in Ⓛ nostril and
		attached to 8 mm Ohio wall
		suction. Esophageal balloon
		inflated to 30 mm Hg and
		clamped. Equal BS bilat. No
		SOB, VSS. Pt. tolerated proce-
		dure. Emotional support given.
		————— Evelyn Sutcliffe, RN

ARTERIAL LINE INSERTION AND REMOVAL

When assisting with the insertion of an arterial line, record the practitioner's name; the time and date; the insertion site; the type, gauge, and length of the catheter; and whether the catheter is sutured in place.

2/5/07	0625	#20G arterial catheter placed in ® radial artery by anesthes. Dr. Mayer on 2nd attempt after + Allen's test. Transducer leveled and zeroed. Readings accurate to cuff pressures. Site w/o redness or swelling. 4" x 4" gauze pad c̄ povidone-iodine ointment applied. ® hand and wrist taped and secured to arm board. Line flushes easily. Good waveform on monitor. Pt.'s hand pink and warm c̄ 2-sec. capillary refill. ———— ———— Lisa Chang, RN

At removal, record the practitioner's name, time and date, length of the catheter, length of time pressure was applied to insertion site, and condition of the insertion site. Be sure to document if any catheter specimens were obtained for culture.

CENTRAL VENOUS LINE INSERTION AND REMOVAL

Typically, when you assist the practitioner who's inserting a central venous (CV) line, you'll need to document the time and date of insertion; the type, length, and location of the catheter; the solution infused; the practitioner's name; and the patient's response to the procedure. Per The Joint Commission's requirements, all medications and solutions must be labeled on and off the sterile field. Document your compliance with this requirement per your facility's policy. Other measures that must be noted include the time of the X-ray study performed to confirm the line's safe and correct placement, the X-ray results, and your notification of the practitioner of the results. Consult your facility's policy regarding timeliness of reporting critical test results and values.

After assisting with a CV line's removal, record the time and date of removal and the type of dressing applied. Note the length of the catheter and the condition of the insertion site. Also document the collection of any catheter specimens for culture or other analysis.

2/24/07	1100	Procedure explained to pt. and consent obtained by Dr. Chavez. Pt. in Trendelenburg position and triple-lumen catheter placed by Dr. Chavez on 1st attempt in ® SC. Cath. sutured in place c̄ 3-0 silk and sterile dressing applied per protocol. All lines flushed c̄ 100 units heparin and portable chest X-ray obtained to confirm line placement. VSS. Pt. tolerated procedure well. ———— ———— Louise Flynn, RN

LUMBAR PUNCTURE

During lumbar puncture, observe the patient closely for such signs and symptoms as a change in LOC, dizziness, or changes in vital signs. Report these observations to the practitioner and document them carefully.

Also record the initiation and completion time of the procedure and the number of test tube specimens of cerebrospinal fluid (CSF) as they're obtained. Document the patient's tolerance of the procedure and any pertinent information about the specimens.

Monitor the patient's condition, and keep him in a flat supine position for 6 to 12 hours. Encourage fluid intake, assess him for headache, and check the puncture site for leaking CSF.

Document all of your observations and interventions.

2/8/07	0900	Procedure explained to patient. Pt. positioned, side lying for lumber puncture. Procedure began at 9am and ended at 9:35am. Pt. draped and prepped by Dr Anne Smith. Specimen obtained on 1st attempt by Dr Smith. Clear straw colored CSF noted. Pt. tolerated procedure without difficulty. Vitals signs stable during procedure. Pt. maintained in supine position as instructed. Due to flat positioning, and NPO status, NSS infusion started at 100 ml/hr. Puncture site dressed by Dr. Smith. Site clean dry and intact. No leakage. Pt. without complaints of headache or dizziness. ———— Jeanette Kane, RN

PARACENTESIS

When caring for a patient during and after paracentesis, be sure to document the date and time of the procedure and the puncture site. Also record the amount, color, viscosity, and odor of the initially aspirated fluid in your notes and the fluid intake and output record.

If you're responsible for ongoing patient care, be sure to keep a running record of the patient's vital signs and nursing activities related to drainage and to dressing changes. The record should indicate the frequency of drainage checks (typically, every 15 minutes for the first hour, every 30 minutes for the next 2 hours, every hour for the next 4 hours, then every 4 hours for the next 24 hours) and the patient's response to the procedure. Continue to document drainage characteristics, including color, amount, odor, and viscosity.

If peritoneal fluid leakage occurs, notify the practitioner and document that you did so. Be sure to include the time and the date.

Also document daily patient weight and abdominal girth measurements before and after the procedure, the number of fluid specimens sent to the laboratory for analysis, and the total volume of fluid removed.

2/12/07	1100	After procedure explained to pt. and consent obtained, Dr. Novello performed paracentesis in RLQ as per protocol. 1500 ml cloudy, pale-yellow fluid drained and sent to lab as ordered. Site sutured with one 3-0 silk suture. Sterile 4" x 4" gauze pad applied. No leakage noted at site. Abd. girth 44" preprocedure and 42 3/4" postprocedure. Pt. tolerated procedure w/o difficulty. VSS before and after procedure as per flow sheet. Emotional support given to pt. ———— Carol Barsky, RN

THORACENTESIS

When assisting with thoracentesis, assess the patient for any sudden or unusual pain, faintness, dizziness, or vital sign changes. Report these observations to the practitioner immediately, and record them as soon as possible. Document the date and time, the name of the practitioner performing the procedure, the amount and quality of fluid aspirated, and the patient's response to the procedure.

If later symptoms of pneumothorax, hemothorax, subcutaneous emphysema, or infection occur, notify the practitioner immediately and document your observations and interventions on the chart. Also note whether you sent a fluid specimen to the laboratory for analysis.

2/10/07	1100	Procedure explained to patient
		and consent obtained by Dr.
		McCall. Pt. positioned over
		secured bedside table. RLL
		thoracentesis performed by Dr
		Garret without incident. Sterile
		4" x 4" dressing applied to site.
		Site clean and dry, no redness
		or drainage present. 900 ml of
		blood-tinged serosanguineous
		fluid aspirated. Specimen sent
		to lab as ordered. Vital signs
		stable. Pt. denies SOB or
		dyspnea. Bilateral breath sounds
		auscultated. Chest X-ray pending.
		———— Ellen Pritchett, RN

Record the dates and times of your interventions in the patient's chart and on the Kardex. Document any breach in an isolation technique, and file an incident report should this occur. If the practitioner prescribes a drug to treat the infection, record this as well.

1/28/07	1300	Wound and skin precautions
		maintained. Pt. temperature
		remains elevated at 102.3° R.
		Tylenol 650 mg suppository given
		as ordered. Amount of purulent
		drainage from the incision has
		increased since yesterday. Dr.
		Levick notified. Repeat C&S
		ordered. Specimen obtained and
		sent to the lab.—— Lynne Kasoff, RN

Infection control

Meticulous record keeping is an important contributor to effective infection control. Various federal agencies require documentation of infections so that the data can be assessed and used to help prevent and control future infections. In addition, the data you record help your health care facility meet national and local accreditation standards.

Typically, you must report to your facility's infection control department any culture result that shows a positive infection and any surgery, drug, elevated temperature, X-ray finding, or specific treatment related to infection. (See *Reportable diseases and infections,* page 282.)

Document to whom you reported the signs and symptoms of suspected infection, instructions received, and treatments initiated. Always follow standard precautions for direct contact with blood and body fluids and the Centers for Disease Control and Prevention (CDC) hand hygiene guidelines, and be sure to document that you've done so.

Teach the patient and his family about these precautions, and document your instructions.

Be sure to communicate the results of any culture and sensitivity studies to the practitioner so that he may prescribe the appropriate drug to treat the infection. Also inform the infection control practitioner. Record the patient's response to this drug. Per The Joint Commission's requirements, your facility must have a policy in place regarding timeliness of reporting critical tests and values. Consult this policy and document your communications accordingly.

Diagnostic tests

Before receiving a diagnosis, most patients undergo testing—as simple as a blood test or as complicated as magnetic resonance imaging.

Begin documenting diagnostic testing with any preliminary assessments you make of a patient's condition. For example, if your patient is pregnant or has certain allergies, record this information because it might affect the test or the test result. If the patient's age, illness, or disability requires special preparation for the test, enter this information in his chart as well.

Reportable diseases and infections

The Centers for Disease Control and Prevention (CDC), the Occupational Safety and Health Administration, The Joint Commission, and the American Hospital Association all require health care facilities to document and report certain diseases acquired in the community or in hospitals and other health care facilities.

Generally, the health care facility reports diseases to the appropriate local authorities. These authorities notify the state health department, which in turn reports the diseases to the appropriate federal agency or national organization.

The list of diseases that appears below is the CDC's list of nationally notifiable infectious diseases for 2007. Each state also keeps a list of reportable diseases appropriate to the region.

▶ Acquired immunodeficiency syndrome (AIDS)
▶ Anthrax
▶ Arboviral neuroinvasive and non-neuroinvasive diseases (California serogroup virus disease, Eastern equine encephalitis virus disease, Powassan virus disease, St. Louis encephalitis virus disease, West Nile virus disease, Western equine encephalitis virus disease)
▶ Botulism (food-borne, infant, other [wound and unspecified])
▶ Brucellosis
▶ Chancroid
▶ *Chlamydia trachomatis,* genital infections
▶ Cholera
▶ Coccidioidomycosis
▶ Cryptosporidiosis
▶ Cyclosporiasis
▶ Diphtheria
▶ Ehrlichiosis (human granulocytic, human monocytic, human [other or unspecified agent])
▶ Giardiasis
▶ Gonorrhea
▶ *Haemophilus influenzae,* invasive disease
▶ Hansen disease (leprosy)
▶ Hantavirus pulmonary syndrome
▶ Hemolytic uremic syndrome, postdiarrheal
▶ Hepatitis, viral, acute (hepatitis A acute, hepatitis B acute, hepatitis B virus perinatal infection, hepatitis C acute)
▶ Hepatitis, viral, chronic (chronic hepatitis B, hepatitis C virus infection [past or present])
▶ Human immunodeficiency virus (adult [≥ 13 years old], pediatric [< 13 years old])

▶ Influenza-associated pediatric mortality
▶ Legionellosis
▶ Listeriosis
▶ Lyme disease
▶ Malaria
▶ Measles
▶ Meningococcal disease
▶ Mumps
▶ Pertussis
▶ Plague
▶ Poliomyelitis (paralytic)
▶ Psittacosis
▶ Q fever
▶ Rabies (animal, human)
▶ Rocky Mountain spotted fever
▶ Rubella (German measles) and congenital syndrome
▶ Salmonellosis
▶ Severe acute respiratory syndrome–associated coronavirus (SARS-CoV) disease
▶ Shiga toxin-producing *Escherichia coli* (STEC)
▶ Shigellosis
▶ Smallpox
▶ Streptococcal disease, invasive, Group A
▶ Streptococcal toxic-shock syndrome
▶ *Streptococcus pneumoniae,* drug resistant, invasive disease
▶ *Streptococcus pneumoniae,* invasive, in children younger than age 5
▶ Syphilis (primary, secondary, latent, early latent, late latent, latent unknown duration, neurosyphilis, late non-neurologic, syphilitic stillbirth)
▶ Syphilis, congenital
▶ Tetanus
▶ Toxic shock syndrome (other than streptococcal)
▶ Trichinellosis (trichinosis)
▶ Tuberculosis
▶ Tularemia
▶ Typhoid fever
▶ Vancomycin intermediate *Staphylococcus aureas* (VISA)
▶ Vancomycin resistant *Staphylococcus aureas* (VRSA)
▶ Varicella (morbidity)
▶ Varicella (deaths only)
▶ Yellow fever

Always prepare the patient for the test, and document any teaching you've done about the test itself and any follow-up care associated with it. Be sure to document the administration or withholding of drugs and preparations, special diets, food or fluid restrictions, enemas, and specimen collection.

2/18/07	0700	24-hour urine test for crea-
		tinine clearance started. Pt.
		taught purpose of this test
		and how to collect urine. Sign
		placed on pt.'s door, over bed,
		and in bathroom. Urine placed
		on ice in bathroom. ———
		———Paul Steadman, RN

Pain control

Pain must be assessed in every patient, although the frequency and criteria for this assessment are developed and specified by each facility. Your primary goal is to eliminate or minimize your patient's pain. Determining its severity can be difficult, however, because pain is subjective. You can use a number of tools to assess pain; when you use them, always document the results. (See *Assessing and documenting pain,* page 284.)

When charting pain levels and characteristics, first determine where the patient feels the pain and whether it's internal, superficial, localized, or diffuse. Also find out whether the pain interferes with the patient's sleep or other activities of daily living. Describe the pain in the patient's own words and enter them in the chart.

Be aware of the patient's body language and behaviors associated with pain. Does he wince or grimace? Does he move or squirm in bed? What positions seem to relieve or worsen the pain? What other measures (heat, cold, massage, drugs) relieve or heighten the pain? All of this information is important in assessing your patient's pain and should be documented.

Enter into the chart whichever interventions you take to alleviate your patient's pain, and doc-

ument the patient's responses to your interventions.

2/19/07	1610	Pt. admitted to room 304 with
		diagnosis of pancreatic cancer
		and severe pain in LLQ. Pt. tak-
		ing Percocet 2 tabs q 4 hr. at
		home without relief at present.
		Dr. Martin notified. Dilaudid
		2 mg. ordered and given I.V. @
		1600 hrs. VS stable. Pt. resting
		at present ———
		——— K. Comerford, RN

PATIENT-CONTROLLED ANALGESIA

Some patients may be receiving opioids via a patient-controlled analgesia (PCA) infusion pump. These pumps allow patients to self-administer boluses of an opioid analgesic I.V., subcutaneously, or epidurally within limits prescribed by the practitioner. To avoid overmedication, an adjustable lockout interval inhibits delivery of additional boluses until the appropriate time has elapsed. PCA increases the patient's sense of control and reduces anxiety, reduces drug use over the postoperative course, and gives enhanced pain control.

Be sure to document the amount of opioids used during your shift, and document the patient's response to the treatment and any patient teaching performed. (See *PCA flow sheet,* page 285.)

Codes

Guidelines established by the American Heart Association direct you to keep a written, chronological account of a patient's condition throughout resuscitative efforts. If you're a designated recorder for a patient's cardiopulmonary arrest record, document therapeutic interventions and the patient's responses to these as they occur. Don't rely on your memory to record the

(*Text continues on page 286.*)

ChartWizard

Assessing and documenting pain

Used appropriately, standard assessment tools, such as the McGill-Melzack Pain Questionnaire and the Initial Pain Assessment Tool (developed by McCaffery and Beebe), provide a solid foundation for your nursing diagnoses and care plans. If your health care facility doesn't use standardized pain questionnaires, you can devise other pain measurement tools, such as the pain flow sheet or the visual and graphic rating scales that appear below. Whichever pain assessment tool you choose, remember to document its use and include the graphic record in your patient's chart.

PAIN FLOW SHEET

Possibly the most convenient tool for pain assessment, a flow sheet provides a standard for reevaluating the patient's pain at ongoing and regular intervals. It's also beneficial for patients and families, who may feel too overwhelmed by the pain experience to answer a long, detailed questionnaire.

If possible, incorporate pain assessment into the flow sheet you're already using. Generally, the easier the flow sheet is to use, the more likely you and your patient will be to use it.

PAIN FLOW SHEET					
Date and time	Pain rating (0 to 10)	Patient behaviors	Vital signs	Pain rating after intervention	Comments
1/16/07 0800	7	Wincing, holding head	186/88 98–22	5	Dilaudid 2 mg I.M. given in R glut.
1/16/07 1200	3	Relaxing, reading	160/80 84–18	2	Tylox ẗ P.O. given

VISUAL ANALOG PAIN SCALE

In a visual analog pain scale, the patient marks a linear scale containing words or numbers that correspond to his perceived degree of pain. Draw a scale to represent a continuum of pain intensity.

Verbal anchors describe the pain's intensity; for example, "no pain" begins the scale and "pain as bad as it could be" ends it. Ask the patient to mark the point on the continuum that best describes his pain.

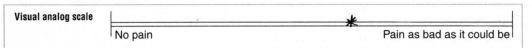

GRAPHIC RATING SCALES

Other rating scales have words that represent pain intensity. Use these scales as you would the

visual analog scale. Have the patient mark the spot on the continuum.

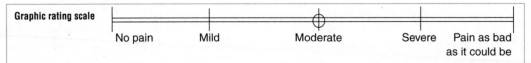

ChartWizard

PCA flow sheet

The form shown below is used to document the use of patient-controlled analgesia (PCA). PCA allows the patient to self-administer an opioid analgesic as needed, yet within limits prescribed by the practitioner.

Date _____ 2/22/07 _____

Medication (Circle one)   Meperidine 300 mg in 30 ml (10 mg/ml)
(Morphine 30 mg in 30 ml (1 mg/ml))

	7–3 Shift				3–11 Shift				11–7 Shift			
Time (enter in box)	1200	1400			1600							
New cartridge inserted	OR											
PCA settings Lockout interval ⎯7⎯ (minutes)		7			7							
Dose volume ⎯1⎯ (ml/dose)												
Four-hour limit 30												
Continuous settings ⎯1⎯ (mg/hr)												
Respiratory rate	18	20			20							
Blood pressure	150/70	130/62			128/70							
Sedation rating 1. Wide awake 2. Drowsy 3. Dozing, intermittent 4. Mostly sleeping 5. Only awakens when stimulated	1	2			3							
Analgesia rts (0 — 10) No Pain – 0 Maximum Pain – 10	7	8			6							
Additional doses given (optional doses)	3ml/OR											
Total ml's delivered (total from ampule)	3	6			15							
ml's remaining	27	24			15							

RN SIGNATURE (7–3 SHIFT) ____ Janet Green, RN ____   Date __ 2/22/07 __

RN SIGNATURE (3–11 SHIFT) ____ Karen Singleton, RN ____   Date __ 2/22/07 __

RN SIGNATURE (11–7 SHIFT) _____   Date _____

sequence of events. (See *Keeping a resuscitation record.*)

If a code is called, you'll complete a *code record,* a form that incorporates detailed information about the code (including observations, interventions, and any drugs given to the patient).

1/24/07	2100	Summoned to the pt.'s room at 2020 hr. by a shout from roommate. Found pt. unresponsive without respirations or pulse. Roommate stated, "He was talking to me; then all of a sudden he started gasping and holding his chest." Code called. Initiated CPR with Ann Barrow, RN. Code team arrived at 2023 hr. and continued resuscitative efforts. (See code record.) Pt. groaned and opened eyes at approx. 2030 hr. (see neurologic flow sheet). Notified Dr. Cooper at home at 2040 hr. and explained situation—will be in immediately. Pt. transferred to ICU @ 2035 hr. Family notified of pt.'s condition and transfer. —Delia Landers, RN

Some health care facilities use a resuscitation critique form to identify actual or potential problems with the resuscitation process. This form tracks personnel responses and response times as well as the availability of appropriate drugs and functioning equipment.

Change in patient's condition

One of your major documentation responsibilities is documenting any change in a patient's condition. Your note should include the patient's complaint, your assessment and interventions, who you notified, what you reported, and what instructions you received. When documenting your observations, avoid using vague words such

as "appears." For example, instead of merely writing "stools appear bloody," describe the stool's characteristics, such as color, amount, frequency, and consistency.

2/28/07	1500	Pt. had moderate sized, soft, dark brown stools positive for blood c̄ a guaiac test. —Jackie Paterno, RN.

Intake and output monitoring

Many patients require 24-hour intake and output monitoring. These include surgical patients, patients receiving I.V. therapy, patients with fluid and electrolyte imbalances, and patients with burns, hemorrhage, or edema.

You'll keep most intake and output sheets at the patient's bedside or by the bathroom door to remind you to measure and document his intake and output. If the patient is incontinent, document this as well as tube drainage and irrigation volumes.

For easy reference, list the volumes of specific containers. Infusion devices make documenting enteral and I.V. intake more accurate. However, keeping track of intake that isn't premeasured—for example, food such as gelatin that's normally fluid at room temperature—requires the cooperation of the patient, family members (who may bring him snacks and soft drinks or help him to eat at the health care facility), and other caregivers. Make sure that everyone understands how to record or report all foods and fluids that the patient consumes orally.

Don't forget to count I.V. piggyback infusions, drugs given by I.V. push, patient-controlled analgesics, and any irrigation solutions that aren't withdrawn. You'll also need to know whether the patient receives any fluids orally or I.V. when he isn't on your unit.

Recording fluid output accurately requires the cooperation of the patient and staff members in any other departments where your pa-

ChartWizard

Keeping a resuscitation record

Here's an example of the completed resuscitation record for inclusion in your patient's chart.

CODE RECORD

Pg. _/_ of _/_

Arrest Date: _4/9/07_
Arrest Time: _0630_
Rm/Location: _431-2_
Discovered by:
C. Brown
☑ RN ☐ MD
☐ Other

Methods of alert:
☑ Witnessed, monitored: rhythm _V fib_
☐ Witnessed, unmonitored
☐ Unwitnessed, unmonitored
☐ Unwitnessed, monitored; rhythm _____
Diagnosis: _Post anterior wall MI_

Condition when needed:
☑ Unresponsive
☐ Apneic
☐ Pulseless
☐ Hemorrhage
☐ Seizure

Ventilation management:
Time: _0635_
Method: _oral ET tube_
Precordial thump: _0631_
CPR initiated at: _0631_

Previous airway:
☐ ET tube
☐ Trach
☑ Natural

James, Anna
556677
DOB 01/06/28

Addressograph

CPR PROGRESS NOTES

	VITAL SIGNS						I.V. PUSH					INFUSIONS				ACTIONS/PATIENT RESPONSE
Time	Pulse CPR	Resp. rate Spont; bag	Blood pressure	Rhythm	Defib (joules)	Atropine	Epinephrine	Lidocaine	NA bicarb	Amiodarone	Lidocaine	Procain.	Amiodarone	Dopamine		Responses to therapy, procedures, labs drawn/results
0631	CPR	Bag	0	V fib			1 mg									No change.
0632		Bag	0	V fib	360											ABGs drawn. Ⓡ fem pressure applied.
0633	CPR	Bag	0	Asystole	360		1 mg									No change
0639	40	Bag	60 palp	SB PVCs				75			✔					Oral intubation by Dr. Hart
0645	60	Bag	80/40	SB PVCs							✔					CCU ready for patient

ABGs & Lab Data

Time Spec Sent	pH	PCO₂	Po₂	HCO₃	Sat%	Fio₂	Other
0633	7.1	76	43	14	80%		

Resuscitation outcome

☑ Successful ☑ Transferred to _CCU_ at _0648_
☐ Unsuccessful — Expired at _____
Pronounced by: _____ MD
Family notified by: _S. Quinn, RN_
Time: _0645_
Attending notified by: _S. Quinn, RN_   Time _0645_
Code Recorder _____ _S. Quinn, RN_
Code Team Nurse _____ _B. Mullen, RN_
Anesthesia Rep. _____ _J. Hanna, RN_
Other Personnel _____ _Dr. Hart_
B. Russo, RT

tient goes. Remind him to use a urinal or a commode if he's ambulatory.

The amount of fluid lost through the GI tract is normally 100 ml or less daily. However, if the patient's stools become excessive or watery, they must be counted as output. Vomiting, drainage from suction devices and wound drains, and bleeding are other measurable sources of fluid loss. (See *Charting intake and output*.)

Skin and wound care

The skin is the largest organ. Along with the hair, nails, and glands, it protects the body from microorganisms, ultraviolet light radiation, fluid loss, and the stress of mechanical forces. Most cuts, scrapes, and other minor wounds heal in a few days. When more serious wounds, such as pressure ulcers, fail to heal quickly and require long-term care and special assessments, careful documentation is essential.

PRESSURE ULCERS

The National Pressure Ulcer Advisory Panel defines a pressure ulcer as "any lesion caused by unrelieved pressure resulting in damage to underlying tissue." When assessing your patient for the potential to develop a pressure ulcer, you need to consider pressure, friction, shearing, and moisture as potential risk factors.

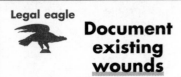

Legal eagle

Document existing wounds

Clearly note in the record whether a patient had a pressure ulcer upon admission or whether the ulcer developed in the health care facility. Be sure to follow your facility's policy when documenting your findings. Failure to document an existing wound on admission may result in legal action.

Because many patients are likely to develop pressure ulcers, always document findings related to the patient's skin condition. (See *Document existing wounds*.)

Many facilities now use assessment tools, such as the Braden Scale, to assess all patients at admission for the presence of or risk of developing pressure ulcers. (See chapter 7, Documentation in Long-Term Care, for an example of the Braden Scale.)

2/10/07	1400	Pt. admitted by stretcher to
		room 418B. Pt. lethargic, skin
		dry. Incontinent of urine. 1"
		wide black pressure ulcer noted
		on ® heel. Purulent, yellow
		drainage noted on ulcer's
		dressing. Dr. Kelly notified.
		Surgical consult ordered for
		debridement of ulcer. ® foot
		elevated on 2 pillows. Heel and
		elbow protectors applied. Skin
		lotion applied. Incontinent
		care given hourly. No other
		skin breakdown noted. Buttocks
		reddened but epidermis intact.
		———— Rachel Moreau, RN

When a chronically ill or immobile patient enters your unit with a pressure ulcer, record its location, appearance, size, depth, and color and the appearance of exudate from that ulcer.

Flow sheets that have defined cues can make your documentation easier. Even if you use a flow sheet, it's a good idea to write a note in the medical record if and when you notify a practitioner about any changes in the wound or surrounding tissue.

If the patient's skin condition worsens during hospitalization, his stay may be extended, in which case you'll need a clear record of skin care and related factors. This is especially important because family members typically think that

ChartWizard

Charting intake and output

As this sample shows, you can monitor your patient's fluid balance by using an intake and output record.

Name: _Josephine Klein_

Medical record #: _49731_

Admission date: _2/13/07_

INTAKE AND OUTPUT RECORD

| | INTAKE (ML) | | | | | | OUTPUT (ML) | | | | |
	Oral	Tube feeding	Instilled	I.V. and IVPB	TPN	Total	Urine	Emesis Tubes	NG	Other	Total
Date _2/15/07_											
0700–1500	250	320	H₂0 50	1100		1720	1355				1355
1500–2300	200	320	H₂0 50	1100		1670	1200				1200
2300–0700	0	320	H₂0 50	1100		1470	1500				1500
24hr total	450	960	H₂0 150	3300		4860	4055				4055
Date											
24hr total											
Date											
24hr total											
Date											
24hr total											

Key: IVPB = I.V. piggyback   TPN = total parenteral nutrition   NG = nasogastric

Standard measures

Styrofoam cup	240 ml	Water (large)	600 ml	Milk (large)	600 ml	Ice cream, sherbet,	
Juice	120 ml	Water pitcher	750 ml	Coffee	240 ml	or gelatin	120 ml
Water (small)	120 ml	Milk (small)	120 ml	Soup	180 ml		

Note: In the subscripts above, H₂0 represents H_2O.

pressure ulcers stem from poor nursing care, although certain risk factors—such as obesity, poor nutritional status, decreased hemoglobin level, immobility, infection, incontinence, and fractures—are equally responsible.

If your health care facility requires you to photograph pressure ulcers found at the time of admission, always date the photographs. You can then evaluate changes in a patient's skin condition by comparing his current skin integrity with previous photographs.

WOUND CARE

Wound assessment and care has changed dramatically in the past 15 years and is continually evolving. One major change has been the shift from dry dressings to moisture-retentive dressings. However, one factor that hasn't changed is the need for good documentation. When documenting a wound assessment, be sure to include all of these points:

▶ wound size, including length, width, and depth in centimeters
▶ wound shape
▶ wound site, drawn on a body plan to document the exact location
▶ wound stage
▶ characteristics of drainage, if any, including amount, color, and presence of odor
▶ characteristics of the wound bed, including description of tissue type, such as granulation tissue, slough, or epithelial tissue, and the percentage of each tissue type
▶ character of the surrounding tissue
▶ presence or absence of eschar
▶ presence or absence of pain
▶ presence or absence of undermining or tunneling (in centimeters).

2/14/07	1330	Pt. admitted to unit for fem-pop
		bypass tomorrow. Pt. has open
		wound at tip of 2nd Ⓛ toe,
		approx. 0.5 cm X 1 cm X 0.5 cm
		deep. Wound is round with even
		edges. Wound bed is pale with
		little granulation tissue. No drain-
		age, odor, eschar, or tunneling
		noted. Pt. reports pain at wound
		site, rates pain as 4/10, on 1-to-10
		scale w/10 being the worst pain
		imaginable. Surrounding skin cool
		to touch, pale, and intact. Pt.
		understands not to cross legs or
		wear tight garments. ———————
		—————————— Mark Silver, RN

Many facilities also have a special form or flow sheet on which to document wounds. (See *Wound and skin assessment tool.*)

Shift reports

Your facility may require an end-of-shift report (sometimes called a *unit report* or *24-hour report*). These documents, which track both conditions and activities on the unit, provide a running record of the patient census, staff-to-patient ratio, bed utilization, patient emergencies or acute changes, patient or family problems, incidents, equipment and supply problems, number of high-risk procedures, and other important data.

These reports are typically reviewed by nursing administrators charged with solving the day-to-day problems of a unit. (See *Documenting the events of your shift,* page 293.)

Personal property

Encourage patients to send home their money, jewelry, and other valuable belongings. If a pa-

ChartWizard

Wound and skin assessment tool

When performing a thorough wound and skin assessment, a pictorial demonstration is often helpful to identify the wound site or sites. Using this wound and skin assessment tool, the nurse has identified the left second toe as having a red partial-thickness wound, vascular ulcer, according to the classification of terms that follow.

PATIENT'S NAME (LAST, MIDDLE, FIRST)		ATTENDING PHYSICIAN		ROOM NUMBER	ID NUMBER
Brown, Ann		Dr. A. Dennis		123-2	01726

WOUND ASSESSMENT:

NUMBER	1	2	3	4	5	6
DATE	2/14/07					
TIME	1330					
LOCATION	Ⓛ second toe					
STAGE	II					
APPEARANCE	G					
SIZE-LENGTH	0.5 cm					
SIZE-WIDTH	1 cm					
COLOR/FLR.	RD					
DRAINAGE	O					
ODOR	O					
VOLUME	O					
INFLAMMATION	O					
SIZE INFLAM.						

KEY

Stage:
   I. Red or discolored
   II. Skin break/blister
   III. Sub 'Q' tissue
   IV. Muscle and/or bone

Appearance:
   D = Depth
   E = Eschar
   G = Granulation
   IN = Inflammation
   NEC = Necrotic
   PK = Pink
   SL = Slough
   TN = Tunneling
   UND = Undermining
   MX = Mixed (specify)

Color of Wound
Floor:
   RD = Red
   Y = Yellow
   BLK = Black
   MX = Mixed (specify)

Drainage:
   O = None
   SR = Serous
   SS = Serosanguinous
   BL = Blood
   PR = Purulent

Odor:
   O = None
   MLD = Mild
   FL = Foul

Volume:
   O = None
   SC = Scant
   MOD = Moderate
   LG = Large

Inflammation:
   O = None
   PK = Pink
   RD = Red

Wound and skin assessment tool *(continued)*

WOUND ANATOMICAL LOCATION:

(circle affected area)

Anterior   Posterior   Left lateral   Right lateral

Left foot   Right foot   Left hand   Right hand

Wound care protocol: *Clean wound with NSS.*

Signature: *Mark Silver, RN*   Date *2/14/07*

tient refuses to do so, make a list of his possessions and store them according to your facility's policy.

The list of the patient's valuables should include a description of each one. To protect yourself and your employer, ask the patient (or a re-

sponsible family member) to sign or witness the list that you compile so that you both understand which items you're responsible for.

Use objective language to describe each item, noting its color, approximate size, style, type, and serial number or other distinguishing feature.

ChartWizard

Documenting the events of your shift

Most health care facilities require the charge nurse to complete an end-of-shift report. The form below is an example of the information most facilities need to know.

Date: 2/26/07   **Charge nurse:** Donna Moriarty, RN   **Shift:** 7–3

Patient census: Start of shift 38   End of shift: 37
Number of admissions 2   Number of transfers 2 in, 3 out
Deaths O   Codes O
Comments
One patient transferred to SICU postop

Staff profile: Start of shift: 9   End of shift: 7
RNs 4   Orientees O   LPNs 3
Students O   Nursing assistants 2
Agency O   Other O
Called in sick Unit clerk – not replaced
Late O   Floated One aide, 1 LPN floated out halfway through shift

Unit workload during shift
Quiet _____   Busy but steady _____   Very busy X   Understaffed X

Equipment and supply problems
I.V. pumps not available. No sterile drsg. kits in supply cart. Not enough linen.

High-risk procedures performed
CVP line insertion, wound debridement, chest tube insertion

Assignment, personnel, or performance problems
Staff floated out 4 hr. into shift to cover sick calls on another unit – increased pt. ratio for rest of staff.

Patient or family problems
Mr. Hale in room 516-B – his condition deteriorated rapidly – developed acute abdomen and required emergency surgery. Family distraught – need time and privacy to speak with doctor and clergy.
Conference room is too small to accommodate more than 10 people (18 family members present). Because room doubles as staff lounge, privacy is difficult to maintain.

Number of incident reports filed: None   **Number of problem logs completed:** None

Don't assess the item's value or authenticity. For example, you might describe a diamond ring as a "clear, round stone set in a yellow metal band."

In addition to jewelry and money, include dentures, eyeglasses or contact lenses, hearing aids, prostheses, and clothing on the list. If your patient is homeless, he may have all of his personal belongings with him. You'll need to identify and tag each item.

2/18/07	1300	Pt. admitted to room 318 with
		one pair of brown glasses, upper
		and lower dentures, a yellow
		metal ring with a red stone, a
		pink bathrobe, and a black radio.
		———— Paul Cullen, RN

Place valuable items in an envelope and other personal belongings in approved containers; then label them with the patient's identification number. Never use garbage containers, laundry bags, or any other unauthorized receptacle for valuables; they could be discarded accidentally.

If the patient refuses to remove a ring, explain that it may have to be cut off if it compromises his circulation. If he decides to leave it on anyway, tape it in place. Be sure to document your conversation and actions.

▶ Challenging patient conditions

Some patient conditions, such as stroke and diabetic ketoacidosis, can be just as challenging to document as they are to provide care for. This section will help you to hone in on essential documentation for some of these challenging patients conditions.

Anaphylaxis

A severe reaction to an allergen after reexposure to the substance, anaphylaxis is a potentially lethal response requiring emergency intervention. Quickly assess the patient for airway, breathing, and circulation, and begin cardiopulmonary resuscitation as necessary. Remain with the patient, and monitor vital signs frequently. If the cause is immediately evident (a blood transfusion, for example), stop the infusion and keep the I.V. line open with a normal saline solution infusion. Contact the practitioner immediately and anticipate orders such as epinephrine injections. When the patient is stable, perform a thorough assessment to identify the cause of the anaphylactic reaction.

Document the date and time the anaphylactic reaction started. Record the events leading up to the anaphylactic response. Document the patient's signs and symptoms, such as anxiety, agitation, flushing, palpitations, itching, chest tightness, light-headedness, throat tightness or swelling, throbbing in the ears, or abdominal cramping. Include such assessment findings as arrhythmias, skin rash, wheals or welts, wheezing, decreased level of consciousness, unresponsiveness, angioedema, decreased blood pressure, weak or rapid pulse, and diaphoresis. Note the name of the practitioner notified, the time of notification, emergency treatments and supportive care given, and the patient's response. If the allergen is identified, note the allergen on the medical record, medication administration record, nursing care plan, patient identification bracelet, practitioner's orders, and dietary and pharmacy profiles. Document that appropriate departments and individuals were notified, including pharmacy, dietary, risk management, and the nursing supervisor. In addition, you may need to fill out an incident report form.

1/15/07	1600	Pt. received Demerol 50 mg I.M. at
		1500 for abdominal incision pain.
		At 1520 pt. was SOB, diaphoretic,
		and c/o intense itching "everywhere."
		Injection site on ® buttock has 4-
		cm erythematous area. Skin is
		blotchy and upper anterior torso
		and face are covered with hives. BP
		90/50, P 140, RR 44 in semi-
		Fowler's position. I.V. of D_5 1/2
		NSS infusing at 125 ml/hr in ®
		hand. O_2 sat. 94% via pulse
		oximetry on room air. O_2 at 2
		L/min via NC started with no
		change in O_2 sat. Dr. Brown
		notified of pt.'s condition at 1525
		and orders noted. Fluid challenge
		of 500 ml NSS over 60 min via ®
		antecubital began at 1535. O_2
		changed to 50% humidified face
		mask with O_2 sat. increasing to
		99%. After 15 min of fluid
		challenge, BP 110/70, P 104, RR 28.
		Benadryl 25 mg P.O. given for
		discomfort after fluid challenge
		absorbed. Allergy band placed on
		pt.'s ® hand for possible Demerol
		allergy. Chart, MAR, nursing plan
		of care, and doctor's orders
		labeled with allergy information.
		Pharmacy, dietary, and nursing
		supervisor, Barbara Jones, RN,
		notified. Pt. told he had what
		appeared to be an allergic reaction
		to Demerol, that he shouldn't
		receive it in the future, and that
		he should notify all health care
		providers and pharmacies of this
		reaction. Recommended that pt.
		wear a Medic Alert ID noting his
		allergic reaction to Demerol. Medic
		Alert order form given to pt.'s
		wife. ———————— Pat Sloan, RN

asymptomatic disturbances requiring no treatment to catastrophic ventricular fibrillation, which requires immediate resuscitation. Arrhythmias are classed according to their origin (ventricular or supraventricular). Their clinical significance depends on their effect on cardiac output and blood pressure. Your prompt detection and response to your patient's arrhythmia can mean the difference between life and death.

2/24/07	1700	While assisting pt. with ambulation
		in the hallway at 1640, pt. c/o
		feeling weak and dizzy. Pt. said he
		was "feeling my heart hammering
		in my chest." Pt. stated he never
		felt like this before. Apical rate
		170, BP 90/50, RR 24, peripheral
		pulses weak, skin cool, clammy, and
		diaphoretic. Denies chest pain or
		SOB. Breath sounds clear bilaterally.
		Pt. placed in wheelchair and
		assisted back to bed without
		incident. Dr. Brown notified at
		1645 and orders noted. Lab called
		to draw stat serum electrolyte and
		digoxin levels. O_2 via NC started
		at 2 L/min. Stat ECG revealed
		PSVT at a rate of 180. I.V.
		infusion of D_5W started in ® hand
		at 30 ml/hour with 18G cannula.
		Placed pt. on continuous cardiac
		monitoring with portable monitor
		from crash cart. At 1650 apical
		rate 180, BP 92/52, and pulses
		weakened all 4 extremities, lungs
		clear, skin cool and clammy. Still
		c/o weakness and dizziness. Patient
		transferred to telemetry unit.
		Report given to Nancy Powell, RN.
		Nursing supervisor, Carol Jones,
		RN, notified. ————————
		———————— Cathy Doll, RN

Arrhythmias

Arrhythmias occur when abnormal electrical conduction or automaticity changes heart rate or rhythm, or both. They vary in severity from mild,

Record the date and time of the arrhythmia. Document events before and at the time of the arrhythmia. Record the patient's symptoms and the findings of your cardiovascular assessment, such as pallor, cold and clammy skin, shortness of breath, palpitations, weakness, chest pain, dizziness, syncope, and decreased urine output. Include the patient's vital signs and heart rhythm (if the patient is on a cardiac monitor, place a rhythm strip in the chart). Note the name of the practitioner notified and time of notification. If ordered, obtain a 12-lead electrocardiogram and report the results. Document your interventions and the patient's response. Include any emotional support and education given.

Brain death

To help practitioners determine death in cases where the patient may be kept alive by medical equipment, such as ventilators, pacemakers, and intra-aortic balloon pumps, an ad hoc committee at Harvard Medical School published a report in 1968 establishing specific criteria for brain death:

▶ failure to respond to the most painful environmental stimuli
▶ absence of spontaneous respiratory or muscular movement
▶ absence of reflexes
▶ flat EEG.

They recommend that all these tests be repeated after 24 hours and that hypothermia and the presence of central nervous system depressants (such as barbiturates) be ruled out. In 1981, the American Medical Association, the American Bar Association, and the President's Commission for the Study of Ethical Problems in Medicine and Behavioral Research derived a working definition of brain death. The Uniform Determination of Death Act (UDODA) was then developed, which defines brain death as the cessation of all measurable functions or ac-

> **Legal eagle**
>
>
>
> # Know your state's laws concerning brain death
>
> In states without laws defining death or without judicial precedents, the common law definition of death (cessation of circulation and respiration) is still used. In these states, practitioners are understandably reluctant to discontinue artificial life support for brain-dead patients. If you're likely to be involved with patients on life-support equipment, protect yourself by finding out how your state defines death.

tivity in every area of the brain, including the brain stem. This definition excludes comatose patients as well as those in a persistent vegetative state.

It's important to know your state's laws regarding the definition of death. Exact criteria may also vary for determining brain death, depending on the facility. (See *Know your state's laws concerning brain death.*)

Your nurse's notes for a patient undergoing testing for brain death should include:

▶ the date and time of each test
▶ the name of the test
▶ the name of the person performing the test
▶ the response of the patient to the test, if any
▶ actions taken in response to the patient, such as your course of action if the patient had gone into ventricular fibrillation
▶ the time and names of any people notified of the results
▶ any support given to family members, if they're present.

In addition, individuals performing the tests, such as the EEG department and respiratory therapy, will need to complete their documentation in appropriate sections of the chart.

2/1/07	0800	ABG results obtained by Michael Burke with pt. on ventilator, respiratory therapist, at 0730. Results pH 7.40, PO_2 100, PCO_2 40. Pt. taken off ventilator by respiratory therapist and placed on 100% flowby. Dr. Brown in attendance. Cardiac monitor showing NSR at a rate of 70, O_2 sat. via continuous pulse oximetry 99%. Within 1 min of testing, heart rate 150 with PVCs, and O_2 sat. dropped to 95%. Pt. without spontaneous respirations. ABGs drawn by respiratory therapy showed pH 7.32, PO_2 60, PCO_2 60. Pt. placed back on ventilator. ———————— Dawn Silfies, RN

Chest pain

When your patient complains of chest pain, you'll need to act quickly to determine its cause. That's because chest pain may be caused by a disorder as benign as epigastric distress (indigestion) or as serious and life-threatening as acute myocardial infarction.

Record the date and time of onset of the chest pain. Question your patient about his pain, and record the responses using the patient's own words when appropriate. Include the following information:

▶ what the patient was doing when the pain started
▶ how long the pain lasted, if it had ever occurred before, and whether the onset was sudden or gradual
▶ whether the pain radiates

▶ factors that improve or aggravate the pain
▶ the exact location of the pain (Ask the patient to point to the pain and record his response. For example, he may move his hand vaguely around his abdomen or may point with one finger to his left chest.)
▶ severity of the pain. (Ask the patient to rank the pain on a 0 to 10 scale, with 0 indicating no pain and 10 indicating the worst pain imaginable.)

Record the patient's vital signs and a quick assessment of his body systems. Perform an electrocardiogram and be sure that it contains the correct patient label, date, and time. Document the time and name of anyone notified, such as the practitioner, nursing supervisor, or admissions department (if the patient is transferred). Record your actions and the patient's responses. Include any patient education and emotional support.

2/9/07	0410	Pt. c/o sudden onset of a sharp chest pain while sleeping. Points to center of chest, over sternum. States, "It feels like an elephant is sitting on my chest." Pain radiates to the neck and shoulders. Rates pain as 7 on a scale of 0 to 10. P 112, BP 90/62, RR 26. Lungs have fine rales in the bases on auscultation. Dr. Romano notified and orders received. Morphine 2 mg I.V. given. O_2 at 4 L/min started by NC. Continuous pulse oximetry started with O_2 sat. 94%. 12-lead ECG and MI profile obtained. ———————— Martha Wolcott, RN
2/9/07	0415	Dr. Romano here to see patient. Pt. states pain is now a 5 on a scale of 0 to 10. Morphine 2 mg I.V. repeated. ECG interpreted by Dr. Romano to show acute ischemia. Pt. prepared for transport to CCU. ———————— Martha Wolcott, RN

Diabetic ketoacidosis

Characterized by severe hyperglycemia, diabetic ketoacidosis (DKA) is a potentially life-threatening condition that most commonly occurs in people with type 1 diabetes (insulin-dependent). An acute insulin deficiency precedes DKA, causing glucose to accumulate in the blood. At the same time, the liver responds to energy-starved cells by converting glycogen to glucose, further increasing blood glucose levels. Because the insulin-deprived cells can't utilize glucose, they metabolize protein, which results in loss of intracellular potassium and phosphorus and excessive liberation of amino acids. The liver converts these amino acids into urea and glucose. The result is grossly elevated blood glucose levels and osmotic diuresis, leading to fluid and electrolyte imbalances and dehydration. Moreover, the absolute insulin deficiency causes cells to convert fats to glycerol and fatty acids for energy. The fatty acids accumulate in the liver, where they're converted to ketones. The ketones accumulate in blood and urine. Acidosis leads to more tissue breakdown, more ketosis and, eventually, shock, coma, and death.

Record the date and time of your entry. Frequently record your patient's blood glucose levels, intake and output, urine glucose levels, mental status, ketone levels, and vital signs, according to the patient's condition or your unit's policy. Depending on the facility, these parameters may be documented on a frequent assessment flow sheet. Record the clinical manifestations of DKA assessed, such as polyuria, polydipsia, polyphagia, Kussmaul respirations, fruity breath odor, changes in level of consciousness, poor skin turgor, hypotension, hypothermia, and warm, dry skin and mucous membranes. Document all interventions, such as fluid and electrolyte replacement and insulin therapy, and record the patient's response. Record any procedures, such as arterial blood gas analysis, blood samples sent to the laboratory, cardiac monitoring, or insertion of an indwelling urinary catheter. Record the results, the name of persons notified, and the time of notification. Include emotional support and patient education in your notes.

2/11/07	0810	Mr. Jones admitted at 0730 with
		serum blood glucose level of 900.
		Pt. c/o nausea, vomiting, and
		excessive urination. Urine positive
		for ketones. P 112, BP 94/58, RR
		28 deep and rapid, oral T 96.8° F.
		Skin warm, dry, with poor skin
		turgor. Mucous membranes dry.
		Resting with eyes closed. Confused
		to time and date. Pt. states, "I
		didn't take my insulin for 2 days
		because I ran out." Dr. Bernhart
		notified and came to see pt. Blood
		sample sent to lab for ABG,
		electrolytes, BUN, creatinine, serum
		glucose, CBC. Urine obtained and
		sent for UA. O₂ 2L via NC started
		with O₂ sat. 94% by pulse oximetry.
		1,000 ml of NSS being infused
		over 1 hr through I.V. line in Ⓡ
		forearm. 100 units I.V. bolus of
		regular insulin infused through
		I.V. line in Ⓛ antecubital followed
		by a cont. infusion of 100 units
		regular insulin in 100 ml NSS at
		5 units/hr. Monitoring blood
		glucose with q1hr fingersticks. Next
		due at 0900. See frequent param-
		eter flow sheet for I/O, VS, and
		blood glucose results. Notified
		diabetes educator, Teresa Mooney,
		RN, about pt.'s admission and the
		need for reinforcing diabetes
		regimen. ——— Louise May, RN

Hypertensive crisis

Hypertensive crisis is a medical emergency in which the patient's diastolic blood pressure suddenly rises above 120 mm Hg. Precipitating factors include abrupt discontinuation of antihypertensive drugs; increased salt consumption; increased production of renin, epinephrine, and norepinephrine; and added stress.

Record the date and time of your entry. Record the patient's blood pressure and the findings of your assessment of the patient's cardiopulmonary, neurologic, and renal systems, such as headache, nausea, vomiting, seizures, blurred vision, transient blindness, confusion, drowsiness, heart failure, pulmonary edema, chest pain, and oliguria. Document the measures you took to ensure a patent airway. Record the name of the practitioner you notified, the time of notification, and orders given, such as continuous blood pressure and cardiac monitoring, I.V. antihypertensive drugs, blood samples, supplemental oxygen, and seizure precautions. Document the patient's response to these interventions. Use the appropriate flow sheets to record intake and output, I.V. fluids, drugs, and frequent vital signs. Include patient teaching and emotional support given.

2/25/07	1500	Pt. arrived in ED with c/o headache,
		blurred vision, and vomiting. BP
		220/125, P 104 bounding, RR 16
		unlabored, oral T 97.4° F. Pt. states,
		"I stopped taking my blood pressure
		pills 2 days ago when I ran out."
		Drowsy, but oriented to place and
		person, knew year but not day of
		week or time of day. No c/o chest
		pain, neck veins not distended, lungs
		clear. Cardiac monitor shows sinus
		tachycardia, no arrhythmias noted.
		—————— Alan Walker, RN
		(continued)

2/25/07 (continued)	1500	Dr. Kelly notified and in to see pt.
		at 1045, orders written. O₂ at 4
		L/min. administered via NC. Dr. Kelly
		explained need for arterial line
		for BP monitoring. Pt. understands
		procedure and signed consent.
		Assisted Dr. Kelly with insertion of
		arterial line in Ⓛ radial artery using
		20G 2½" arterial catheter, after
		a positive Allen's test. Catheter
		secured with 1 suture. 4" X 4" gauze
		pad with povidone-iodine ointment
		applied. Ⓛ hand and wrist secured
		to arm board. Transducer leveled
		and zeroed. Initial readings
		238/124 mean arterial pressure
		162 mm Hg with pt.'s head at 30
		degrees. Readings accurate to cuff
		pressures. Line flushes easily. Pt.
		tolerated procedure well. I.V. line
		inserted in Ⓡ forearm with 18G
		catheter. Nitroprusside sodium
		50 mg in 250 ml D₅W started at
		0.30 mcg/kg/min. See frequent vital
		sign flow sheet for frequent vital
		signs. Blood sent to lab for stat CBC,
		ABG, electrolytes, BUN, creatinine,
		blood glucose level. Stat ECG and
		portable CXR done, results pending.
		Foley catheter inserted, urine sent
		for UA. Side rails padded, bed in
		low position, airway taped to
		headboard of bed, suction equipment
		placed in room. All procedures
		explained to pt. and wife. ———
		—————— Alan Walker, RN

Hypotension

Defined as blood pressure below the patient's normal, hypotension reduces perfusion to the tissues and organs of the body. Severe hypotension is a medical emergency that may progress to shock and death.

Record the date and time of your entry. Record the patient's blood pressure and other vital signs. Document your assessment findings, such as bradycardia; tachycardia; weak pulses; cool, clammy skin; oliguria; reduced bowel sounds; dizziness; syncope; reduced level of consciousness; and myocardial ischemia. Note the name of the practitioner notified, the time of notification, and any orders given, such as continuous blood pressure and cardiac monitoring, obtaining a 12-lead electrocardiogram, administering supplemental oxygen, and inserting an I.V. line for fluids and vasopressor drugs. Describe other interventions, such as lowering the head of the bed, inserting an indwelling urinary catheter, and assisting with insertion of hemodynamic monitoring lines. Document adherence to advanced cardiac life support protocols, using a code sheet to record interventions, if necessary. Use the appropriate flow sheets to record intake and output, I.V. fluids, drugs, and frequent vital signs. Record the patient's responses to these interventions. Include any emotional support and patient teaching.

2/1/07	1235	Pt. c/o dizziness at 1220. P 48, RR
		18, BP 86/48, oral T 97.6° F.
		Peripheral pulses weak, skin cool
		and diaphoretic, normal bowel
		sounds, clear breath sounds, alert
		and oriented to time, place, and
		person, no c/o chest pain.
		Continuous cardiac monitoring via
		portable monitor shows failure of
		permanent pacemaker to capture.
		Rhythm strip mounted below. Dr.
		King called at 1225, came to see
		pt., and orders given. 12-lead ECG
		done and confirms failure to
		capture. Placed on O2 2L by NC.
		—————— Kathy Thompson, RN

2/1/07	1235	(continued)
(continued)		Heparin lock started in ® forearm
		with 18G catheter. VS recorded
		q5min on frequent VS sheet. Stat
		portable CXR done at 1230.
		Explained pacemaker malfunction
		to pt. Assured her that she's being
		monitored and that a temporary
		pacemaker is available, if needed.
		Dr. King called pt.'s husband and
		told him of situation. ———————

Koller, Johanna   2/1/07   1235

2/1/07	1240	Dr. King explained that CXR
		showed a lead fracture in
		pacemaker wire requiring
		replacement. Procedure explained
		by doctor and informed consent
		signed. Pt. still c/o dizziness. P 46,
		R 20, BP 88/46. Preoperative
		teaching performed. Pt. states she
		remembers the procedure from
		last year when the pacemaker was
		inserted. Report called to Sally
		Lane, RN, in operating room.
		—————— Kathy Thompson, RN

Hypoxemia

Defined as a low concentration of oxygen in the arterial blood, hypoxemia occurs when the partial pressure of arterial oxygen (PaO_2) falls below 60 mm Hg. Hypoxemia causes poor tissue perfusion and may lead to respiratory failure.

Record the date and time of your entry. Record your patient's PaO_2 level and cardiopulmonary assessment findings, such as change in level of consciousness, tachycardia, increased blood pressure, tachypnea, dyspnea, mottled skin, cyanosis and, in patients with severe hypoxemia, bradycardia and hypotension. Chart the name of the practitioner notified, the time of notification, and any orders given. Record your interventions, such as measuring oxygen saturation by pulse oximetry, obtaining arterial blood gas values, providing supplemental oxygen, positioning the patient in a high Fowler position, assisting with endotracheal intubation, monitoring mechanical ventilation, and providing continuous cardiac monitoring. Document the patient's responses to these interventions. Use the appropriate flow sheets to record intake and output, I.V. fluids, drugs, and frequent vital signs. Include any emotional support and patient teaching.

2/19/07	1400	Pt. restless and confused, SOB, skin
		mottled. P 112, BP 148/78, RR 32
		labored, rectal T 97.4° F. Dr. Bou-
		chard notified and came to see pt.
		ABGs drawn by Dr. Tara Aims and
		sent to lab. Pulse oximetry 86% on
		O₂ 3 L/min by NC. Placed on O₂
		100% via nonrebreather mask with
		pulse oximetry 92%. Pt. positioned
		in high Fowler's position. Continuous
		cardiac monitoring shows sinus
		tachycardia at 116, no arrhythmias
		noted. Radiology called for stat
		portable CXR. Dr. Bouchard notified
		wife of change in husband's status.
		——————— Donna Damico, RN

Intracerebral hemorrhage

Intracerebral hemorrhage is the result of the rupture of a cerebral vessel that causes bleeding into the brain tissue. This type of hemorrhage usually causes extensive loss of function and has very slow recovery and poor prognosis. The ef-

fects of the hemorrhage depend on the site and extent of the bleeding. Intracerebral hemorrhage may occur in patients with hypertension or atherosclerosis. Other causes include aneurysm, arteriovenous malformation, tumors, trauma, or bleeding disorders.

Record the date and time of your entry. Evaluate the patient's airway, breathing, and circulation, and document your findings, actions taken, and the patient's response. Record your neurologic assessment (such as reduced level of consciousness, confused, restless, agitated, lethargic, comatose), pupillary changes (including unequal size, sluggish or absent response to light), headache, seizures, focal neurologic signs, increased blood pressure, widened pulse pressure, bradycardia, decorticate or decerebrate posturing, and vomiting. Document the name of the practitioner notified, the time of notification, and the orders given. Record your actions, such as drug and fluid administration, assisting with intracranial pressure monitoring insertion, administering oxygen, assisting intubation, and maintaining mechanical ventilation. Chart the patient's responses to these interventions. Record any patient and family teaching and support given.

Assess your patient frequently and record the specific time and results of your assessments. Use the appropriate flow sheets to record intake and output, I.V. fluids, drugs, and frequent hemodynamic measurements and vital signs. A critical care flow sheet also may be used to document frequent assessments. A neurologic flow sheet that includes the Glasgow Coma Scale or the National Institutes of Health Stroke Scale may be used to record your frequent neurologic assessments.

2/1/07	0810	Pt. found in bed at 0735
		unresponsive to verbal stimuli but
		grimaces and opens eyes with
		painful stimuli. PERRL. Moving ®
		side of body but not Ⓛ. Airway is
		patent, with unlabored breathing.
		BP 100/60, P 72 reg, RR 16, rectal
		T 98° F. Breath sounds clear,
		normal heart sounds. Skin cool,
		dry. Peripheral pulses palpable. Dr.
		Martinez notified at 0740 and
		orders given. Administering O₂ at
		2L/min by NC. I.V. infusion
		started in ® forearm with 18G
		catheter. NSS infusing at 30 ml/
		hour Foley catheter inserted. MRI
		scheduled for 0900. Dr. Martinez
		in to see pt. at 0750. Dr. called
		family to notify them of change in
		pt.'s condition. Family consented to
		MRI. Glasgow score of 7. See
		Glasgow Coma Scale, I.V., I/O, and
		VS flow sheets for frequent
		assessments. — Juanita Perez, RN

Myocardial infarction, acute

A myocardial infarction (MI) is an occlusion of a coronary artery that leads to oxygen deprivation, myocardial ischemia and, eventually, necrosis. The extent of functional impairment depends on the size and location of the infarct, the condition of the uninvolved myocardium, the potential for collateral circulation, and the effectiveness of compensatory mechanisms.

Mortality is high when treatment for MI is delayed; however, prognosis improves if vigorous treatment begins immediately. Therefore, prompt recognition of MI and nursing interventions to relieve chest pain, stabilize heart rhythm, reduce cardiac workload, and revascularize the coronary artery are essential to preserving myocardial tissue and preventing complications, including death.

Record the date and time of your entry. Describe the patient's symptoms of MI, using his own words whenever possible. Record your assessment findings, such as feelings of impending doom, chest pain, anxiety, restlessness, fatigue, nausea, vomiting, dyspnea, tachypnea, cool extremities, weak peripheral pulses, diaphoresis, third or fourth heart sounds, a new murmur, pericardial friction rub, low-grade fever, hypotension or hypertension, bradycardia or tachycardia, and crackles on lung auscultation.

Document the name of the practitioner you notified, the time of notification, and the orders given, such as transfer to the coronary care unit, continuous cardiac monitoring, supplemental oxygen, 12-lead electrocardiogram, I.V. therapy, cardiac enzymes (including troponin and myoglobin), nitroglycerin (sublingual or via an I.V. line), thrombolytic therapy, aspirin, morphine, bed rest, antiarrhythmics, beta-adrenergic blockers, angiotensin-converting enzyme inhibitors, and heparin.

Document your actions and the patient's response to these therapies. Use the appropriate flow sheets to record intake and output, hemodynamic parameters, I.V. fluids, drugs, and frequent vital signs. Record what you teach the patient, such as details about the disease process, treatments, drugs, signs and symptoms to report, exercise, sexual activity, proper nutrition, smoking cessation, support groups, and cardiac rehabilitation programs. Include emotional support given to the patient and family in your documentation.

1/30/07	2310	Pt. c/o severe crushing midsternal
		chest pain with radiation to Ⓛ arm
		at 2240. Pt. pointed to center of
		chest and stated, "I feel like I have
		an elephant on my chest." Rates pain
		at 9 on a 1 to 10 scale w/ 10 being
		worst pain imaginable. Pt. is restless
		in bed and diaphoretic, c/o nausea.
		P 84 and regular, BP 128/82, RR 24,
		oral T 98.8° F. Extremities cool,
		pedal pulses weak, normal heart
		sounds, breath sounds clear. Dr.
		Boone notified of pt.'s chest pain
		and physical findings at 2245 and
		came to see pt. and orders given.
		O₂ started at 2 L by NC. 12-lead
		ECG obtained; showed ST-segment
		elevation in anterior leads. Pt.
		placed on portable cardiac monitor.
		I.V. line started in Ⓛ forearm with
		18 G catheter with NSS at 30ml/
		hour. Lab called for stat cardiac
		enzymes, troponin, myoglobin, and
		electrolytes. Nitroglycerin 1/150 gr
		given SL, 5 minutes apart X 3 with
		no relief. Explaining all procedures
		to pt. Assuring him that he's being
		monitored closely and will be
		transferred to CCU for closer
		monitoring and treatment. Dr.
		Boone called wife and notified her
		of husband's chest pain and
		transfer. Report called to CCU at
		2255 and given to Laurie Feldman,
		RN. ——— Patricia Silver, RN

Pulmonary edema

Pulmonary edema is a diffuse extravascular accumulation of fluid in the tissues and airspaces of the lungs due to increased pressure in the pulmonary capillaries. Normally, fluid that crosses the capillary membrane and enters the lung is removed by the pulmonary lymphatic system. If the left ventricle fails, blood backs up into the pulmonary vasculature, and capillary pressure increases. Fluid crosses the membrane in amounts greater than the lymphatics can drain. Fluid builds up in the interstitial tissues, then in the alveoli. Pulmonary edema can occur as a chronic condition, or it can develop quickly and rapidly become fatal.

2/17/07	0300	Pt. discovered lying flat in bed at
		0230 trying to sit up and stating,
		"I can't breathe." Pt. coughing and
		bringing up small amount of pink
		frothy sputum. Skin pale, lips
		cyanotic, sluggish capillary refill, +1
		ankle edema. Lungs with crackles
		½ way up bilaterally, S₃ heard on
		auscultation of heart. P 120 and
		irregular, BP 140/90, RR 30 and
		shallow, tympanic T 98.8° F. Pt.
		restless, alert, and oriented to
		time, place, and person. Dr. Green
		notified of assessment findings at
		0235 and came to see pt. at
		0245. Pt. placed in sitting position
		with legs dangling. O₂ via NC at 2
		L/min changed to nonrebreather
		mask at 12 L/min. Explained to pt.
		that mask would give her more O₂
		and help her breathing. O₂ sat. by
		pulse oximetry 81%. Stat portable
		CXR done. 12-lead ECG shows sinus
		tachycardia with occasional PVCs.
		CBC and electrolytes drawn and
		sent to lab stat. Morphine,
		furosemide, and digoxin I.V.
		ordered and given through saline
		lock in Ⓛ forearm. See MAR.
		Indwelling urinary catheter
		inserted to straight drainage,
		drained 100 ml on insertion. Pt.
		encouraged to cough and deep
		breathe. Explained all procedures
		and drugs to pt. See flow sheets
		for documentation of frequent
		VS, I/O, and lab values. ———
		——— Rachel Moreau, RN

Record the date and time of your entry. Document your assessment findings of pulmonary edema, such as dyspnea, orthopnea, use of accessory muscles, pink frothy sputum, diaphoresis, cyanosis, tachypnea, tachycardia, adventitious breath sounds (such as crackles, wheezing, or rhonchi), pleural rub, neck vein distention, and increased intensity of the pulmonic component of S_2 and S_3 heart sounds. Note the name of the practitioner notified, time of notification, and orders given, such as oxygen and drug administration. Record your interventions, such as positioning the patient with legs dangling, inserting I.V. lines, administering oxygen and drugs, assisting with the insertion of hemodynamic monitoring lines, and suctioning. Chart the patient's responses to these interventions. Use flow sheets to record your frequent assessments, vital signs, hemodynamic measurements, intake and output, I.V. therapy, and laboratory and arterial blood gas values. Include patient teaching and emotional care given.

Stroke

Stroke is a sudden impairment of cerebral circulation in one or more of the blood vessels supplying the brain. A stroke interrupts or diminishes oxygen supply and commonly causes serious damage or necrosis in brain tissues. Clinical features of stroke vary with the artery affected and, consequently, the portion of the brain it supplies, the severity of damage, and the extent of collateral circulation. Stroke may be caused by thrombosis, embolus, or intracerebral hemorrhage and may be confirmed by computed tomography or magnetic resonance imaging. Treatment options vary, depending on the cause of the stroke.

The sooner you detect signs and symptoms of a stroke, the sooner your patient can receive treatment and the better his prognosis may be.

Record the date and time of your nurse's note. Record the events leading up to the suspected stroke and the signs you noted. If the patient can communicate, record symptoms using his own words. Evaluate the patient's airway, breathing, and circulation. Document your findings, actions taken, and the patient's response. Record your neurologic and cardiovascular assessments, actions taken, and patient response. Document the name of the practitioner notified, the time of notification, and whether orders were given.

2/10/07	2030	When giving pt. her medication at
		2015, noted drooping of Ⓛ eyelid
		and Ⓛ side of mouth. Pt. was in bed
		breathing comfortably with RR 24,
		P 112, BP 142/72, axillary T 97.2°
		F. PEARLA, awake and aware of her
		surroundings, answering yes and no
		by shake of head, speech slurred
		with some words inappropriate.
		Follows simple commands. Ⓛ hand
		grasp weaker than Ⓡ hand grasp. Ⓛ
		foot slightly dropped and weaker
		than Ⓡ. Glasgow score of 13. See
		Glasgow Coma Scale flow sheet for
		frequent assessments. Skin cool,
		dry. Peripheral pulses palpable.
		Brisk capillary refill. Called Dr. Lee
		at 2020. Stat CT scan ordered.
		Administered O_2 at 2 L/min by NC.
		I.V. infusion of NSS at 30 ml/
		hour started in Ⓡ forearm with
		18G catheter. Continuous pulse
		oximetry started with O_2 sat. of
		96% on 2 L O_2. Dr. Lee in to see
		pt. at 2025. Pt. being prepared
		for transfer to ICU. Dr. Lee will
		notify family of transfer. ————
		———————— Luke Newell, RN

ChartWizard

Using the N.I.H. Stroke Scale

CATEGORY	DESCRIPTION	SCORE	BASELINE DATE/TIME	DATE/TIME
1a. Level of consciousness (LOC)	Alert Drowsy Stuporous Coma	0 1 2 3	2/15/07 1100 1	
1b. LOC questions (Month, age)	Answers both correctly Answers one correctly Incorrect	0 1 2	0	
1c. LOC commands (Open/close eyes, make fist, let go)	Obeys both correctly Obeys one correctly Incorrect	0 1 2	1	
2. Best gaze (Eyes open — patient follows examiner's finger or face.)	Normal Partial gaze palsy Forced deviation	0 1 2	0	
3. Visual (Introduce visual stimulus/threat to patient's visual field quadrants.)	No visual loss Partial hemianopia Complete hemianopia Bilateral hemianopia	0 1 2 3	1	
4. Facial palsy (Show teeth, raise eyebrows, and squeeze eyes shut.)	Normal Minor Partial Complete	0 1 2 3	2	
5a. Motor arm — left (Elevate extremity to 90 degrees and score drift/movement.)	No drift Drift Can't resist gravity No effort against gravity No movement Amputation, joint fusion (explain)	0 1 2 3 4 9	4	
5b. Motor arm — right (Elevate extremity to 90 degrees and score drift/movement.)	No drift Drift Can't resist gravity No effort against gravity No movement Amputation, joint fusion (explain)	0 1 2 3 4 9	0	

Using the N.I.H. Stroke Scale *(continued)*

CATEGORY	DESCRIPTION	SCORE	BASELINE DATE/TIME		DATE/ TIME	
6a. Motor leg — left (Elevate extremity to 30 degrees and score drift/movement.)	No drift Drift Can't resist gravity No effort against gravity No movement Amputation, joint fusion (explain)	0 1 2 3 4 9	4			
6b. Motor leg — right (Elevate extremity to 30 degrees and score drift/movement.)	No drift Drift Can't resist gravity No effort against gravity No movement Amputation, joint fusion (explain)	0 1 2 3 4 9	0			
7. Limb ataxia (Finger-nose, heel down shin)	Absent Present in one limb Present in two limbs	0 1 2	0			
8. Sensory (Pinprick to face, arm, trunk, and leg — compare side to side.)	Normal Partial loss Severe loss	0 1 2	R L 0 2		R L	
9. Best language (Name items; describe a picture and read sentences.)	No aphasia Mild to moderate aphasia Severe aphasia Mute	0 1 2 3	1			
10. Dysarthria (Evaluate speech clarity by patient repeating listed words.)	Normal articulation Mild to moderate dysarthria Near to unintelligible or worse Intubated or other physical barrier	0 1 2 9	1			
11. Extinction and inattention (Use information from prior testing to identify neglect or double simultaneous stimuli testing.)	No neglect Partial neglect Complete neglect	0 1 2	0			
		Total	17			

Individual Administering Scale: *Helen Hareson, RN*

Assess the patient frequently, and record the specific time and results of your assessments. Avoid using block charting. Use a frequent vital sign assessment sheet to document vital signs. A neurologic flow sheet such as the N.I.H. Stroke Scale may be used to record your frequent neurologic assessments. (See *Using the N.I.H. Stroke Scale,* pages 305 and 306.)

Common charting flaws

Ideally, every chart you receive from the nurse on the previous shift will be complete and accurate. Unfortunately, this isn't always the case. Although you can't necessarily affect what other nurses do, you can try to make your own charting flawless so it doesn't mislead other caregivers.

Blank spaces in chart or flow sheet

Follow your facility's policy regarding blank spaces on forms. A blank space may imply that you failed to give complete care or assess the patient fully.

Because flow sheets have increased in size (sometimes to four to six pages), nurses may be required to fill in only those fields or prompts that apply to their patient. It's now common for health care facilities to have a written policy on how to complete such forms correctly. For example, if information requested on a form doesn't apply to a particular patient, your facility's policy may require you to write "N/A" (not applicable) or draw a line through empty spaces.

2/9/07	1500	20 y/o male admitted to room 418B by wheelchair. #20 angiocath inserted in ℝ antecubital vein with I.V. of 1,000 ml D5-½NSS infusing at 125 ml/hr. O₂ at 2 L/min. via NC. Demerol 50 mg given I.M. for abdominal pain. Relief reported.————
		———————— David Dunn, RN

This leaves no doubt that you addressed every part of the record. It also prevents others from inserting information that could change the meaning of your original documentation.

Care given by someone else

Unless you document otherwise, anyone reading your notes assumes that they're a firsthand account of care provided. In some settings, nursing assistants and technicians aren't allowed to make formal charting entries. If this is the case in your facility, determine what care was provided, assess the patient and the task performed (for example, a dressing change), and document your findings. Be sure to record the full names and titles of unlicensed personnel who provided care; don't record just their initials.

1/23/07	0600	Morning care provided by Kevin Lawson, NA, who stated that patient moaned when being turned.————
		————Camille Dunn, RN

If your facility allows unlicensed personnel to chart, you may have to countersign their notes. If your facility's policy states that the unlicensed person must provide care in your presence, don't countersign unless you actually witness her actions. If the policy says that you don't have to be there, your countersigning indicates that the note describes care that the other person had the authority and competence to perform and that you verified that the procedure was performed.

You can specifically document that you reviewed the notes and consulted with the technician or assistant on certain aspects of care. Of course, you must document any follow-up care you provide. (For more information on countersigning, see chapter 12, Legally Perilous Charting Practices.)

Late entries

Late entries are appropriate in several situations:
▶ if the chart was unavailable when you needed it—for example, when the patient was away from the unit (in X-ray or physical therapy)
▶ if you need to add important information after completing your notes
▶ if you forgot to write notes on a particular chart.

| 2/14/07 | 0900 | (Chart not available 2/13/07 1500 hr.) On 2/13 @ 1300 hr., pt. stated she felt faint when getting OOB on 2/13 @ 1200 hr and fell to the floor. States she did not hurt herself and did not think she had to tell anyone about this until her husband encouraged her to report it. No bruises or lacerations noted. Pt. denies pain. Dr. Muir examined pt. at 1320 hr on 2/13. ————— Elaine Kasmer, RN |

Legal eagle

Avoid late additions

If the court uncovers alterations in a patient's chart during the course of a trial, suspicions may be aroused. The court may logically infer that additional alterations were made. In such situations, the value of the entire medical record may be brought into question.

That's what happened to a nurse who failed to chart her observations of a postoperative patient for 7 hours, during which time the patient died. The patient's family later sued the hospital, charging the nurse with malpractice. The nurse insisted that she had observed the patient, but because her particular unit was understaffed and overpopulated, she wasn't able to record her observations. She explained that the assistant director of nursing later instructed her about the hospital's policy on charting late additions. The nurse subsequently added her observations to the patient's medical record.

However, the court wasn't convinced that the nurse had indeed observed the patient during the postoperative period. Suspicious of the altered record, it ruled that the nurse's failure to chart her observations at the proper time supported the plaintiff's claim that she had made no such observations.

Keep in mind, however, that a late or altered chart entry can arouse suspicions and can be a significant problem in the event of a malpractice lawsuit. (See *Avoid late additions.*)

If you must make a late entry or alter an earlier entry, find out if your facility has a protocol for doing so. If it doesn't, the best approach is to add the entry to the first available line and label

ChartWizard

Correcting a charting error

When you make a mistake documenting on the medical record, correct it by drawing a single line through it and writing the words "mistaken entry" above or beside it. Follow these words with your initials and the date. If appropriate, briefly explain the necessity for the correction.

Make sure that the mistaken entry is still readable. This indicates that you're only trying to correct a mistake, not cover it up.

Date	Time	Progress notes
1/19/07	0900	Mistaken entry J.M. 1/19/07 ~~Pt. walked to bathroom.~~
		~~States he experienced no~~
		~~difficulty urinating.~~
		——————— John Mora, RN

it "late entry" to indicate that it's out of sequence. Then record the time and date of the entry and, in the body of the entry, record the time and date it should have been made.

Corrections

When you make a mistake on a chart, correct it promptly. Never erase, cover, completely scratch out, or otherwise obscure an erroneous entry because this may imply a cover-up. If the chart ends up in court, the plaintiff's attorney will be looking for anything that may cast doubt on the chart's accuracy. Erasures or the use of correction fluid or heavy black ink to obliterate an error are red flags. (See *Correcting a charting error.*)

Patient noncompliance

It isn't unheard of for a patient to refuse to comply with nursing or medical interventions—for example, a patient may violate such common instructions as "Follow your diet," "Don't get out of bed without assistance," "Take your medicine as directed," or "Keep your practitioner's appointment for a checkup." Beyond re-explaining the importance of following such instructions after an incident occurs, there's little you can do. However, you must chart the noncompliance.

In the chart, describe any patient behavior that goes against your instructions, and report the problem to the appropriate person. Note any attempts to encourage the patient's compliance, even if unsuccessful. If the patient's care is questioned later, the record will be an important factor in your defense. Below you'll find examples of specific types of noncompliance.

Dietary restrictions

If your patient is on dietary restrictions and you discover unauthorized food or beverages at his bedside, point out to him the need to follow his prescribed dietary plan. Document the noncompliance and your patient teaching, and notify the patient's practitioner.

2/17/07	1400	Pt. found with milkshake and
		cookies at bedside. Discussed
		with pt. his need to maintain
		1,800-calorie ADA diet. Pt. re-
		fused to remove these foods,
		stating, "I'll eat what I want."
		Dr. Mayer notified that pt. is
		not complying with prescribed
		diabetic diet. Dietitian called to
		meet with pt. and wife. ————
		———— Claire Bowen, RN

Out of bed against advice

Even after you've told a patient that he must not get out of bed alone and that he must call you for help, you may go to his room and find him climbing over the bed rails or discover relatives helping him to the bathroom because they don't want to disturb you.

Either scenario puts the patient at risk for a fall and you at risk for a lawsuit. What can you do? You can clearly document your instructions and anything that the patient does in spite of them. Be sure to include any devices being used to ensure patient safety, such as bed alarms or leg alarms. This shows that you recognized the potential for a fall and that you tried to prevent it.

2/10/07	0300	Assisted pt. to bathroom. Weak,
		unsteady on feet. States she
		gets dizzy when she stands. In-
		structed pt. to call for assis-
		tance to get OOB. Side rails up.
		Call button within reach. ————
		———— Joseph Romano, RN
2/10/07	0430	Found pt. walking to bathroom.
		Stated she got OOB by herself.
		Reminded her to call for assis-
		tance. Said she understood. ———
		———— Joseph Romano, RN

Medication abuse or refusal

If the patient refuses or abuses prescribed medication, describe the event in his chart. Here are some examples of situations that need careful documentation:

▶ You discover unprescribed drugs at the patient's bedside. Document the type of medication (pills or powders), the amount, and its appearance (color and shape).

▶ You find a supply of his prescribed drugs in his bedside table, indicating that he's hoarding his medication instead of swallowing each dose. Record the type of medication that you found and the amount.

▶ You try to give the patient prescribed medications but he refuses. Document his refusal and the reason for it, assuming he tells you. Also be sure to name the medications. Taking these steps will ensure that the patient's refusal isn't misinterpreted as an omission or a medication error on your part.

▶ You observe that the patient's behavior suddenly changes after he has visitors, and you suspect the visitors of providing him with contraband (opioids or other drugs, for example). Document how the patient appeared before and after the visitors came to see him.

1/2/07	1100	Visitor present at bedside. Pt.
		alert, oriented. I.V. D₅¹/₂NSS
		infusing at 125 ml/hr. ————
		————Eileen Sullivan, RN
1/2/07	1125	Upon entering room, I found
		pt. lethargic. Pupils were con-
		stricted, speech was slurred. Pt.
		stated, "My friend gave me
		something to help with the
		pain." Dr. Ettingoff notified
		and told of lethargy, slurred
		speech, and pinpoint pupils.
		———— Eileen Sullivan, RN
1/2/07	1130	Dr. Ettingoff in to see pt. Nar-
		can administered as ordered.
		———— Eileen Sullivan, RN

Discharge instructions

At discharge, review the discharge instructions and discuss the date on which the patient will have a follow-up evaluation. If the patient will make the appointment himself, encourage him to do so, explaining the need for ongoing medical care.

Document the date on which the patient is expected to return for a follow-up visit and the date on which you discussed the appointment with him. This protects you from claims that you neglected to inform him of the need to return for medical care.

Also document any related patient teaching that you performed and any written instructions that you provided. Be sure to document that you provided the patient with a complete and accurate list of his discharge medications, per The Joint Commission requirements.

If feasible, mail a reminder letter with a return receipt requested. If you should be accused of negligence related to follow-up care, you can then point to tangible evidence of your attempt to encourage the patient's compliance.

1/12/07	1300	Pt. notified to return to see
		Dr. Bonn on 1/26/07 at 0900.
		Discussed this with pt. and his
		wife. ————————————————
		———— Laura E. Cray, RN

Refusing treatment

Refusing treatment isn't just an important patient care and safety issue—it's a critical documentation concern as well.

Any mentally competent adult can refuse treatment. And in most cases, the health care personnel who are responsible for the patient's care can remain free of legal jeopardy as long as they fully inform the patient about his medical condition and the likely consequences of refusing treatment. The courts recognize a competent adult's right to refuse medical treatment, even when that refusal will clearly result in his death.

When your patient refuses treatment, inform him of the risks involved in making such a decision. If possible, inform him in writing. If he continues to refuse, notify the practitioner, who will then decide on the most appropriate plan of action.

2/8/07	2000	Pt. refusing to have I.V. inser-
		ted, stating that he's "sick and
		tired of being stuck." Explained
		to pt. the need for I.V. fluids
		and antibiotics and risks of
		refusing treatment. Dr. Eisen-
		berg notified. Dr. Eisenberg spent
		time with pt. Pt. still refusing
		I.V. Orders written to force
		fluids, repeat electrolytes in
		morning, and give amoxicillin P.O.
		———— Barbara Tyson, RN

Make sure that you document the patient's exact words in the chart. To protect yourself legally, document that you didn't provide the prescribed treatment because the patient refused it. Then ask the patient to sign a refusal-of-treatment release form.

If the patient refuses to sign the release form, document this refusal in the progress notes. For additional protection, your facility's policy may require you to ask the patient's spouse or closest relative to sign another refusal-of-treatment release form. Document whether the spouse or another relative does this. (See chapter 2, Legal and Ethical Implications of Documentation.)

Interdisciplinary communication

Because health care involves teamwork, all inter-departmental and interdisciplinary communication about the patient must be documented. This includes calls from the laboratory informing you of a patient's test results, calls you make to the practitioner about the patient's condition, and calls from patients requesting advice. In addition, you may on occasion have to give a patient's family bad news over the telephone, and this too must be noted in the chart.

Information from other departments

When a department, such as the laboratory or X-ray department, notifies your unit of a patient's test results, you must notify the practitioner of any abnormal results and then document your notification, including the practitioner's name and the time he was notified. Consult your facility's policy for specific requirements regarding reporting critical test values and results.

1/4/07	1400	Laboratory technician Donald Boyle called floor to report pt.'s random blood glucose level of 486. Dr. Somers notified. Stat blood glucose ordered. Pt. being monitored until results available. ———— Peggy Irwin, RN

Reports to practitioners

You've just phoned the practitioner to tell him about his patient's deteriorating condition. He listens as you give laboratory test results and the patient's signs and symptoms, thanks you for the information, and hangs up—without giving you an order. Unless you properly document your

conversation with him, the practitioner could claim he wasn't notified, should this patient's care subsequently come into question. (See *Ensuring clear communication.*)

Nurses commonly write, "Notified practitioner of patient's condition." This statement is too vague. In the event of a malpractice suit, it allows the plaintiff's lawyer (and the practitioner) to imply that you didn't communicate the essential data. The chart should include exactly what you told the practitioner.

2/15/07	2215	Called Dr. Spencer regarding
		increased serous drainage
		from pt.'s Ⓛ chest tube. Dr.
		Spencer's order was to ob-
		serve the drainage for 1 more
		hr and then call him. ————
		————Danielle Bergeron, RN

Telephone advice to patients

Nurses, especially those working in hospital emergency departments (ED), commonly get requests to give advice to patients by telephone. A hospital has no legal duty to provide a telephone-advice service, and you have no legal duty to give advice to anyone who calls.

The best response to a telephone request for medical advice is to tell the caller to come to the hospital because you can't assess his condition or treat him over the phone. As with all rules, however, this one has its exceptions—for example, a life-threatening situation when someone needs immediate care, treatment, or referral.

ACCEPTING RESPONSIBILITY

If you dispense advice over the phone, keep in mind that a legal duty arises the minute you say, "Okay, let me tell you what to do." You now have a nurse-patient relationship, and you're responsible for any advice you give. After you start to give advice by telephone, you can't decide midway through that you're in over your head and simply hang up; that could be considered abandonment. You must give appropriate advice or a referral—for example, "After listening to you, I strongly suggest that you come to the emergency department or call your practitioner."

If the caller is a patient you cared for recently, you may choose to give him advice. For example, if the practitioner prescribed medication and gave him an instruction sheet, you probably told him to call if he had any questions. Obviously, you wouldn't refuse to answer his questions if he called. However, you may prefer to direct some questions to the practitioner, especially if the patient's symptoms have changed.

If you do decide to give telephone advice, establish a system of documenting such calls—with a telephone log, for example. The log should include the date and time of the call, name of the caller, address of the caller, caller's request or chief complaint, disposition of the call, and name of the person who made that disposition.

2/6/07	1615	Louis Chapman phoned asking
		how big a cut has to be to re-
		quire stitches. I asked him to
		describe the injury. He describ-
		ed a 4" gash in his Ⓛ leg from
		a fall. I recommended that he
		apply pressure to the cut and
		come into the ED to be assessed.
		————Claire Bowen, RN

The disposition will depend on the request. For example, you may give the caller a poison-control number or suggest that he come to the ED for evaluation. Document whatever information you give.

Some nurses hesitate to use a telephone log because they assume that if they don't document, they won't be responsible for the advice they give. This assumption is faulty. A patient may make only one call to the hospital, usually about something important to him. He'll remember that; you may not.

The telephone log can provide evidence and refresh your recollection of the event. It may remind you that you didn't tell the patient to take two acetaminophen tablets to lower his fever of 105° F (40.6° C). Instead, you told him to come to the ED.

When you log such information, the law presumes that it's true because you wrote it in the course of ordinary business.

Giving bad news by phone

Sometimes you may have the unpleasant task of telephoning a patient's family member with news of a patient's deteriorating condition or death. Be sure to chart the date, time, and name of the family member notified.

Practitioner's orders

Most patient treatments require practitioner's orders; therefore, careful and accurate documentation of these orders is crucial.

Written orders

No matter who transcribes a practitioner's orders—a registered nurse, licensed practical nurse, or unit secretary—a second person needs to double-check the transcription for accuracy. Your unit should have a method of checking for transcription errors, such as performing 8-hour or 24-hour chart checks.

Night-shift nurses usually do the 24-hour check by placing a line across the order sheet to indicate that all orders above the line have been checked. They also sign and date the sheet to verify that they have done the 24-hour medication check. The nurse caring for the patient will perform the 8-hour check.

When checking a patient's order sheet, always make sure that the orders were written for the intended patient. Occasionally, an order sheet stamped with one patient's ID plate will inadvertently be placed in another patient's chart. By double-checking, you'll avoid potential mistakes.

If an order is unclear, ask the practitioner who wrote it for clarification. If a practitioner is known to have poor handwriting, ask him to read his orders to you before he leaves the unit.

PREPRINTED ORDERS

Many health care facilities use preprinted order forms to make practitioner's orders easier to read and interpret. If this is the case in your facility, don't automatically assume that a preprinted order is a flawless document in the medical record; it isn't. You may still need to clarify its meaning with the practitioner who filled it out. (See *Avoiding pitfalls of preprinted order forms.*)

COMPUTERIZED PHYSICIAN ORDER ENTRY

Many health care facilities have clinical information systems that include the computerized physician order entry (CPOE). Computerized orders are typically easier to read and interpret. If your facility uses an electronic system, you still must review the orders for accuracy. Some facilities have policies that require a 24-hour review of all CPOE orders.

Verbal orders

Errors made in the interpretation or documentation of verbal orders can lead to mistakes in patient care and liability problems for you. Clearly, verbal orders can be a necessity—especially if you're providing home health care. However, in a health care facility, try to take verbal orders only in an emergency when the practitioner can't immediately attend to the patient. For both verbal

Avoiding pitfalls of preprinted order forms

When documenting the execution of a practitioner's preprinted order, make sure that you've interpreted and carried out the order correctly. Even though these forms aim to prevent problems (caused by illegible handwriting, for example), they may still be misread. Here are some considerations for using preprinted forms.

INSIST ON APPROVED FORMS

Use only preprinted order forms that have your health care facility's approval and seal of approval by the medical records committee. Most facilities stamp or print an identification number or code on the form. When in doubt, call the medical records department—the practitioner may be using a form he developed or one provided by a drug manufacturer.

REQUIRE COMPLIANCE WITH POLICIES

To enhance communication and continuity, a preprinted order form needs to comply with facility policies and other regulations. For example, a postoperative preprinted order form shouldn't say, "Renew all previous orders" if facility policy requires specific orders. It also shouldn't allow you to select a drug dose from a range ("meperidine 50 to 100 mg I.M. q 4 h," for example) if that's prohibited in your state. Alert your nurse-manager if any order form requires you to perform duties that are outside your scope of practice.

MAKE SURE THAT THE FORM IS COMPLETED CORRECTLY

Many preprinted order forms list more orders than the practitioner wants you to follow, so he'll need to indicate which specific interventions he's ordering. For example, he may check the appropriate orders, put his initials next to them, or cross out the ones he doesn't want.

ASK FOR CLARITY AND PRECISION

Make sure that the practitioner orders drug doses in the unit of measure in which they're dispensed. For example, make sure that the form uses the metric system instead of the error-prone apothecary system. Report any errors to your nurse-manager.

PROMOTE PROPER NOMENCLATURE

Ask practitioners to use generic drug names, especially when more than one brand of a generic drug is available (for example, "acetaminophen" instead of "Tylenol"). If only one brand of a drug is available, its name can be included in parentheses after the generic name—for example, "sitagliptin phosphate (Januvia)."

TAKE STEPS TO AVOID MISINTERPRETATION

Unapproved, potentially dangerous abbreviations and symbols—such as q.d., U, and q.o.d.—don't belong on preprinted order forms. Improper spacing between a drug name and its dosage can also contribute to medication errors. For example, a 20-mg dose of Inderal written as "Inderal20 mg" could be misinterpreted as 120 mg. Be sure you're familiar with your facility's list of abbreviations to avoid, and notify the appropriate individual if you find a preprinted order form that contains any item on that list.

ENSURE THAT THE COPY IS READABLE

If your facility uses a no-carbon-required form, make sure that the bottom copy contains an identical set of preprinted orders; this is the copy that goes to the pharmacy. All lines on the bottom copy should also appear on the top copy—extra lines on the pharmacy copy can hide decimal points (making 1.5 look like 15, for example) and the tops of numbers (making 7 look like 1 and 5 look like 3).

and telephone orders, the complete order must be verified by having the person receiving the order read back the complete order per The Joint Commission's requirements.

In most cases, verbal orders shouldn't include do-not-resuscitate (DNR) or no-code orders.

Carefully follow your facility's policy for documenting a verbal order, and use a special form if one exists. Usually, you'll follow this procedure:

▶ If time and circumstances allow, have another nurse read the order back to the practitioner.

▶ Record the order on the practitioner's order sheet as soon as possible. Note the date and time, and then record the order verbatim.

▶ On the next line, write "V.V.O." for verified verbal order. Then write the practitioner's name and the name of the nurse who read the order back to the practitioner.

▶ Sign your name and draw a line for the practitioner to sign.

▶ Draw lines through any spaces between the order and your verification of the order.

▶ Record the type of drug, the dosage, the time you gave it, and any other information your facility's policy requires.

2/23/07	1500	Digoxin 0.125 mg P.O. now and
		daily in a.m. Furosemide 40
		mg P.O. now and daily starting
		in a.m. V.V.O. Dr. Blackstone
		taken by ————————
		———— Judith Schilling, RN, &
		———————— Carla Roy, RN

Make sure that the practitioner countersigns the order within the time limits set by your facility's policy. Without this countersignature, you may be held liable for practicing medicine without a license.

Telephone orders

Your patient is having trouble breathing. Your assessment findings include bilateral crackles on auscultation and dependent edema. The practitioner, who's busy in an emergency, gives you a telephone order for oxygen.

Normally, you should accept only written orders from a practitioner. However, in a situation such as this, when the patient needs immediate treatment and the practitioner isn't available to write an order, telephone orders are acceptable.

Telephone orders may also be taken to expedite care when new information is available that doesn't require a physical examination (such as laboratory data). Keep in mind that telephone orders are for the patient's well-being and not strictly for convenience. They should be given directly to you, rather than through a third party.

Carefully follow your facility's policy for documenting a telephone order. Generally, you'll follow this procedure:

▶ When you receive the telephone order from the practitioner, read back the entire order to confirm all details and ensure accuracy.

▶ Record the order on the practitioner's order sheet as soon as possible. Note the date and time, then write the order verbatim. On the next line, write "V.T.O." for verified telephone order. (Don't use "P.O." for phone order; that abbreviation could be misinterpreted to mean "by mouth.") Then write the practitioner's name and sign your name. If another nurse listened to the order with you, have her sign the order as well.

2/4/07	1100	M.S. Contin 30 mg P.O. now
		and q 12 hr for pain. Bisacodyl
		suppos. † PR now. May repeat
		x 1 if no results. ————
		– V.T.O. Dr. Kaufman/Jane Goddard, RN,
		———————— & Carol Barsky, RN

Smarter charting

Advantages of faxing orders

Most hospital units now have a facsimile, or fax, machine at their disposal. Faxing has two main advantages: It speeds the transmittal of practitioner's orders and test results to different departments, and it reduces the likelihood of errors.

SPEEDS COMMUNICATION
Faxing allows practitioners to back up phone orders in writing for the patient's chart. Orders can be faxed to you on the unit and also to the pharmacy, radiology department, and other relevant departments. The results: no more time wasted calling the department and waiting to get through and no more time spent waiting for orders to be picked up.

In return, the receiving department gets a copy of the original order (needed for filling the order and for department files). If an order can't be filled, the receiving department can contact the practitioner for clarification or for a new order, again reducing delays in filling orders and wasting your time as a go-between. An additional advantage comes from the fax machine itself, which prints the date and time the order was sent and the department it came from.

Faxing also allows staff members to transmit exact copies of X-rays, laboratory test results, and electrocardiogram strips in a matter of seconds.

Be sure to limit the faxing of protected health information (PHI) to situations when the information is needed immediately and more secure transmission methods aren't feasible. When faxing PHI, use a cover sheet and verify receipt of the fax by the appropriate person. Consult your facility policy for any further instructions.

REDUCES ERRORS
Using a fax network helps you and other staff members prevent errors by checking one another's work and consulting the practitioner directly about unresolved problems. In addition, faxing provides printed accounts, promoting accurate documentation.

▶ Draw lines through any blank spaces in the order.

▶ Make sure that the practitioner countersigns the order within the set time limits. Without his signature, you may be held liable for practicing medicine without a license.

To save time and avoid errors, consider asking the practitioner to send a copy of the order by fax machine. (See *Advantages of faxing orders.*)

Clarifying practitioner's orders
Although unit secretaries may transcribe orders, the nurse is ultimately responsible for the accuracy of the transcription. Only you have the authority and knowledge to question the validity of orders and to spot errors.

Follow your health care facility's policy for clarifying orders that are vague or possibly erroneous. If you don't have a policy to cover a particular situation, contact the prescribing practitioner, and always document your actions. Then ask your nursing administrator for a step-by-step policy to follow so you'll know what to do if the situation ever recurs.

An order may be correct when issued but improper later because of changes in the patient's status. When this occurs, delay the treatment until you've contacted the practitioner and clarified the situation. Follow your facility's policy for

When in doubt, question orders

Always question a practitioner's order if it doesn't seem appropriate.

In *Poor Sisters of Saint Francis Seraph of the Perpetual Adoration, et al. v. Catron* (1982), a hospital was held liable for negligence because a nurse failed to question a physician's order about an endotracheal tube.

The physician ordered that the tube be left in the patient's trachea for an excessively long period: 5 days instead of the standard 2 to 3 days. The nurse knew that 5 days was exceptionally long, but instead of clarifying the physician's order and documenting her actions, she followed the order.

As a result, the patient's voice box was irreparably damaged, and the court ruled the hospital negligent.

1/19/07	1900	DO NOT RESUSCITATE THIS PATIENT.— Deepak Patel, MD

clarifying an order. (See *When in doubt, question orders.*)

Clarify ambiguous orders with the practitioner. Document your efforts to clarify the order, and document whether the order was carried out. If you believe a practitioner's order is in error, you must refuse to carry it out until you receive clarification. Keep a record of your refusal together with the reasons and an account of all communication with the practitioner. Inform your immediate supervisor. If the order is correct as written, initial and check off each line. Below the practitioner's signature, sign your name, the date, and the time.

DNR ORDERS

When a patient is terminally ill and his death is expected, his practitioner and family (and the patient if appropriate) may agree that a DNR, or *no-code*, order is appropriate. The physician writes the order, and the staff carries it out when the patient goes into cardiac or respiratory arrest.

Because DNR orders are recognized legally, you'll incur no liability when a patient you don't try to resuscitate later dies. You may, however, incur liability if you initiate resuscitation counter to the DNR order.

Every patient with a DNR code should have a written order on file. The order should be consistent with the facility's policy, which often requires that such orders be reviewed every 48 to 72 hours.

If a terminally ill patient without a DNR order tells you orally that he doesn't want to be resuscitated in a crisis, document his statement as well as his degree of awareness and orientation. Then contact the patient's practitioner and your nurse-manager, and ask for assistance from administration, legal services, or social services.

Increasingly, patients are deciding in advance of a crisis whether or not they want to be resuscitated. Health care facilities must provide written information to patients concerning their rights under state law to make decisions regarding their care, including the right to refuse medical treatment and the right to formulate an advance directive. (See chapter 2, Legal and Ethical Implications of Documentation.)

This information must be provided to all patients, usually upon admission. You must also document that the patient received this informa-

Documenting advance directives

Spurred by patients' requests and the passage of self-determination laws in many states, more and more health care facilities are requiring documentation of advance directives or lack of the same.

An *advance directive* is a legal document by which a person tells his medical caregivers how he prefers to be treated in an illness from which he can't reasonably expect to recover. Advance directives also include *living wills* (which instruct the practitioner to administer no life-sustaining treatment) and *durable powers of attorney* (which name another person to act in the patient's behalf for medical decisions in the event that the patient can't act for himself).

Because these laws vary from state to state, be sure to find out how your state's law applies to your practice and to the medical record.

PREVIOUSLY EXECUTED DIRECTIVE

If a patient has previously executed an advance directive, request a copy of it for his chart and make sure that his practitioner is aware of it. Some health care facilities routinely make this request a part of admission or preadmission procedures.

Also, be sure to document the name, address, and phone number of the person entrusted with decision-making power.

PRESENTLY EXECUTED DIRECTIVE

If a patient wants to execute an advance directive during his stay in your facility, he can do so as long as he's a competent adult. In such a case, the record should include documented proof of competence (usually the responsibility of the medical, legal, social services, or risk management department) along with the signed and witnessed, newly executed advance directive.

DIRECTIVES ABOUT NUTRITION AND HYDRATION

If you practice in an area with laws related to artificial nutrition and hydration (nourishment provided by invasive tubes and I.V. lines), record the patient's wishes if these issues aren't addressed in his advance directive.

REVOCATION OF THE DIRECTIVE

Legally, the patient can revoke an advance directive at any time either orally or in writing. In such a case, include a copy of the written revocation in the record, or sign and date a statement in the patient's medical record explaining that the patient made the request orally. Consult your facility's policy and state laws pertaining to living wills and advance directives; revocation statements may need to be countersigned.

tion and whether he brought a written advance directive with him. (See *Documenting advance directives.*) In some instances, you can file a photocopy of the directive in the patient's record.

As a nurse, you have a responsibility to help the patient make an informed decision about continuing treatment. If the patient's wishes differ from those of his family or practitioner, make sure that the discrepancies are thoroughly documented in the chart.

Incidents

A patient injury—typically referred to as an *incident*—is a serious situation. It may be the result of patient action, staff action, or equipment failure. Chart all patient injuries caused by falls, restraints, burns, or other factors. Then file an incident report in compliance with your health care facility's procedure. Also file an incident report whenever a patient insists on being discharged against medical advice.

An incident report serves two functions. First, it informs the administration of the incident, allowing the risk management team to consider changes that might prevent similar incidents in the future. Second, it alerts the administration and the health care facility's insurance company to a potential claim and the need for further investigation.

Only a person with firsthand knowledge of an incident should file a report, and only the person making the report should sign it. Never sign a report describing circumstances or events that you didn't witness. Each person with firsthand knowledge should fill out and sign a *separate* report. Your report should:

▶ identify the person involved in the incident

▶ document accurately and objectively any unusual occurrences that you witnessed

▶ record details of what happened and the consequences for the persons involved; include sufficient information so that administrators can decide whether the matter requires further investigation

▶ avoid opinions, judgments, conclusions, or assumptions about who or what caused the incident

▶ avoid making suggestions about how to prevent the incident from happening again.

Detailed statements from witnesses and descriptions of remedial action are normally part of an investigative follow-up; don't include them in the incident report itself. Although the incident report isn't part of the patient's chart, it may be used later in litigation. Don't note in the chart that you filed an incident report, but do include the clinical details of the incident in the chart. Make sure that the descriptions in the incident report are consistent with those in the chart. (See chapter 2, Legal and Ethical Implications of Documentation.)

After it's filed, the incident report may be reviewed by the nursing supervisor, the practitioner called to examine the patient, appropriate department heads and administrators, the health care facility's attorney, and the insurance company. (See *What happens to an incident report.*)

Falls

Current research shows that falls—involving patients, visitors, and staff—constitute most of the incidents reported on clinical units. Among the events qualifying as falls are slips, slides, knees giving way, faints, or tripping over equipment.

Consequences of falls include prolonged hospitalization, increased hospital costs, and liability problems.

RISK ASSESSMENT AND PREVENTION

Because falls raise so many problems, your health care facility may require an all-out risk assessment and prevention effort. If so, you'll need to document your role in this activity. For example, if your facility requires a risk assessment form for patients, complete it and keep it in the patient's chart. (See *Determining a patient's risk of falling,* page 322.)

Avoiding falls

There are no foolproof ways to prevent every patient from falling, but the following strategies may help. Review your facility's fall reduction program per The Joint Commission's requirements. Document the following safety interventions, as required by your health care facility:

▶ Keep the bed's side rails raised or lowered, when indicated, and include your decision to do so in the chart as part of your interventions for addressing the nursing diagnosis of "Risk for trauma."

▶ Monitor the patient regularly—continuously, if his condition requires it—and document your findings.

ChartWizard

What happens to an incident report

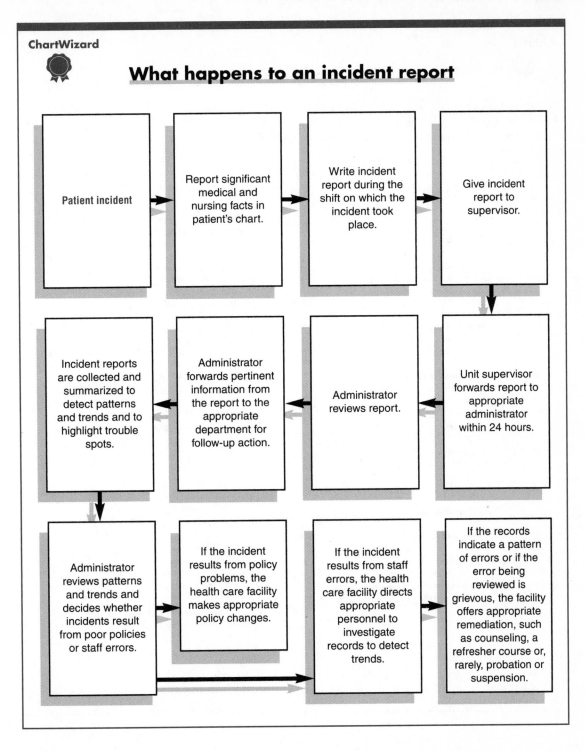

Patient incident	Report significant medical and nursing facts in patient's chart.	Write incident report during the shift on which the incident took place.	Give incident report to supervisor.

Incident reports are collected and summarized to detect patterns and trends and to highlight trouble spots.

Administrator forwards pertinent information from the report to the appropriate department for follow-up action.

Administrator reviews report.

Unit supervisor forwards report to appropriate administrator within 24 hours.

Administrator reviews patterns and trends and decides whether incidents result from poor policies or staff errors.

If the incident results from policy problems, the health care facility makes appropriate policy changes.

If the incident results from staff errors, the health care facility directs appropriate personnel to investigate records to detect trends.

If the records indicate a pattern of errors or if the error being reviewed is grievous, the facility offers appropriate remediation, such as counseling, a refresher course or, rarely, probation or suspension.

ChartWizard

Determining a patient's risk of falling

Certain patients have a greater risk of falling than others. Using a chart such as the one below, which was developed for use with older patients, can help you determine the extent of the risk. To use the chart, check each applicable item and total the number of points. A score of 10 or more indicates a risk of falling.

POINTS	PATIENT CATEGORY
	Age
1	70 to 79 years old
2 ✔	80 or older
	Mental state
0	Oriented at all times or comatose
2	Confused periodically
4 ✔	Confused at all times
	Duration of hospitalization
0 ✔	0 to 3 days
2	Over 3 days
	Falls within the past 6 months
0	None
2 ✔	1 or 2
5	3 or more
	Elimination
0 ✔	Independent and continent
1	Uses catheter, ostomy, or both
3	Needs help with elimination
5	Independent and incontinent
1 ✔	**Visual impairment**
3	**Confinement to chair**
2	**Blood pressure** Drop in systolic pressure of 20 mm Hg or more between lying and standing positions

POINTS	PATIENT CATEGORY
	Gait and balance Assess gait by having the patient stand in one spot with both feet on the ground for 30 seconds without holding onto something. Then have him walk straight ahead and through a doorway. Next, have him turn while walking.
1	Wide base of support
1 ✔	Loss of balance while standing
1	Balance problems when walking
1	Diminished muscle coordination
1	Lurching or swaying
1	Holds on or changes gait when walking through a doorway
1	Jerking or instability when turning
1	Needs an assistive device such as a walker
	Medications How many different drugs is the patient taking?
0	None
1	1
2 ✔	2 or more

___	Alcohol	___ Cathartics
___	Anesthetics	___ Diuretics
___	Antihistamines	___ Opioids
✔	Antihypertensives	___ Psychotropics
___	Antiseizure drugs	___ Sedative hypnotics
✔	Antidiabetics	___ Other drugs (specify)
___	Benzodiazepines	

1 ✔   Check if the patient has changed drugs, dosage, or both in the past 5 days.

_13_   **TOTAL**

- Offer a bedpan or commode regularly, and chart this care measure.
- Provide an adequately lighted, clean, and clutterfree environment.
- Make sure that someone helps and supports the patient whenever he gets out of bed and that he has proper footwear for walking safely.
- Make sure that adequate staff members are available to transfer him, if necessary.
- Apply restraints or mechanical devices as ordered that provide a warning signal when a patient tries to climb out of bed.
- Suggest that a relative or friend stay with the patient.
- A patient taking a medication that causes orthostatic hypotension, central nervous system depression, or vestibular toxicity needs special nursing care when a practitioner's order requires him to be in a chair for meals. If you can't supervise such a patient while he's sitting, make sure that another member of the health care team does.

Charting falls

If a patient falls despite precautions, be sure to chart the event and file an incident report. Check the patient for bruises, lacerations, or abrasions. Note any pain or deformity in the extremities, particularly the hip, arm, leg, or lumbar spine. Assess blood pressure while the patient is lying down and sitting up. Look for a drop of 20 to 30 mm Hg in the systolic reading, which may indicate orthostatic hypotension. Perform a neurologic assessment. Check for slurred speech, weakness in the extremities, or a change in mental status. Notify the patient's practitioner, who should assess the patient.

2/6/07	1400	Pt. found on floor beside her
		bed and chair. Pt. c/o pain in
		her Ⓡ hip area and difficulty
		moving Ⓡ leg. No abrasions or
		lacerations noted. BP elevated
		at 158/94; P, 94; R, 22. Pt.
		states she fell trying to get to
		her chair. Mental status un-
		changed. Dr. Dayoub notified.
		Pt. returned to bed. Hip X-ray
		reveals fractured Ⓡ hip. Pt.
		medicated for hip pain. Family
		notified by Dr. Dayoub. Pt.
		assessed hourly. Discussed the
		need for side rails with pt.
		Instructed her in use of call
		button. Side rails up at pres-
		ent. ———— Beverly Katsur, RN

Restraints

Restraints are defined as any method of physically restricting a person's freedom of movement, physical activity, or normal access to his body. Restraints can cause numerous problems, including limited mobility, skin breakdown, impaired circulation, incontinence, and strangulation.

Restraints are "prescriptive devices"—you can't use them unless you have a physician's order. (Some states may authorize other licensed health care professionals to prescribe restraints.) In most facilities, the physician must renew the order every 24 hours. (See *Physical restraint order,* page 324.) You'll need to consult your facility's policy for the correct protocol to follow in emergencies—for example, when the patient's safety is at risk and you've no time to obtain an order.

Institutional restraint policies, procedures, and protocols should be based on professional practice standards and then approved by appropriate committees. Depending on the institution involved, the committee will include members

ChartWizard

A form such as the one shown here must be in the patient's chart before physical restraints are applied.

Physical restraint order

Date: _2/12/07_   **Time:** _0315_

Reason for restraint use (circle all that apply):
To prevent:
1. High risk for self-harm
2. High risk for harm to others
(3.) High potential for removing tubes, equipment, or invasive lines
   ® subclavian CV line
4. High risk for causing significant disruption in the treatment environment

Duration of restraint: (Not to exceed 24 hr)   _24 hr_

Type of restraint (circle all that apply):
Vest
(Left mitt)   (Right mitt)
Left wrist   Right wrist
Left ankle   Right ankle
Other _____

Practitioner's signature _Cynthia Brown, MD_

---

of the medical staff, nursing staff, and safety committee. Policies and protocols must specify your facility's definition of restraints, who is authorized to carry out the order, and how the order will be conveyed.

If you're ordered to use restraints on a patient, avoid causing pain or injury to the patient by applying them in a safe manner. (See *Using restraints safely.*)

The medical record of all restrained patients must show evidence of the following:
▶ written orders for restraint or seclusion
▶ name of the licensed independent practitioner who ordered the restraint

▶ reason for the restraint
▶ type of restraint
▶ attempted alternatives to restraints, if any
▶ reassessment by a licensed independent practitioner for a continuation of the original order
▶ monitoring and reassessment of the patient in restraints. (See *Quality assurance outcome monitor for soft restraints,* page 326.)

If a competent patient makes an informed decision to refuse restraints, the facility may require the patient to sign a release that would absolve the facility of liability should injury result from the patient's refusal to be restrained.

Burns

Burns are another common cause of injury to patients. Patients are burned by spilled hot food or liquids, hot baths, and electrical equipment. Always assess the risk of burns and take appropriate precautions.

Patients who have hand tremors should be cautioned not to handle hot foods or liquids by themselves. Patients with decreased sensation in their feet or hands should be taught to test bathwater with an unaffected extremity. Explain to patients taking medications that cause drowsiness that they may be more prone to burns and need to be cautious. Document these instructions and the patient's response to this information in your notes.

If a patient in your care does burn himself, always document the injury in his chart.

1/8/07	1100	Pt. dropped hot cup of tea on
		℞ thigh. Area slightly pink, sen-
		sitive to touch, with no edema.
		Dr. Adler notified. Cold com-
		presses ordered and applied.
		Pt. tolerates cold compress
		well. Tylenol Extra-Strength
		500 mg X 1 given with relief.
		———— Colleen Cameron, RN

Discharge AMA

Although a patient can choose to leave a health care facility against medical advice (AMA) at any time, the law requires clear evidence that he's mentally competent to make that choice. In most facilities, an AMA form serves as a legal document to protect you, the practitioners, and the facility, should any problems arise from a patient's unapproved discharge.

Legal eagle

Using restraints safely

Improperly restraining a patient can leave you vulnerable to a host of legal charges, such as negligence, professional malpractice, false imprisonment, and battery. The case discussed below is about a nurse who failed to use restraints effectively.

THE PATIENT WHO SLIPPED AWAY
In *Robison v. Micheline Faine and Catalano's Nurse Registry, Inc.* (1987), the nurse, Micheline Faine, was required to restrain the patient, Ms. Robison, before leaving her hospital room. With the time for lunch break approaching, Faine tied the patient in a restraining device and left to find a relief nurse. After the relief nurse entered the room, Faine left for lunch.

When Faine returned 20 minutes later, she found that Ms. Robison was gone, although the restraining device was still attached to the bed and the side rails were up. While Faine had been at lunch, Ms. Robison had slipped out of the restraint, left the hospital through an emergency stairway leading to the roof, and attempted to jump to a nearby tree. She fell to the ground and sustained serious injuries.

NO EXEMPTION FROM LIABILITY
At the malpractice trial, the judge instructed the jury to exempt Ms. Faine from liability. However, an appeals court disagreed. It ruled that Ms. Faine wasn't automatically exempt from liability because the patient would have been unable to free herself if the restraining device had been tied correctly. The appeals court ordered a new trial for Ms. Faine to determine whether she was negligent.

ChartWizard

Quality assurance
outcome monitor for soft restraints

This form lists criteria for the use of soft restraints and for ensuring that interventions are properly documented.

Date: _1/30/07_   **Department:** _Nursing_

Room No.: _325_   **Staff signature:** _Pamela Petrakis, RN_

Criteria: Soft restraint: Any use of soft restraints (padded mitts, cloth wrist or ankle restraints, cloth vests)	Satisfactory	Unsatisfactory
1. Is there documentation of clinical justification for restraint?	✓	
2. Does the documentation show that less restrictive measures were attempted prior to restraints?	✓	
3. Is a clinical assessment documented prior to the use of restraint by an RN?	✓	
4. Is there a practitioner's order for each incident of restraint documented within appropriate time limit of restraints according to patient's age? Signed within 24 hours?	✓	
5. Is the time of going into restraint specified in the practitioner's order?	✓	
6. Is the practitioner's order time limited? Use "Not to exceed 24 hours" instead of "up to."	✓	
7. Is there an RN progress note written describing this incident? (Prior to and after discontinue of restraint)	✓	
8. Does the restraint documentation reflect that the patient's needs were not neglected? (Review flow sheet.)	✓	
9. Does documentation reflect interventions of staff with patient after restraint?	✓	
10. Is the restraint record complete?	✓	
11. Does the documentation reflect the physical status of the patient prior to use of restraint and after removal of restraint?	✓	
12. Is the order renewed every 24 hours?	✓	

Comments:

The AMA form should clearly document that the patient knows he's leaving against medical advice, that he's been advised of the risks of leaving and understands them, and that he knows he can come back. If a patient refuses to sign the AMA form, document this refusal on the form and enter it in his chart. Use the patient's own words to describe his refusal.

Include the following information on the AMA form:

▶ patient's reason for leaving AMA
▶ names of relatives or others notified of the patient's decision and the dates and times of the notifications
▶ explanation of the risks and consequences of the AMA discharge, as told to the patient, including the name of the person who provided the explanation
▶ instructions regarding alternative sources of follow-up care given to the patient
▶ list of those accompanying the patient at discharge and the instructions given to them
▶ patient's destination after discharge.

Document any statements and actions reflecting the patient's mental state at the time he chose to leave the facility. This will help protect you, the practitioners, and the facility against a charge of negligence. The patient may later claim that his discharge occurred while he was mentally incompetent and that he was improperly supervised while he was in that state.

Also check your facility's policy regarding incident reports. If the patient leaves without anyone's knowledge or if he refuses to sign the AMA form, you'll probably be required to complete an incident report.

1/4/07	1455	Pt. found in room packing his clothes at 1400. When asked why he was dressed and packing, he stated, "I'm tired of all these tests. They keep doing tests, but they still don't know what's wrong with me. I can't take any more. I'm going home." Dr. Giordano notified and came to speak with pt. Pt.'s wife notified and she came to the hospital. She was unable to persuade husband to stay. Pt. willing to sign AMA form. AMA form signed. Pt. told of possible risks of his leaving the hospital with headaches and hypertension. Pt. agrees to see Dr. Giordano in his office in 2 days. Discussed appointment with pt. and wife. Pt. going home after discharge. Accompanied patient in wheelchair to main lobby, with wife. Pt. left at 1445 hr. ——— Lynn Nakashima, RN

Missing patient

Suppose the same patient never said anything about leaving, but on rounds you discover he's missing. First, of course, try to find him in the building. Attempt to contact his home. If he's gone, notify your nurse-manager, the patient's practitioner, and the police, if necessary. The police are usually called if there's a possibility of the patient's hurting himself or others, especially if he has left the facility with any medical devices.

In the chart, note the time that you discovered the patient missing, your attempts to find him, and the people notified. Include any other pertinent information.

Selected references

Austin, S. "'Ladies & Gentlemen of the Jury, I Present ... the Nursing Documentation,'" *Nursing* 36(1):56-62, January 2006.

Balas, M.C., et al. "Frequency and Type of Errors and Near Errors Reported by Critical Care Nurses," *Canadian Journal of Nursing Research* 38(2):24-41, June 2006.

Banet, G.A., et al. "Effects of Implementing Computerized Practitioner Order Entry and Nursing Documentation on Nursing Workflow in an Emergency Department," *Journal of Healthcare Information Management* 20(2):45-54, Spring 2006.

Deans, C. "Medication Errors and Professional Practice of Registered Nurses," *Collegian* 12(1):29-33, January 2005.

Dimond, B. "Prescription and Medication Records," *British Journal of Nursing* 14(22):1203-205, December 2005–January 2006.

Dock, B. "Improving the Accuracy of Specimen Labeling," *Clinical Laboratory Science* 18(4):210-12, Fall 2005.

Drendel, A.L., et al. "Pain Assessment for Pediatric Patients in the Emergency Department," *Pediatrics* 117(5):1511-18, May 2006.

Gugerty, B. "Progress and Challenges in Nursing Documentation, Part I," *Journal of Healthcare Information Management* 20(2):18-20, Spring 2006.

Karkkainen, O., and Eriksson, K. "Recording the Content of the Caring Process," *Journal of Nursing Management* 13(3):202-208, May 2005.

Kleinbeck, S.V., and Dopp, A. "The Perioperative Nursing Data Set—A New Language for Documenting Care," *AORN Journal* 82(1):51-57, July 2005.

O'Dell, K. "Allergy Documentation: Strategies for Patient Safety," *Oklahoma Nurse* 51(2):16, June-August 2006.

Odwazny, R., et al. "Organizational and Cultural Changes for Providing Safe Patient Care," *Quality Management in Health Care* 14(3):132-43, July-September 2005.

Poissant, L., et al. "The Impact of Electronic Health Records on Time Efficiency of Physicians and Nurses: A Systematic Review," *Journal of the American Medical Informatics Association* 12(5):505-16, September-October 2005.

Rosenthal, K. "Documenting Peripheral I.V. Therapy," *Nursing* 35(7):28, July 2005.

Smith, L.S. "Documenting an Adverse Drug Reaction," *Nursing* 35(10):22, October 2005.

Wagner, L.M., et al. "Impact of a Falls Menu-Driven Incident-Reporting System on Documentation and Quality Improvement in Nursing Homes," *Gerontologist* 45(6):835-42, December 2005.

DOCUMENTATION IN SELECTED CLINICAL SPECIALTIES

11

Many nursing documentation guidelines employed in the workplace today are relevant to all nurses, regardless of their clinical specialty. There are, however, certain areas of nursing practice that use specialized guidelines and forms. If you work in one of these specialized areas, you need to know what to document, when to document, and what forms to document with. This chapter covers special aspects of documentation for six selected clinical specialties: critical care nursing, emergency department (ED) nursing, maternal-neonatal nursing, pediatric nursing, psychiatric nursing, and surgical nursing.

Critical care nursing

As with any nursing specialty area, critical care has its own unique documentation requirements based on the nature of the patient's condition, equipment used, and internal standards. In general, nurses working in intensive care units (ICUs) have fewer patient assignments than in medical-surgical units. Because more intensive care, as well as increased monitoring and documentation, are needed, the workload is similar to that of nurses with larger patient assignments.

Some facilities have developed specific documentation forms or flow sheets for the ICU staff to use. These forms allow the nurse to document all aspects of care on one form, rather than using multiple forms. Because critical care patients require frequent monitoring, ICU flow sheets are designed to document more frequent assessments than in medical-surgical units, at time intervals dictated by the patient's condition and the facility's policy.

These ICU flow sheets also contain documentation items specific to critical care, and many include special locations on them to document such assessments as:

▶ Ramsey scale sedation

▶ pulmonary artery catheter readings, such as pulmonary artery systolic and diastolic pressure, pulmonary artery wedge pressure, central venous pressure, cardiac output, cardiac index, and systemic vascular resistance

▶ insertion dates, locations, and care associated with arterial lines, pulmonary artery catheters, central venous pressure (CVP) lines, and indwelling urinary catheters

▶ intake, including medicated infusions, I.V. fluids, I.V. medications, blood products, and gastric feedings

▶ frequent laboratory test results, including blood glucose levels used to manage insulin infusion protocols (see *Insulin infusion protocol*)

▶ respiratory status, including ventilator settings and arterial blood gas values

▶ neurologic status, such as pupil size and reaction to light, Glasgow Coma Scale score, upper and lower extremity strength, intracranial pressure (ICP), and cerebral perfusion pressure (CPP)

▶ maintenance for specialty beds or equipment (such as traction, braces, splints, and venous boots)

▶ dressings and wound care

▶ maintenance for arterial lines, central lines, tracheostomies, tubes, drains, and temporary pacemakers.

Special considerations in critical care

As a critical care nurse, you're responsible for assessing the patient's condition, monitoring his status, and documenting based on internal standards. There are several areas, including vital signs; respiratory, cardiac, and neurologic status; patient comfort; organ donation; and code documentation that require special consideration in critical care patients.

VITAL SIGNS

Temperature, heart rate, respiratory rate, and blood pressure are generally taken more frequently in the critical care setting. Vital signs may be taken as often as every 5 to 10 minutes, depending on the patient's condition and your facility's policy. The use of monitors and automatic blood pressure cuffs may facilitate this process.

RESPIRATORY STATUS

Along with the patient's respiratory rate, his respiratory status must be monitored closely, especially if he has respiratory compromise. If the patient is on a mechanical ventilator, you should assess and document these items early in your shift and as your patient's condition warrants:

▶ endotracheal (ET) tube size, reference mark on the tube that coincides with the patient's lip, and location (oral or nasal) or if via tracheostomy

▶ presence and character of bilateral breath sounds and coughing

▶ ventilator settings, including mode, tidal volume, set rate, percentage of inspired oxygen, patient's respiratory rate, PEEP (positive expiratory end pressures), pressure support, and end-tidal carbon dioxide ($ETCO_2$) measurements

▶ suctioning attempts, secretions obtained, and patient response

▶ SaO_2 (arterial oxygen saturation of hemoglobin) and amount of inspired oxygen

▶ patient's tolerance of the ventilator

▶ use of restraints

▶ weaning attempts, mode used (CPAP—continuous positive airway pressure—or bilevel ventilation), and patient's tolerance and response.

In addition to these assessment items, the patient with a tracheostomy has some additional requirements. Document the condition of the skin around the stoma, tracheostomy care you

Smarter charting

Insulin infusion protocol

Doctor's Order Sheet Berkshire Medical Center Berkshire Health System 725 North St., Pittsfield, MA 01201	Patient label:

Insulin Infusion Protocol
[FOR USE ONLY IN THE CRITICAL CARE UNITS]
(not for patients with diabetic ketoacidosis/hyperosmolar nonketotic hyperglycemia)

Date	Time	Transcriber

Feeding
- Patient must be receiving constant feeding by (i) standard intravenous, (ii) TPN, or (iii) tube feeding.
- Feedings must provide 5 – 10 grams of carbohydrate/hr (e.g., 100 – 200 ml/hr D_5W).
- If the rate of tube feeding is changed or discontinued, *notify the physician on call.*

Frequency of fingerstick blood sugars
- Check blood sugars q 1 hour until patient reaches the target range.
- When blood sugar in range for 4 consecutive hours, check blood sugars q 2 hours.
- When blood sugar in range for a second 4-hour period, check blood sugars q 4 hours.
- If blood sugar increases above target range, begin checking blood sugars q 1 hour again.
- If blood sugar in hypoglycemia range, follow hypoglycemia protocol below & resume checking blood sugars q 1 hour.

Target Blood Glucose: 80 – 150 mg/dL [FOR THIS PROTOCOL ONLY!]

Insulin: Regular insulin 100 units in 100 ml 0.9% Sodium Chloride. [1 Unit/ml]

Steroids: *If steroids are started, stopped or the dosage increased or decreased,* notify the physician on call immediately.

Initial Insulin Infusion Rate: *Select desired algorithm below.*
- ☐ Start Algorithm 1 **[Most patients will start with Algorithm 1.]**
- ☐ Start Algorithm 2 **[Start here if patient is on 80 units or more of insulin daily or has started steroids]**

Match the patient's blood glucose to the corresponding insulin infusion rate in the appropriate algorithm column.

Insulin Infusion Protocol Adjustments: *CALL MD STAT IF PATIENT NOT CONTROLLED WITH ALGORITHM 4.*
- Move up to the next higher algorithm *if:* blood glucose is higher than target range *&* the blood glucose fell < 60 mg/dL over 1 hour.
- Move down to the next lower algorithm *if:* blood glucose is < 70 mg/dL for 2 consecutive hours.

BLOOD GLUCOSE	ALGORITHM 1	ALGORITHM 2	ALGORITHM 3	ALGORITHM 4
Mg/dL	Units/hr	Units/hr	Units/hr	Units/hr
< 70	Off	Off	Off	Off
70 – 79	0.2	0.5	1	1.5
80 – 120	0.5	1	2	3
121 – 150	1	1.5	3	5
151 – 179	1.5	2	4	7
180 – 209	2	3	5	9
210 – 239	2.5	4	6	12
240 – 269	3	5	8	16
270 – 299	3.5	6	10	20
300 – 329	4	7	12	24
330 – 359	4.5	8	14	28
≥ 360	6	12	16	

Treatment of hypoglycemia (BG < 60 mg/dL)
- Discontinue insulin drip AND *if patient awake* give $D_{50}W$ 25 ml (½ amp) IV × 1 OR *if patient not awake* give $D_{50}W$ 50 ml (1 amp) IV × 1.
- Recheck blood glucose q 20 min. and repeat 25 ml $D_{50}W$ IV if blood glucose < 60 mg/dL. Notify physician. After blood glucose > 70 mg/dL on 2 successive 20 minute checks, resume insulin infusion at the next lower algorithm.

Notify the physician for: *CALL MD STAT IF PATIENT NOT CONTROLLED WITH ALGORITHM 4.*
- Any blood glucose > 360 mg/dL.
- A change in blood glucose that is > 100 mg/dL in any one hour.
- Hypoglycemia that persists > 20 minutes

Transitioning from Insulin Infusion Protocol
- Change to fixed rate insulin infusion or intermittent insulin administration per ICU team for patients well controlled with protocol and for transfer to medical/surgical units.
- Order SC insulin online or via Doctors Order Sheet. Start SC insulin 2 hours before stopping insulin infusion.

Physician Signature:	Pager #:
Pilot 060613 DRAFT	Storeroom #:	Valid until:

Adapted from John Rogers, Hospital Counsel Berkshire Health System, Inc., 725 North Street, Pittsfield, MA 01201, with permission.

have performed, suctioning attempts, whether the cuff is inflated, and what type of oxygen the patient is receiving.

If sputum and secretions are present, describe each, noting the color, consistency, and quantity (approximate in teaspoons or some other common measurement). Careful examination may alert you to changes in the patient's condition. For example, the patient who develops pink, frothy sputum is most likely experiencing pulmonary edema. A specimen may be needed for sputum analysis to diagnose respiratory disease, identify the cause of pulmonary infection, or to identify abnormal lung cells. If so, document the sputum collection techniques used and follow up by promptly obtaining laboratory results.

Although pulse oximetry may be performed intermittently, most ICU patients are monitored continuously. Pulse oximetry is a simple, noninvasive procedure used to measure arterial oxygen saturation. It works by placing a photodetector (also called a *sensor* or *transducer*) over the patient's finger, toe, or earlobe, which then calculates saturation based on the amount of color absorbed by arterial blood when red and infrared light are sent through the vascular bed. The arterial oxygen saturation value is documented with the symbol SpO_2 when pulse oximetry is used, and SaO_2 when measured invasively via arterial blood gas (ABG) analysis. A normal reading is 95% to 100%, and should be within 2% of ABG values. Follow your facility's policy for proper site rotation and documentation.

ABG analysis is another tool to evaluate oxygenation and is used to detect how much oxygen is available to peripheral tissues. In most critical care units, a practitioner, respiratory therapist, or specially trained ICU nurse draws ABG samples, usually from an arterial line if the patient has one. Before obtaining an ABG sample from the radial artery, perform an Allen test to determine the presence of collateral circulation and docu-

ment the results. Be sure to specify that you or another health care provider drew the sample, at which time, and from which site (including if drawn from an arterial line). Note the amount of inspired oxygen being given to the patient and whether or not he's attached to a ventilator. When the results are obtained, document the PaO_2 and $PaCO_2$ (respectively, partial pressures of oxygen and carbon dioxide dissolved in arterial blood); pH (hydrogen ion concentration, reflecting acidity or alkalinity); HCO_3^- (serum bicarbonate); and SaO_2. It's also important to note if the patient is experiencing any compensation, and if so, whether it's respiratory or metabolic.

Some ICU patients also have one or more chest tubes in place. If your patient has a chest tube, in addition to documenting his respiratory status, also make note of the condition of the dressing at the insertion site, any tidaling noted in the tube itself and the drainage collection device, the suction settings, and the amount and character of drainage.

CARDIAC STATUS

Nearly all ICU patients are connected to cardiac monitors during their hospitalization. This may be according to your facility's protocol or it may be specifically warranted by the patient's condition. Without exception, if your patient is connected to a cardiac monitor, you should print out a rhythm strip at the beginning of your shift to use as comparison with the patient's previous rhythms and to any subsequent rhythms or abnormalities that may be experienced during your shift.

If the monitor doesn't do so automatically, label each rhythm strip with the patient's name, medical record number, date, and time. Also measure and document the patient's:
▶ cardiac rate and rhythm
▶ PR interval (the start of the P wave to the start of the QRS complex)

▶ QRS duration (the end of the PR interval to the end of the S wave)

▶ QT interval (the number of squares between the beginning of the QRS complex and the end of the T wave multiplied by 0.04 seconds).

Also check for ST segment abnormalities, ectopic beats, and other abnormalities. Note your findings, and interpret them by naming the rhythm strip according to the origin of the rhythm, the rate characteristics, and the rhythm abnormalities.

For patients diagnosed with heart failure or pulmonary edema, pressures within the pulmonary or cardiac systems may rise. Inspecting the jugular veins can provide information about blood volume and pressure in the right side of the heart. Normally, the highest pulsation occurs no more than 1½ " (4 cm) above the sternal notch, so if the patient's pulsations appear higher, this indicates elevation in central venous pressure and jugular vein distention. Note the level of distention in fingerbreadths above the clavicle or in relation to the jaw or clavicle. Document the distention as mild, moderate, or severe, and note the amount of distention in relation to the patient's head elevation.

If the patient has had a myocardial infarction (MI) or other cardiac event, document his symptoms, exactly as he describes them. Most facilities use a 0 to 10 scale for rating pain, with 10 being the worst pain imaginable. You should also use the same terms used by the patient—for example, sharp, dull, pressure, or tightness. Document the drugs given for chest pain and note their effectiveness.

Some ICU patients may receive continuous invasive hemodynamic monitoring via a pulmonary artery catheter. If this is the case with your patient, describe the appearance and location of the insertion site. Depending on the practitioner's orders or your facility's protocol, you may be required to document the frequency of zeroing and leveling the device. Also, list the measurements obtained—CVP; pulmonary artery pressure (PAP), including systolic and diastolic readings; pulmonary artery wedge pressure (PAWP); cardiac output (CO), cardiac index (CI), and systemic vascular resistance (SVR). (See *Hemodynamic variables,* page 334.)

NEUROLOGIC STATUS

Facilities may use different scales to measure neurologic status in ICU patients, but the Glasgow Coma Scale (GCS) is universally accepted as a basic tool for mental status evaluation. The GCS incorporates the assessment of eye opening, best verbal and motor responses, giving each a rating and then combining their scores into a total. (See the entry "Neurologic assessment," in chapter 5, for an example of the GCS.)

The patient's extremity strength may also be tested separately from the GCS but is often reported concurrently. However, this may be more subjective and, therefore, less helpful in getting a true assessment of the patient. This is an example of a strength rating scale:

5 – full strength

4 – lifts and resists

3 – lifts and holds

2 – lifts and falls behind

1 – moves on bed

0 – no movement

Pupillary response to light is also an important assessment tool in the patient with brain injury or neurologic impairment. Document the size of the patient's pupils in darkness as well as the response to light (measured in millimeters). Note the briskness of the reaction and whether the pupils respond equally.

Patients with head injuries may also have intracranial pressure (ICP) monitors and drains in place. Per your facility's protocol, document the location and appearance of the site, the amount and character of drainage, and ICP readings. You may also need to document the cerebral perfu-

Hemodynamic variables

PARAMETER	NORMAL VALUE
Mean arterial pressure (MAP) = $\dfrac{\text{Systolic blood pressure (BP)} + 2\,(\text{diastolic BP})}{3}$	70 to 105 mm Hg
Central venous pressure (CVP); right atrial pressure (RAP)	2 to 6 cm H_2O; 2 to 8 mm Hg
Right ventricular pressure	20 to 30 mm Hg (systolic) 0 to 8 mm Hg (diastolic)
Pulmonary artery pressure (PAP)	20 to 30 mm Hg (systolic; PAS) 8 to 15 mm Hg (diastolic; PAD) 10 to 20 mm Hg (mean; PAM)
Pulmonary artery wedge pressure (PAWP)	4 to 12 mm Hg
Cardiac output (CO) = Heart rate (HR) $\times$ stroke volume (SV)	4 to 8 L/min
Cardiac index (CI) = $\dfrac{CO}{\text{Body surface area}}$	2.5 to 4 L/min/m^2
Stroke volume (SV) = $\dfrac{CO}{HR}$	60 to 100 ml/beat
Stroke volume index	30 to 60 ml/beat/m^2
Systemic vascular resistance	900 to 1,200 dynes/sec/cm^{-5}
Systemic vascular resistance index	1,360 to 2,200 dynes/sec/cm^{-5}/m^2

sion pressure (CPP), which indicates the level of perfusion to the brain. CPP is determined by subtracting the ICP from the patient's mean arterial pressure. If possible, print out a strip from the ICP monitor during your shift so that it may be used for future comparison, as needed.

PATIENT COMFORT

The ICU patient often receives different pain and sedation medications than the medical-surgical patient. For instance, the patient on a ventilator frequently requires higher levels of sedation than other patients. In addition to standard documentation requirements for medication administration, you should be prepared to describe the patient's comfort level. The Ramsay scale is one scale used to assess restlessness and agitation. It's used to determine the patient's level of sedation, which is especially helpful during ventilator weaning or when trying to reduce medication levels. These levels are assessed as:

Level 1 – anxious and agitated or restless, or both

Level 2 – cooperative, oriented, and tranquil

Level 3 – response to commands only

Level 4 – brisk response to light glabellar tap or loud auditory stimulus

Level 5 – sluggish response to light glabellar tap or loud auditory stimulus

Level 6 – no response to light glabellar tap or loud auditory stimulus

Pain assessment is another important aspect of patient care in the ICU. The numerical rating scale is perhaps the most commonly used pain rating scale. To use this scale, simply ask the patient to rate his pain from 0 to 10, with 0 representing no pain and 10 representing the worst pain imaginable.

Some ICU patients, however, are unable to verbalize their pain or discomfort. These patients may be able to communicate their level of pain by selecting a number on a numeric rating scale, by selecting 1 of 6 faces representing pain severity, or by marking a line along the 10-cm visual analog scale. Additionally, some facilities use an alternative pain scale for nonverbal adults. (See *Adult nonverbal pain scale,* page 336.)

ORGAN DONATION

The Uniform Anatomical Gift Act governs organ and tissue donation. In addition, most states have legislation governing the procurement of organs and tissues. Some require medical staff to ask about organ donation upon every death. Other states require staff to notify a regional organ procurement agency that then approaches the family. As a critical care nurse, you should become familiar with the state's laws and facility's policies in which you practice.

Patients who are candidates for organ and tissue donation have highly specialized care needs, and the documentation required for their care is quite specific as well. It's imperative that hemodynamic variables and electrolyte values be kept within tight ranges for successful organ transplantation. Urine output must be assessed and documented hourly to detect diabetes insipidus. In order to assess organ function such laboratory results as complete blood count, liver and renal function tests, and electrolyte levels are closely monitored.

Any patient who donates an organ must first be declared brain dead. Death was previously defined as the cessation of respiratory and cardiac function, but with developments in technology, this definition has become obsolete. Specified brain death criteria now are used to determine death of an individual. For instance, the apnea test is widely accepted as a standard in determining death by brain criteria. If this test is performed, it's important for the nurse to document the person or persons present and conducting the test; ventilator settings before starting the test; and preliminary test results. Other tests performed should also be reported, such as corneal or gag reflex testing, the cold water caloric test, response to painful stimuli, and the doll's eye test. Many states are required to send an end-of-life summary to their affiliated organ bank describing the patient's condition at admission and the circumstances surrounding his death.

When the decision is made to donate a patient's organs and tissues, extensive documentation is required regarding family discussions, protocols, and authorization permits. It's important to study your facility's policies as well as those of the associated organ bank to ensure that all requirements are met.

Adult nonverbal pain scale

CATEGORIES	0	1	2
Face	No particular expression or smile	Occasional grimace, tearing, frowning, wrinkled forehead	Frequent grimaces, tearing, frowning, wrinkled forehead
Activity (movement)	Lying quietly, normal position	Seeking attention through movement or slow, cautious movement	Restless, excessive activity and/or withdrawal reflexes
Guarding	Lying quietly, no positioning of hands over areas of body	Splinting areas of the body, tense	Rigid, stiff
Physiology	Stable vital signs	Change in SBP greater than 20 mm Hg or heart rate greater than 20 beats per minute	Change in SBP greater than 30 mm Hg or heart rate greater than 25 beats per minute
Respiratory	Baseline respiratory rate/SpO$_2$ Compliant with ventilator	Respiratory rate greater than 10 above baseline or 5% decrease in SpO$_2$ Asynchrony with ventilator	Respiratory rate greater than 20 breaths/minute above baseline or 10% decrease in SpO$_2$ Severe asynchrony with ventilator

© Strong Memorial Hospital, University of Rochester Medical Center. Source: Wegman D. Tool for pain assessment. *Crit Care Nurse.* Available at: http://www.findarticles.p/com/articles/mi_mONUC/is_1_25/ai_n9545015. Accessed July 21, 2006.

CODE DOCUMENTATION

As discussed in chapter 10, cardiopulmonary arrest is an occurrence that requires detailed, written, and chronological documentation. Once a code is called, the designated recorder must document therapeutic interventions and the patient's responses as they occur. Most facilities use a resuscitation (or *code*) record for this purpose. (See chapter 10, Documentation of Everyday Events, for an example of a completed resuscitation record). It's critical to note the precise time for each intervention. For instance, the American Heart Association recommends a dosing interval of 3 to 5 minutes when giving epinephrine during an arrest. Documentation should support whether this protocol as well as others were followed.

Emergency department nursing

It's imperative that ED nurses keep careful and accurate documentation. Thorough documentation contributes to quality patient care by providing a physical record of the care you give. It also acts as a legal safeguard against allegations of negligence and litigation, which is why EDs across the country are developing their own specialized documentation forms and systems. Some recent additions to routine ED nursing documentation include:

▶ documenting barriers to learning
▶ documenting nutritional risk factors
▶ pain assessment
▶ screening for domestic violence.

The Standards of Emergency Nursing Practice, last updated in 1999, also influence your documentation practices by stating that the nursing plan, patient evaluation, interventions, patient assessment data, and nursing diagnoses must be documented in a retrievable form. Of course, meeting these standards of care and documenting them may not prevent litigation, but they act as a medical and legal record of your nursing care, should litigation arise.

Special considerations

As an ED nurse, you're responsible for many different facets of patient care, and no one aspect of care is more or less important than any other. Let's look more in depth at some of the unique features of ED documentation.

OBTAINING INFORMED CONSENT IN AN EMERGENCY SITUATION

A patient must sign a consent form before most treatments and procedures. Informed consent means the patient understands the proposed therapy, alternate therapies, the risks, and the hazards of not undergoing treatment at all.

However, in specific circumstances, emergency treatment (to save a patient's life or to prevent loss of organ, limb, or a function) may be done without first obtaining consent. If the patient is unconscious or a minor who can't give consent, emergency treatment may be performed without first obtaining consent. The presumption is the patient would have consented if he had been able, unless there's a reason to believe otherwise. For example, to sustain the life of unconscious patients in the emergency department, intubation has been held to be appropriate even if no one is available to consent to the procedure.

Courts will uphold emergency medical treatment as long as reasonable effort was made to obtain consent and no alternatives were available to save life and limb.

2/21/07	1000	Pt. arrived in ED at 0940 via ambulance following MVA. Pt. not responding to verbal commands, opens eyes and pushes at stimulus in response to pain, making no verbal responses. Pt. has bruising across upper chest, labored breathing, skin pale and cool, normal heart sounds, reduced breath sounds throughout ® lung, normal breath sounds Ⓛ lung, no tracheal deviation. P 112, BP 88/52, RR 26. Dr. Mallory called at 0945 and came to see pt. I.V. line inserted in Ⓛ antecubital with 20G catheter. 1,000 ml NSS infusing at 125 ml/hr. 100% oxygen given via nonrebreather mask. Stat CXR ordered to confirm pneumothorax. Pt. identified by driver's license and credit cards as Michael Brown of 123 Maple St., Valley View. Doctor called house to speak with family about need for immediate chest tube and treatment, no answer, left message on machine. Business card of Michelle Brown found in wallet. Company receptionist confirms she is wife of Michael Brown, but she's out of the office and won't return until this afternoon. Left message for wife to call doctor.
		———————— Sandy Becker, RN
2/21/07	1015	Tracheal deviation to Ⓛ side, difficulty breathing, cyanosis of lips, and mucous membranes, distended neck veins, absent breath sounds in ® lung, muffled heart sounds. P 120, BP 88/58, RR 32. Neurologic status unchanged. Dr. Mallory called pt.'s home and wife's place of business but was unable to speak with her. Again, left messages. Because of pt.'s deteriorating condition, pt.'s inability to give consent, and inability to reach wife, Dr. Mallory has ordered chest tube to be inserted on ® side to relieve tension pneumothorax. ————————
		———————— Sandy Becker, RN

TRIAGE

Your documentation of patient triage—deciding which patients should be treated before others and where the treatment should take place—is crucial. You need to obtain the most important components of this initial patient assessment (such as obtaining a focused history of the patient's chief complaint, performing a limited physical examination, and classifying the patient's problem for urgency) as quickly as possible. When your assessment is complete, you'll be better able to determine patient acuity, prioritize care needs, and make appropriate room placement. (See *Triage assessment principles.*) Most ED documentation forms have a triage space for this important information.

If the patient must wait in the waiting room for an extended period of time, reevaluate him according to your facility's policy and document your findings.

TRAUMA

Many EDs are designated trauma centers and must document specific data to demonstrate that they're providing the level of trauma care that they're licensed to deliver. Specific criteria that must be documented for the trauma patient includes:

▶ arrival time in the ED
▶ time the trauma alert was activated
▶ time the trauma surgeon arrived
▶ treatment before arrival
▶ primary survey (assessing airway, breathing, circulation, and cervical spine control)
▶ secondary survey (a more detailed assessment by body system).

Most trauma centers have trauma flow sheets used for patients meeting trauma alert criteria. (See *Trauma flow sheet,* pages 340 to 342.)

An important consideration during the care of many trauma patients is forensics. Suppose a patient arrives in your ED after sustaining a gun-shot or stab wound and, in order to fully assess him, you need to cut the clothes off his body. This process isn't as simple as it might seem. In order to refrain from contaminating possible evidence, you must avoid cutting through any puncture holes in the clothes. (Be sure to chart the name of the person to whom you gave the patient's clothing and other belongings, usually a local law enforcement officer.)

SEXUAL ASSAULT

Sexual assault, commonly called *rape,* refers to sexual contact without the person's consent. It includes many behaviors including physical and psychological coercion and force that result in varying degrees of physical and psychological trauma. Most information related to sexual assault is derived from statistics involving women who have been sexually assaulted; however, men and children can also be victims.

A person who has been sexually assaulted or has experienced an attempted sexual assault may develop rape-trauma syndrome, which refers to the victim's short- and long-term reactions to the trauma and to the methods used to cope with it. The prognosis is good if the victim receives physical and emotional support and counseling.

EDs commonly see and treat sexual assault victims, and while many facilities have a Sexual Assault Response Team or a Sexual Assault Nurse Examiner, some don't. If you're responsible for the care of one of these patients, make sure that your documentation is clear and accurate. Assist with the history-taking and physical examination. Obtain the date and time of the assault; where it occurred and the surroundings; body areas penetrated, including the use of foreign objects; and other sexual acts. Also ask about injuries occurring during the assault; actions after the assault, such as showering, urinating, douching, or changing clothing; recent gyne-

(*Text continues on page 343.*)

Triage assessment principles

To make triage decisions effectively, you must gather and interpret both subjective and objective data rapidly and accurately. Follow this rule: "When in doubt, triage up." That is, if you're uncertain as to the seriousness of a patient's condition, treat it as more, rather than less, serious. Triage activity consists of:

▶ obtaining a focused history of the patient's chief complaint
▶ performing a limited physical examination
▶ classifying the patient's problem for urgency
▶ reassuring the patient that he'll receive definitive medical care as soon as possible.

OBTAIN A HISTORY

Focus on the patient's chief complaint. Record it in his own words, using quotation marks, if possible. Have him qualify his complaint as precisely as he can, using the PQRST acronym (Provocative/Palliative, Quality/Quantity, Region/Radiation, Severity scale, Timing) or a similar device.

▶ Also record the patient's age, current medications (including over-the-counter and herbal remedies as well as vitamins) and time of last dose, allergies, date of last tetanus toxoid inoculation, and any other medical history, such as height, weight, and last menstrual period.

PERFORM A PHYSICAL EXAMINATION

Observe the patient's general appearance and assess vital signs and level of consciousness (LOC).

▶ Take oral or tympanic temperature as appropriate. Rectal temperature is the most accurate; take this as indicated and if you can ensure the patient's privacy.
▶ Check radial or apical pulse. Note rate, rhythm, and quality. While assessing the pulse, check skin temperature and capillary refill time.
▶ Check blood pressure as quickly and accurately as possible.
▶ Note rate, depth, symmetry, and quality of respirations. Also note skin color and turgor, facial expression, accessory muscle use, and any audible breath sounds.
▶ Assess LOC using a scale such as the Glasgow Coma Scale, or make a notation indicating whether the patient is oriented to time, place, and person.

CLASSIFYING EMERGENCY CONDITIONS

These lists help you determine which conditions to treat first.

Emergent conditions: A patient with the following conditions must receive immediate medical attention. Start lifesaving measures and call the practitioner immediately if you find:

▶ respiratory distress or arrest
▶ cardiac arrest
▶ severe chest pain with dyspnea or cyanosis
▶ seizures
▶ severe hemorrhage
▶ severe head injury
▶ coma
▶ poisoning or drug overdose
▶ open chest or abdominal wounds
▶ profound shock
▶ multiple injuries
▶ hyperpyrexia (temperature over 105° F [40.6° C])
▶ emergency childbirth or complications of pregnancy.

Urgent conditions: Although serious, the following conditions don't immediately threaten the patient's life or organ functions. You can delay treatment for 20 minutes to 2 hours, if necessary, if you find:

▶ chest pain not associated with respiratory symptoms
▶ back injury
▶ persistent nausea, vomiting, or diarrhea
▶ severe abdominal pain
▶ temperature of 102° to 105° F (38.9° to 40.6° C)
▶ panic
▶ bleeding from any orifice.

ChartWizard

Trauma flow sheet

The following form is an example of a trauma flow sheet. Notice that the Trauma Nursing Assessment section covers the primary and secondary surveys to make charting easier.

Trauma Flow Sheet
Trauma Nursing Assessment

Arrival time: _1420_   Date: _2/2/07_
Mechanism of injury: _Dog bite_
Via: ☐ Ambulance   Transferred from: _____
   ☒ Private vehicle   Allergies: _NKDA_
Sex: ☒ M   ☐ F   Current meds: _None_

Treatment prior to arrival (PTA):
☐ CPR ☐ Intubation ☐ C-spine ☐ Oxygen
☐ Mast ☐ Splints ☐ IV ☐ Other: _____
   ☐ Inflated ☐ Chest tube _____
   ☐ Deflated ☐ R ☐ L _____

Primary survey
AIRWAY | Interventions: | Oxygen:
☒ Open | ☐ Oral airway | ☐ Nasal canula
☐ Compromised | ☐ Endo/naso/cryco | ☐ Simple mask
  | ☐ Trach | ☐ Nonrebreathing
  | ☒ None | ☐ Ambu-bag
  | | _____ Liters

C-SPINE
☐ Immobilized PTA   Type: _____
☐ Immobilized in ED
Time: _____   Type: _____

BREATHING
☒ Spontaneous | Breath sounds: | Respiratory effort:
☐ Bagged | ☒ Clear bilateral | ☒ Unlabored
 | ☐ Diminished | ☐ Labored
 | ☐ L ☐ R |
 | ☐ Absent |
 | ☐ L ☐ R |

CIRCULATION
Pulse: ☒ Present/rate: _106_
   ☐ Absent/CPR-time: _____
Skin: | External hemorrhage:
☐ Warm/dry ☒ Pale/cool | Location: _Ⓡ hand_
☐ Diaphoretic ☐ Cyanotic | Intervention: _See progress note_

Secondary survey

HEAD	Yes	No
Ear/nose bleeding	☐	☒

Blood glucose level: _98_

	Yes	No
Battles sign	☐	☒
Facial asymmetry	☐	☒

Wounds/deformities
   Scalp: _N/A_
   Face: _N/A_

NECK	Yes	No
Trachea deviated	☐	☒
Subcutaneous emphysema	☐	☒
Jugular vein distention	☐	☒

Wounds/deformities: _N/A_ _____
_____

CHEST	Yes	No
Asymmetrical movement	☐	☒
Crepitus/subcutaneous air	☐	☒

Heart sounds:
   ☒ Clear ☐ Muffled
Wounds/contusions: _N/A_

ABDOMEN	Yes	No
Tender	☐	☒
Rigid	☐	☒
Distended	☐	☒
Obese	☐	☒

Wounds/contusions: _N/A_

PELVIS/GU
Pelvis:
   ☒ Stable ☐ Unstable
Blood at meatus:
   ☐ Yes ☒ No

EXTREMITIES

	Pulses	Movement	Wounds/ deformities
R. arm	☒ Pres ☐ Abs ☐ Dec	☒ Yes ☐ No	_Puncture wound_
L. arm	☒ Pres ☐ Abs ☐ Dec	☒ Yes ☐ No	_N/A_
R. leg	☒ Pres ☐ Abs ☐ Dec	☒ Yes ☐ No	_N/A_
L. leg	☒ Pres ☐ Abs ☐ Dec	☒ Yes ☐ No	_N/A_

POSTERIOR SURVEY:
Wounds/deformities: _N/A_ _____
_____

Rectal tone: ☐ Present ☐ Absent ☒ Deferred

GLASGOW COMA SCALE (GCS)

EYES OPENING		
Spontaneously	④
To Speech	3
To Pain	2
None	1

VERBAL	Adult		Infant/child	
	Oriented	⑤	Coos/babbles	5
	Confused	4	Irritable/cries, consolable	4
	Inappropriate	3	Cries to pain	3
	Incomprehensible	2	Moans to pain	2
	None	1	None	1

MOTOR				
	Obeys commands	⑥	Spontaneous movements	6
	Localizes	5	Withdraws to touch	5
	Withdraws	4	Withdraws to pain	4
	Flexion	3	Flexion	3
	Extension	2	Extension	2
	None	1	None	1

REVISED TRAUMA SCORE

A: SPONT. RESP.		
10-24	④
25-35	3
> 35	2
< 10	1
0	0

B: SYSTOLIC BP		
> 90	④
70-89	3
50-69	2
< 50	1
0	0

C: CONVERT GCS		
13-15	④
9-12	3
6-8	2
4-5	1
3-0	0

Revised trauma score:
A + B + C = _12_

Trauma flow sheet (continued)

Trauma Flow Sheet
Page 2 of 3

Trauma alert called: _____	☐ PTA ☐ ED		
		TRAUMA TEAM	
	Name		Arrival time
Trauma surgeon			
ED MD	Jacob Smiling, MD		1430
Other			
Primary RN	Frances Baldwin, RN		1420
Secondary RN			

			R	L	R	L	R	L	R	L	R	L	R	L	R	L	R	L	R	L	R	L	R	L	R	L	R	L
Time	1420	1435																											
BP	100/60	102/68																											
Pulse	106	103																											
Resp (S=Spont.)	20 S	22 S																											
Temp	98.8	/																											
Cardiac rhythm	NSR	NSR																											
Pulse oximeter	98%	99%																											
Pupils	B-S	B-S	B-S	B-S																									
LOC	/	/																											

LOC
1 - Alert/oriented 4 - Responds to pain
2 - Disoriented 5 - Unresponsive
3 - Responds to verbal 6 - Chemically paralyzed

PUPIL REACTION KEY:
S - Sluggish
B - Brisk
N - Nonreactive

Pupil size in mm:
1 2 3 4 5 6 7 8

FLUIDS Fluid warmer used: ☐ Yes ☒ No

Time	Solution	Amount	Location	Rate/hr	Cath size	Additive	Amount infused	Initials
1500	NSS	1000ml	@ arm	75/hr	18G	—		FB

MEDICATIONS

Time 15/0	Tetanus	0.5 cc	I.M.	Lot #: 426718 Expires: 12/05

Time	Med.	Dose	Route	Site	Initials
1515	Demerol	25 mg	I.V.	@ arm	FB
1530	Rocephin	250 mg	I.V.	@ arm	FB

BLOOD ADMINISTRATION

Time	Unit number	Blood type	Total infused

	INTAKE			OUTPUT	
Oral	250	cc	Urine	550	cc
IV/IVPB	600	cc	NG/emesis	—	cc
NG	—	cc	Feces	—	cc
Other	—	cc	Other	—	cc

(continued)

Trauma flow sheet *(continued)*

Trauma Flow Sheet

Page 3 of 3

TREATMENTS AND PROCEDURES

Intubated by: _____ / _____ / _____
Size — Inserted by — Time

NG tube: _____ / _____ / _____
Size — Inserted by — Time

Chest tube: ☐ Left _____ / _____ / _____
Size — Inserted by — Time

☐ Right _____ / _____ / _____
Size — Inserted by — Time

Drainage: _____ / _____
Amount — Time

Foley catheter: *14 Fr* / *F. Baldwin, RN* / *1500* / *Yellow* Dip: ☐ Pos. ☒ Neg.
Size — Inserted by — Time — Color

Peritoneal lavage: _____ / _____
Performed by — Timer

Grossly positive? ☐ Yes ☐ No

Warm blankets ☐

Thoracotomy: _____ / _____
Performed by — Timer

Warm fluids ☐

Central line: _____ / _____ / _____ / _____
Size — Inserted by — Time — Location

MAJOR INJURIES

Puncture wound to Ⓡ hand from dog bite.

Time	Progress Notes
1420	12-year-old white male with dog bite arrived to ED via private vehicle. Alert and oriented X3. Puncture wound to dorsal aspect of Ⓡ hand. Moderate bleeding. ——— Frances Baldwin, RN
1440	Wound irrigated c̄ NS and betadine. ——————————— F. Baldwin, RN
1500	I.V. placed Ⓛ arm with 18G jelco. 1,000 ml NSS hung and infusing at 75 ml/hr. F. Baldwin, RN
1510	0.5 ml tetanus shot given I.M. ———————————— F. Baldwin, RN
1515	25 mg Demerol given I.V. push. ————————————— F. Baldwin, RN
1530	250 mg Rocephin in 100 ml NSS given IVPB. ————————— F. Baldwin, RN

Police agency: *Georgetown sheriff* ☒ Notified: *1520* ☐ Arrived: _____

Time transfer initiated: _____ Time accepted: _____

FAMILY	PATIENT DISPOSITION:	SIGNATURES:	INITIALS
☒ Present	Admitted to: _____ Expired: _____	*F. Baldwin, RN*	*FB*
☐ Not present but notified	Report called: _____ / _____ Time / Person		
☐ Unable to contact	Transported by: _____ Name		

2/10/07	2250	Pt. admitted to ED accompanied by police officers John Hanson (badge #1234) and Teresa Collins (badge #5678). Pt. states, "I was attacked in the supermarket parking lot. I think it was about 9 p.m. He pulled me into the bushes and raped me. When he ran away, I called 911 from my cell phone." Pt. trembling and crying but able to walk into ED on her own. Placed in private room. Police officers waited in waiting room. Pt. denies being pregnant, drug allergies, and recent illnesses including venereal disease. LMP 1/28/07. States she didn't wash or douche before coming to the hospital. Chain of evidence maintained for all specimens collected (see flow sheet). After obtaining written consent and explaining procedure, Dr. Smith examined pt. Pt. has reddened areas on face and anterior neck and blood on lips. Bruising noted on inner aspects of both thighs; some vaginal bleeding noted. See dr.'s note for details of pelvic exam. Specimens for venereal disease, blood, and vaginal smears collected and labeled. Evidence from fingernail scraping and pubic hair combing collected and labeled. Photographs of injuries taken. Stayed with pt. throughout exam, holding her hand and offering reassurance and comfort. Pt. cooperated with exam but was often teary. After explaining the need for prophylactic antibiotics to pt., she consented and ceftriaxone 250 mg I.M. was administered in Ⓡ dorsogluteal muscle. Pt. declined morning-after pill. Pt. consented to blood screening for HIV and hepatitis. Blood samples drawn, labeled, and sent to lab. Pt. understands need for f/u tests for HIV, hepatitis, and venereal disease. States she will f/u with family dr. ———— Susan Rose, RN
2/10/07	2330	June Jones, MSW, spoke with pt. at length. Gave pt. information on rape crisis center and victim's rights advocate. Pt. states, "I'll call them. Ms. Jones told me they can help me deal with this." Pt. phoned brother and sister-in-law who will come to hospital and take pt. to their home for the night. Police officers interviewed pt. with her permission regarding the details of the event. At pt.'s request Ms. Jones and myself remained with pt. ———— ———————————————— Susan Rose, RN
2/10/07	2350	Pt.'s brother, John Muncy and his wife, Carol Muncy, arrived to take pt. to their house. Pt. will make appt. tomorrow to f/u with own doctor next week or sooner, if needed. Pt. has names and phone numbers for rape crisis counselor, victim's rights advocate, Ms. Jones, ED, and police dept. ——— ———————————————— Susan Rose, RN

cologic treatment or surgery; and a history of sexual intercourse within the past 72 hours. Make sure the chain of custody for all evidence collected is maintained and logged according to your facility's protocol. Document all information completely, including the date and time that the evidence was given to law enforcement officers. Include the names of all individuals involved in the medical record.

REPORTABLE SITUATIONS
Reportable situations, which are occurrences that must be reported to the appropriate agency, vary by state. Documentation of the notification of appropriate agencies should be included in the patient's ED record. (See *Reportable situations in the ED,* page 344.)

Learn the reportable situations in the state in which you work as well as the agencies to which they should be reported.

PATIENT REFUSAL OF EMERGENCY TREATMENT
A competent adult has the right to refuse emergency treatment. His family can't overrule his decision, and his practitioner isn't allowed to give the expressly refused treatment, even if the patient becomes unconscious.

In most cases, the health care personnel who are responsible for the patient can remain free from legal jeopardy as long as they fully inform the patient about his medical condition and the likely consequences of refusing treatment. The courts recognize a competent adult's right to refuse medical treatment, even when that refusal will clearly result in his death. If the patient understands the risks but still refuses treatment, notify the nursing supervisor and the patient's practitioner.

The courts recognize several circumstances that justify overruling a patient's refusal of treatment. These include when refusing treatment endangers the life of another, when a parent's

Reportable situations in the ED

The following chart gives examples of reportable situations in the emergency department (ED) and the agencies to which they should be reported. Be aware that mandatory reporting may vary by state.

REPORTABLE SITUATION	AGENCY
Homicide	▶ Coroner ▶ Law enforcement
Suicide	▶ Coroner ▶ Law enforcement
Altercations and assaults	▶ Law enforcement
Motor vehicle crashes	▶ Law enforcement
Deaths	▶ Coroner ▶ Local organ procurement (in most states)
Child abuse	▶ Child protective services
Elder abuse	▶ Adult protective services
Communicable diseases	▶ Varies by state
Animal bites	▶ Animal control

1/23/07	1300	Pt. brought to ED by ambulance
		with chest pain, radiating to Ⓛ
		arm. Pt. sitting up in bed, not in
		acute distress. Skin pale, RR 28,
		occasionally rubbing Ⓛ arm. Pt.
		refusing physical exam, blood work,
		and ECG. States "I didn't want to
		come to the hospital. My coworkers
		called an ambulance without telling
		me. I'm fine, my arm's just sore
		from raking leaves. I'm leaving."
		Explained to pt. that chest and
		arm pain may be symptoms of a
		heart attack and explained the
		risks of leaving without treatment,
		including death. Pt. stated, "I told
		you, I'm not having a heart attack.
		I want to leave." Notified Mary
		Colwell, RN, nursing supervisor,
		and Dr. Lowell. Dr. Lowell explained
		the need for diagnostic tests to
		r/o MI and the risks involved in
		not having treatment. Pt. still
		refusing treatment but did agree
		to sign refusal of treatment
		release form. Explained signs and
		symptoms of MI to pt. Encouraged
		pt. to seek treatment and call 911
		if symptoms persist. Pt. discharged
		with ED # to call with questions.
		———————— Melissa Worthing, RN

decision threatens the child's life, or when despite refusing treatment the patient makes statements that indicate he wants to live. If none of these grounds exist, then you have an ethical duty to defend your patient's right to refuse treatment. Try to explain the patient's choice to his family. Emphasize that the decision is his as long as he's competent.

ADMISSION TO THE FACILITY

When patients are admitted to a floor in the facility, it's important to document certain essential information. Chart the time that the patient was admitted and the time the admitting practitioner was notified. After giving the report to the receiving nurse, document where the patient is going, the name of the nurse taking report, mode of transfer to the floor, and the condition of the patient upon transfer.

Consult your facility's policy for hand-off communication during all patient transfers, which should include passing on the most current information about the patient's treatment, care, condition, and anticipated changes. Document this interactive communication appropriately.

TRANSFER TO ANOTHER FACILITY

At times it becomes necessary to transfer ED patients to other facilities. You need to be particularly aware of documentation requirements for patients being transferred in order to demonstrate compliance with the Emergency Medical Treatment and Active Labor Act (EMTALA). EMTALA was designed to prevent inappropriate transfers ("dumping") of patients seeking emergency care or those who are in active labor, but it actually applies to any patient seeking medical care anywhere on hospital property.

EMTALA requirements include:

▶ An appropriate medical screening examination. Assessment by the triage nurse doesn't constitute an appropriate medical screening examination. Any services that normally would be included, such as laboratory tests or radiology, must be included in this examination.

▶ The examination can't be delayed to ask about insurance or method of payment.

▶ An attempt to stabilize the patient before transfer must be demonstrated.

If your patient is going to be transferred, make sure that the following has been documented:

▶ a qualified practitioner's signature certifying that the transfer is medically necessary

▶ the name of the receiving practitioner (this may be the ED physician at the receiving facility)

▶ that the receiving hospital has agreed to accept the patient

▶ that medical records are being sent with the patient

▶ the patient's or a relative's signature

▶ consent to release copies of the patient's medical record, signed by the patient or a family member

▶ that the patient was transferred with qualified personnel and appropriate equipment.

Failure to properly comply with EMTALA requirements could result in significant fines for the facility, the potential loss of Medicare provider status, and the potential for civil liability.

DISCHARGE INSTRUCTIONS

It's important to chart the patient's condition at the time of discharge or transfer to another facility. You must also document discharge instructions that you gave to the patient and his family as well as evidence of their understanding. Many EDs have preprinted discharge instructions. These are usually written at a fourth- to sixth-grade reading level and may come in different languages. Make sure that you individualize these preprinted instructions for your patient. Include instructions for follow-up with other health care providers if needed. To comply with The Joint Commission's Patient Safety Goals, you also must provide the patient with a complete list of his medications upon discharge. Obtain the signature of the patient or family member, and sign the discharge instructions yourself, as they become a part of the medical record.

Maternal-neonatal nursing

Maternal-neonatal nursing takes place in a variety of settings. Traditionally, maternal-neonatal nurses worked in only one of the following areas: outpatient offices or clinics caring for the pregnant woman, hospital labor and delivery units, postpartum units, neonatal nurseries and intensive care units, or high-risk antepartum units. The current trend is for the maternal-neonatal nurse to be competent to give care in multiple settings. Most hospitals have eliminated the traditional well-baby nursery, which means that nurses are often responsible for the mother and neonate from the time of delivery until the time of discharge. In smaller hospitals, a nurse may be caring for high-risk antepartum women, laboring women, and postpartum women and their infants. You must be prepared to care for and document the care of women and infants in these multifunctional settings.

Documentation in maternal-neonatal nursing is especially sensitive and critical for two reasons that don't exist in other areas of nursing documentation:

▶ You're often caring for two patients at once, whose best interests may be in conflict.

▶ In the case of a pregnancy, labor, or birth injury, the parents or the child have until the child reaches the age of majority plus 18 months to sue.

The Association for Women's Health, Obstetric, and Neonatal Nurses (AWHONN) primarily sets the standards of care for women and neonates. Standards set by the American Nurses Association, the American College of Obstetricians and Gynecologists, and the American Academy of Pediatrics may also apply, but those are most likely reflected in AWHONN standards. Remember that the policies of each health care facility may differ slightly from general guidelines and that the best advice is to always follow the most stringent guidelines. When patient circumstances indicate the need for more frequent assessments and documentation, assess as frequently as needed to ensure the best possible outcome for the patient.

Also, keep in mind these three important points when providing care in a maternal-neonate setting:

▶ The nurse is expected to be thoroughly familiar with pregnancy, labor, postpartum, and neonate care.

▶ The nurse is expected to recognize deviations from normal assessment findings.

▶ The nurse is expected to implement measures to maintain the patient's well-being and correct problems expediently.

Your careful documentation of observations and interventions assures your patient quality care and provides you with the best legal protection available.

Labor and delivery

Many institutions have a checklist or form for physical assessment of the mother on admission and another checklist or form for ongoing assessment during labor. You also should be familiar with the specific procedures or protocols of your practice setting, your state's nurse practice act, and applicable national standards.

A woman who's in labor will usually call her health care provider to let him know that she's on her way to the hospital. Although not always possible to accomplish before the woman arrives, try to review the prenatal record (the foundation for care and documentation during the hospital stay) for the following information (or obtain it once the woman arrives if there's no existing record):

▶ gravidity (number of pregnancies), parity (number of live births), and abortions (spontaneous or therapeutic)

▶ estimated due date

▶ weeks gestation and the frequency of visits for prenatal care

▶ medical, surgical, psychiatric, and obstetric history

▶ laboratory results

▶ ultrasound or other diagnostic procedures

▶ allergies

▶ medications, including prenatal vitamins

▶ use of alcohol, tobacco, and illicit drugs

▶ complementary therapies or supplements.

In addition to this preliminary information, you'll need to obtain more comprehensive infor-

Initial assessment on admission to labor and delivery

For your initial assessment of the patient on admission to labor and delivery, evaluate and document the following information.
▶ The patient's reason for coming to the labor and delivery unit. This will determine the speed of the assessment and prioritize what needs to be done as well as facilitate correct documentation. For a woman in early labor or one who's being admitted for a pregnancy-related problem, there will be plenty of time to ask questions and document as you go along. If the woman is in active labor, especially if birth is imminent, ask the most important questions, do the examination quickly, and finish the paperwork later. You're never expected to sacrifice patient care in order to do paperwork.
▶ Ask the patient if she has a birth plan or what her birth plans and desires are, including positions for labor, support people, and use of medications.
▶ If the patient is in labor—or if she thinks she's in labor—ask her to describe the onset of contractions, the timing and strength of contractions, and her pain level.

▶ Ask the patient if there's anything else you should know in order to provide her with the best possible care.
 Question the patient about the following:
▶ gravidity, parity, and weeks of gestation
▶ symptoms of gestational hypertension, diabetes, or other medical problems such as asthma
▶ status of membranes.
 If it's available, verify this information with the prenatal record and enter it into the hospital record (typically on an admission flow sheet, labor flow sheet, and delivery record).
 Finish your assessment with a physical examination, including:
▶ baseline vital signs, understanding that there may be circumstances existing that have already changed the patient's normal vital signs (such as labor, pain, infection, gestational hypertension, or diabetes)
▶ a vaginal examination, including the documentation of dilation, effacement, presenting part, and station.

mation from the patient upon her admission. (See *Initial assessment on admission to labor and delivery.*)

From the perspective of the woman and her family, the most important factors in her care are your perceived competency and caring attitude. You're far less likely to get sued if you greet the woman warmly, make her and her family feel welcomed and cared for, and elicit the woman's perceptions and expectations about giving birth, than if you portray yourself as superbly competent, yet cold and uncaring.

MEDICATIONS
The four most common medications used in labor are antibiotics, magnesium sulfate, oxytocin,

and pain relievers. When a patient receives any of these medications, make sure that you document the medication's administration, timing, and dose as well as the patient's response.

WHERE TO DOCUMENT
In labor and delivery, you have to document your action in numerous places. Documentation is required on the chart, which usually contains one or more flow sheets; nurse's notes; the delivery record; and on the monitor tracing. In addition, you must carefully transcribe appropriate information from the prenatal record to these documents. A seemingly small error on your part, such as transcribing a negative rather than the

Frequency of documentation

The chart below shows documentation intervals for the patient in labor that meet the Association for Women's Health, Obstetric, and Neonatal Nurses standards.

STAGE OF LABOR	UNCOMPLICATED LABOR WITH NO MEDICATIONS	COMPLICATED LABOR	PITOCIN-INDUCED OR AUGMENTED LABOR
Latent	Every 60 minutes	Every 30 minutes	At a minimum, before every dose increase
Active	Every 30 minutes	Every 15 minutes	At a minimum, before every dose increase
Second stage	Every 15 minutes	Every 5 minutes	At a minimum, before every dose increase

correct positive Rh factor, can have serious consequences for the mother and fetus.

In general, evaluate and document fetal heart rate and contractions according to your facility's policy. (See *Frequency of documentation*.)

DOCUMENTING FETAL WELL-BEING
Assessing the fetus is equally as important as assessing the mother. First, determine whether there have been fetal problems identified during the pregnancy by reviewing the prenatal record and by asking the patient. Then apply electronic fetal monitoring, which can be done internally or externally. External fetal monitoring is used for most women and consists of a fetal heart rate (FHR) monitor and a tocotransducer. These devices trace FHR and uterine contraction data on the same printout paper. Internal fetal monitoring assesses fetal response to uterine contractions by providing an electrocardiogram of the FHR. It precisely measures intrauterine pressure, tracks labor progress, and allows evaluation of short- and long-term FHR variability. (See *Reading a fetal monitor strip*.)

Whether using internal or external monitoring, you must first label the monitoring strip, or enter into the computer, the patient's identification information, the date, maternal vital signs and position, the paper speed, and the number of the strip paper. During a time when numerous events are occurring, the fetal monitor strip may be the best place to document. However, keep three factors in mind when documenting on the monitor strip: First, don't obscure any part of the tracing with writing; second, write legibly; third, don't draw attention to problems (for example, by circling an FHR deceleration). If significant events are documented on the monitor strip, they can be easily transferred to the chart later.

When the patient or fetal condition requires notification of the practitioner or midwife who isn't present on the unit, you need to document complete information, not just "Dr. Barnett notified." Complete documentation includes the

Reading a fetal monitor strip

Presented in two parallel recordings, the fetal monitor strip records the fetal heart rate (FHR) in beats/minute in the top recording and uterine activity (UA) in mm Hg in the bottom recording. You can obtain information on fetal status and labor progress by reading the strips horizontally and vertically.

Reading horizontally on the FHR or the UA strip, each small block represents 10 seconds. Six consecutive small blocks, separated by a dark vertical line, represent 1 minute.

Reading vertically on the FHR strip, each block represents an amplitude of 10 beats/minute. Reading vertically on the UA strip, each block represents 8.33 mm Hg of pressure.

Assess the baseline FHR—the "resting" heart rate—between uterine contractions when fetal movement diminishes. This baseline FHR (normal range: 120 to 160 beats/minute) pattern serves as a reference for subsequent FHR tracings produced during contractions.

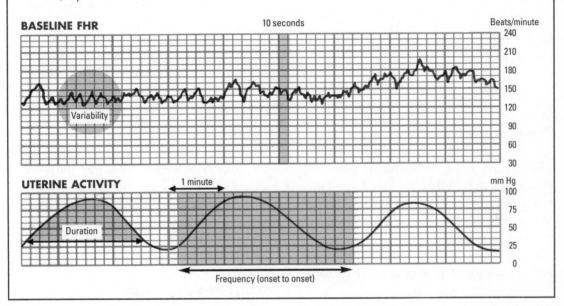

exact time the practitioner or midwife was notified, what information he was given, and his response.

Here's an example of a notification that's documented correctly:

"At 1000, Dr. Barnett was notified of the patient's 102.4° F temperature with other vital signs as noted on flow sheet, fetal tachycardia of 180 to 194 beats/minute, and moderate amount of foul-smelling amniotic fluid leaking from vagina. Dr. Barnett ordered Unasyn 2 g I.V. q 4 hours, was reminded of patient's allergy to penicillin, and changed the order to clindamycin 900 mg I.V. q 8 hours." This information documented incorrectly may look like this: "MD notified of maternal fever and fetal tachycardia. Antibiotics ordered."

Also, document the time you administered the medication as well as the patient's response.

Recording the Apgar score

Use this chart to determine the neonatal Apgar score at 1 minute and 5 minutes after birth. For each category listed, assign a score of 0 to 2, as shown. A total score of 7 to 10 indicates the neonate is in good condition; 4 to 6, fair condition (the neonate may have moderate central nervous system depression, muscle flaccidity, cyanosis, and poor respirations); 0 to 3, danger (the neonate needs immediate resuscitation, as ordered).

SIGN	0	1	2
Heart rate	Absent	Less than 100 beats/minute	More than 100 beats/minute
Respiratory effort	Absent	Slow, irregular	Good crying
Muscle tone	Flaccid	Some flexion and resistance to extension of extremities	Active motion
Reflex irritability	No response	Grimace or weak cry	Vigorous cry
Color	Pale, cyanosis	Pink body, blue extremities	Completely pink

Postpartum care

Assess each assigned patient as soon as possible after your shift begins. In smaller hospitals, the labor and delivery nurse may also care for the patient throughout her postpartum stay. Intrapartum and postpartum care overlap during the fourth stage of labor.

In general, the guidelines for assessment frequency are determined by your facility's policy. However, assessments must be done and documented more frequently if any of the assessment parameters are found to be abnormal. Pertinent teaching also must be given and documented.

Neonatal documentation

Neonatal assessment includes initial and ongoing assessment as well as a thorough physical examination, all of which must be carefully documented. Special areas of neonatal documentation include Apgar scoring and the initial physical assessment.

APGAR SCORING

The Apgar scoring system provides a way to evaluate the neonate's cardiopulmonary and neurologic status. The assessment is performed at 1 and 5 minutes after birth and repeated every 5 minutes (up to 20 minutes) if the Apgar score at 5 minutes is less than 7. (See *Recording the Apgar score.*)

NEONATAL ASSESSMENT

Perform a thorough visual and physical examination of the neonate, being sure to include each body part. This assessment is important in identifying whether congenital anomalies or other abnormalities exist. Health care facilities develop their own neonatal assessment forms arranged by body system; most follow the same general guidelines to ensure that the assessment is complete. (See *General guidelines for neonatal assessment.*)

Smarter charting

General guidelines for neonatal assessment

When performing the initial neonatal assessment, these guidelines will help you make sure that your examination and documentation are complete.

INTEGUMENTARY SYSTEM
▶ Assess the general appearance. Is there cyanosis or duskiness?
▶ Assess the quality of skin turgor.
▶ Assess skin temperature.
▶ Check for lacerations or abrasions. Note the location and degree if present.
▶ Observe for anomalies, such as birth marks, forcep marks, or Mongolian spots.
▶ Observe for the presence of erythema toxicum, lanugo, milia, petechia, or vernix, and note the location and degree if present.

HEAD
▶ Assess the anterior and posterior fontanelles. Are they sunken, soft, tense, or bulging? What's their size?
▶ Assess the scalp. Look for the presence of bruising, caput, cephalhematoma, lacerations, and scalp electrode placement marking. Also, measure the head circumference.
▶ Assess the sutures. Are they overlapping, separated (indicate in cm), fused, or soft?
▶ Assess the ears. Observe their form and positioning and check their degree of recoil. Also check for the presence of vernix, tags, or pits.
▶ Assess the eyes. Are the lids fused? Is there periorbital edema? If the eyes are open, assess for pupil reaction, red reflex, and scleral hemorrhages. If there's conjunctivitis, describe drainage.
▶ Assess the face. Observe its general appearance for color, eye spacing, and symmetry. Look for the presence of birthmarks, edema, forceps marks, malformations, paralysis, and skin tags.
▶ Assess the nose. Is each nasal passage patent? Observe for nasal flaring.
▶ Assess the mouth and lips. Observe chin size and the integrity of the lips (cleft lip present?).

Open the mouth and look for the presence of teeth. Observe the mucous membranes for color, moisture, and the presence of lesions. Assess the suck reflex, and follow the roof of the mouth with your finger to assess for cleft palate.
▶ Assess the neck. Is it supple with normal range of motion? Is the trachea aligned? Is there webbing, crepitus, or palpable glands or masses? Assess each clavicle for fracture.

CARDIOVASCULAR SYSTEM
▶ Assess capillary refill time (normally less than 3 seconds).
▶ Assess for edema. Note its location and whether it's pitting or nonpitting.
▶ Assess heart rate and rhythm. Are they regular? Are heart sounds muffled or distant?
▶ Assess for murmurs. If present, describe the location and intensity.
▶ Assess peripheral pulses (brachial and femoral, bilaterally). Are they equal and regular, or bounding, weak, or thready?
▶ Assess the location of the point of maximal impulse (normally located at the 5th intercostal space).

RESPIRATORY SYSTEM
▶ Assess rate and rhythm of respirations. Are they shallow or rapid? Is the pattern regular? Are there periods of apnea? Does the chest expand symmetrically?
▶ Assess breath sounds. Are they equal, clear, and audible in all lobes? Listen for crackles, rhonchi, or wheezes.
▶ Assess for the presence of grunting or retracting.
▶ Measure the chest's circumference.
▶ Assess the shape of the chest as well as the placement and number of nipples. Assess breast development.

(continued)

General guidelines for neonatal assessment *(continued)*

GI SYSTEM
▶ Assess the umbilical cord. Note its appearance and the number of vessels.
▶ Observe the abdomen for general appearance. Is it round, distended, flat, or scaphoid? Is ascites present? Auscultate for bowel sounds.
▶ Gently palpate the abdomen. Note masses, organomegaly, or tenderness.
▶ Measure abdominal circumference.
▶ Record the first passage of meconium.
▶ Assess the anus for patency.

GENITOURINARY SYSTEM
Male
▶ Assess the penis. Is gender obvious or is it questionable? Note the placement of the urethral meatus. (Is there epispadias or hypospadias?)
▶ Assess the scrotum for edema, masses, the amount of rugae, and for herniation.
▶ Assess the testes. Are both descended or are they still in the inguinal canal?

Female
▶ Assess for masses or herniation.
▶ Assess the clitoris and labia for size. Is gender obvious or is it questionable?
▶ Assess the vagina for discharge. If present, describe it.

General
▶ Record the first void.

NEUROMUSCULAR SYSTEM
▶ Assess general activity. Is the neonate active, lethargic, or paralyzed? Is he jittery, tremulous, or having seizures?
▶ Assess the spine for limited range of motion.
▶ Assess the sucking, rooting, grasping, Moro, and Babinski reflexes.
▶ Assess tone. Is he hypotonic or hypertonic?

EXTREMITIES
▶ Assess for range of motion.
▶ Assess hips for clicks and check gluteal fold and thigh length symmetry.
▶ Assess the number of digits and check for webbing, extra digits, clubbing, or cyanosis.
▶ Assess the soles of the feet for normal creases.
▶ Check the palms for simian creases.
▶ Observe for gross abnormalities.

PSYCHOSOCIAL
▶ Assess the mother's status: Is she single, married, divorced, separated, widowed? Are there siblings?
▶ Determine the primary caregiver: mother, father, grandparent?
▶ Note if breast or bottle feeding.

Pediatric nursing

If you're a nurse who works with children, you have special challenges. Helping a child achieve and maintain an optimal level of health means working with the child and his family. Clear and accurate documentation is necessary because it allows information regarding the patient to be passed on to multiple members of the health care team in a way that oral communication can't, which may serve to protect you many years later.

We live in a litigious society, and the courts give children special consideration when it comes to lawsuits. For nurses working with the pediatric population, liability from malpractice may extend for years. This differs from the adult population that typically has only a few years from the date or discovery of an injury to file a lawsuit. With children, however, the time requirement or statute of limitations is suspended until the age of majority (18 years), and then the adult statute of limitations period begins. Therefore, a nurse theoretically can be held liable for care given 20 years before to a child who was 2 years old at the time in question. Following the filing of the suit, it may be another 2 to 3 years before the case is actually brought to court. After that length of time, the chart is usually all that one has to recall the patient and the care that was given. (See *Documenting thoroughly.*)

Special issues in pediatric nursing documentation

Special aspects for the documentation of nursing care for children include growth and development, psychosocial considerations, and child abuse and neglect.

GROWTH AND DEVELOPMENT

Working with children requires a certain amount of skill and flexibility in providing care to a wide range of ages and developmental stages. A toddler is vastly different from an adolescent; the care given and subsequent documentation must reflect that. While the format of the documentation tool that's used might be similar for all age groups, including adults, it must have the capacity to include the different stages that children go through. The documentation tool used to evaluate children needs to have been developed using national standards and should include current recommendations for physical assessment and health guidance.

Bright Futures provides guidelines that meet these criteria. This project is a national child

---

Smarter charting

Documenting thoroughly

A good rule of thumb to follow is to document so thoroughly, completely, and accurately that another person, reviewing your work 2 years or more later, can see exactly what you saw and follow your train of thought in providing the nursing care and interventions that you performed. This includes your care of the child as well as your care and support of the family.

---

health promotion and disease prevention initiative that was launched in 1990 as part of the National Center for Education in Maternal and Child Health. The guidelines provide a framework that health care professionals can use for health assessment for the recommended 29 health supervision visits, from neonatal visits until the child is age 21. The information focuses on the physical aspects of health as well as the social, cognitive, and emotional well-being of children and adolescents in the context of family and community.

Developmental screening

Multiple screening tools exist to assess a child's development. These tools assess gross and fine motor skills, personal and social behaviors, language abilities, and other components of development. One of the most commonly used tools is the Denver-II, formerly known as the Denver Developmental Screening Test II (DDST II). This screening tool assesses the developmental level of children ages 1 month to 6 years; however, it isn't a diagnostic tool or intelligence test. It employs a series of developmental tasks to determine whether a child's development is within the normal range.

The Denver-II looks at four domains: personal-social, fine motor adaptive, language, and gross motor skills. It's easy to administer, has been used by health care professionals for years, provides a good indication of where the child is developmentally, and is helpful in providing guidance to parents. If the child's development is questionable in any of the four areas (compared with normal standards), referral for an in-depth evaluation is recommended.

Other tools have been developed or adapted and may be used by your health care facility. Follow the recommended procedures for administering the tool and completely document your findings.

Growth charts

All growth parameters should be followed sequentially on the appropriate growth charts. Growth is a continuous process that must be evaluated over time. Evaluating a child's growth provides useful information for the early detection of abnormalities and provides reassurance to the parents and health care providers that the child is growing normally.

Document growth using the most recent Centers for Disease Control and Prevention growth charts, developed by the National Center for Health Statistics and adopted by the World Health Organization (WHO) for international use in 1977 (although the WHO launched the new Child Growth Standards in 2006, which may be used worldwide once officially adopted by individual countries.) These 16 revised charts (8 for boys, 8 for girls) include weight-for-age, length/stature-for-age, and weight-for-length/stature percentile charts. These charts represent revisions to the previous charts and use the body mass index (BMI).

The BMI is a number calculated from a person's weight and height measurements, and it helps to determine if a person is overweight or underweight. With children, the interpretation of BMI depends on the child's age because as a child grows, his percentage of body fat changes. It's also important to remember that BMI is plotted for age on sex-specific charts because girls differ from boys in their percentage of body fat as they mature. (See *Using pediatric growth grids.*)

Obesity commonly begins in childhood and is associated with multiple diseases and chronic conditions. It can be extremely difficult to treat, so prevention is the most effective solution. Tracking BMI allows you and other health care providers to detect early on those at risk for becoming overweight. Sixty percent of children and teens with a BMI-for-age above the 95th percentile have at least one risk factor, while 20 percent have two or more risk factors for cardiovascular disease.

PSYCHOSOCIAL ASSESSMENT

Psychosocial assessment, which includes topics such as behavior, school performance, and family dynamics, is a vital part of the evaluation that is, unfortunately, commonly forgotten. When performing a psychosocial assessment of a child, be sure to assess and record information regarding the child's relationships with his siblings and friends. Also, note the child's typical behavior and reactions to stressors. Because illness and hospitalization is a crisis for families, you'll also need to assess and chart how the rest of the family copes with stressful situations. Other information, such as current living situations, recent losses, or other ongoing or acute crises, can provide you and others caring for the child with valuable information.

ChartWizard

Using pediatric growth grids

Use a growth grid to correlate the child's height with his age and his weight with his height and age. You can also determine the child's body mass index (BMI), which is then plotted on another grid. There are charts for boys and girls. The sample forms below show the growth of a girl tracked over a number of years. Note how her BMI was calculated and then plotted on the BMI grid.

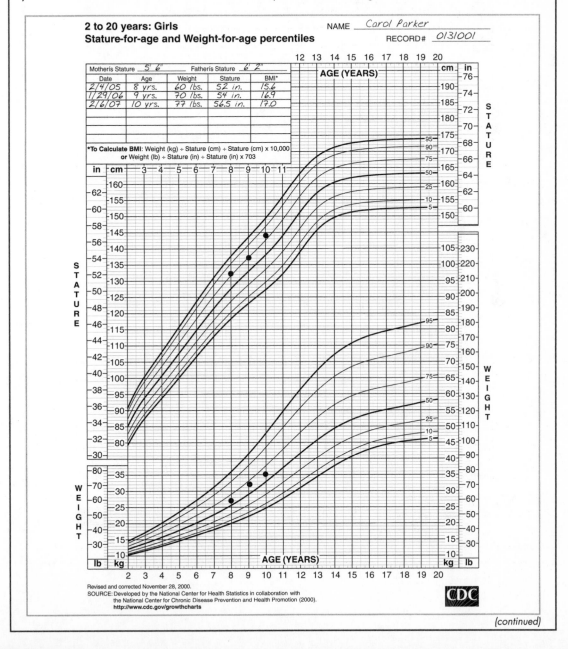

2 to 20 years: Girls
Stature-for-age and Weight-for-age percentiles

NAME _Carol Parker_
RECORD# _0131001_

Mother's Stature	_5' 6"_	Father's Stature	_6' 2"_	
Date	Age	Weight	Stature	BMI*
2/4/05	8 yrs.	60 lbs.	52 in.	15.6
1/29/06	9 yrs.	70 lbs.	54 in.	16.9
2/6/07	10 yrs.	77 lbs.	56.5 in.	17.0

*To Calculate BMI: Weight (kg) ÷ Stature (cm) ÷ Stature (cm) x 10,000
or Weight (lb) ÷ Stature (in) ÷ Stature (in) x 703

Revised and corrected November 28, 2000.
SOURCE: Developed by the National Center for Health Statistics in collaboration with the National Center for Chronic Disease Prevention and Health Promotion (2000).
http://www.cdc.gov/growthcharts

CDC

(continued)

Using pediatric growth grids *(continued)*

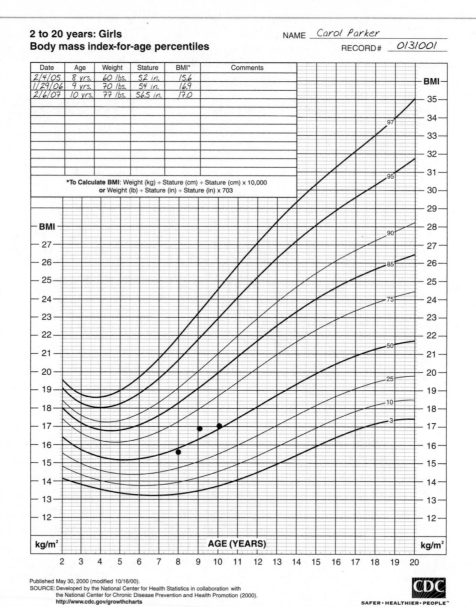

2 to 20 years: Girls
Body mass index-for-age percentiles

NAME *Carol Parker*

RECORD# *013/001*

Date	Age	Weight	Stature	BMI*	Comments
2/4/05	8 yrs.	60 lbs.	52 in.	15.6	
1/29/06	9 yrs.	70 lbs.	54 in.	16.9	
2/6/07	10 yrs.	77 lbs.	56.5 in.	17.0	

*To Calculate BMI: Weight (kg) ÷ Stature (cm) ÷ Stature (cm) x 10,000
or Weight (lb) ÷ Stature (in) ÷ Stature (in) x 703

AGE (YEARS)

kg/m² ... kg/m²

Published May 30, 2000 (modified 10/16/00).
SOURCE: Developed by the National Center for Health Statistics in collaboration with
the National Center for Chronic Disease Prevention and Health Promotion (2000).
http://www.cdc.gov/growthcharts

CDC
SAFER · HEALTHIER · PEOPLE™

Common signs of neglect and abuse

If your assessment reveals any of the following signs, consider neglect or abuse as a possible cause and document your findings. Be sure to notify the appropriate people and agencies.

NEGLECT
► Failure to thrive in infants
► Malnutrition
► Dehydration
► Poor personal hygiene
► Inadequate clothing
► Severe diaper rash
► Injuries from falls
► Failure of wounds to heal
► Periodontal disease
► Infestations, such as scabies, lice, or maggots in a wound

ABUSE
► Recurrent injuries
► Multiple injuries or fractures in various stages of healing
► Unexplained bruises, abrasions, burns, bites, damaged or missing teeth, strap or rope marks
► Head injuries or bald spots from pulling hair out
► Bleeding from body orifices

► Genital trauma
► Sexually transmitted diseases in children
► Pregnancy in young girls or those with physical or mental handicaps
► Verbalized accounts of being beaten, slapped, kicked, or involved in sexual activities
► Precocious sexual behaviors
► Exposure to inappropriately harsh discipline
► Exposure to verbal abuse and belittlement
► Extreme fear or anxiety

ADDITIONAL SIGNS
► Mistrust of others
► Blunted or flat affect
► Depression or mood changes
► Social withdrawal
► Lack of appropriate peer relationships
► Sudden school difficulties, such as poor grades, truancy, or fighting with peers
► Nonspecific headaches, stomachaches, or eating and sleeping problems
► Clinging behavior directed toward health care providers
► Aggressive speech or behavior toward adults
► Abusive behavior toward younger children and pets
► Runaway behavior

CHILD ABUSE AND NEGLECT
Child abuse (including physical, sexual, emotional, and psychological abuse) and neglect are two of the leading causes of pediatric hospital admissions. They may be suspected in any age group, cultural setting, or environment.

In most states, a nurse is required by law to report signs of abuse. (See *Common signs of neglect and abuse.*) Use appropriate channels for your facility and report your suspicions to the appropriate administrator and agency. Document suspicions on the appropriate form for your facility or in your nurse's notes. When interviewing

the family, interview the child alone and try to interview caregivers separately to note inconsistencies with histories. An injunction can be obtained to separate the abuser and the abused so that the patient may be safe until the circumstances can be investigated.

Remember that certain cultural practices that produce bruises or burns, such as coin rubbing in Vietnamese groups, may be mistaken for child abuse. However, regardless of cultural practices, the department of social services and the health care team judge what is and what isn't abuse. (See *Your role in reporting abuse,* page 358.)

Your role in reporting abuse

As a nurse, you play a crucial role in recognizing and reporting incidents of suspected abuse. While caring for patients, you can readily note evidence of apparent abuse. When you do, you must pass the information along to the appropriate authorities. In many states, failure to report actual or suspected abuse constitutes a crime.

If you've ever hesitated to file an abuse report because you fear repercussions, remember that the Child Abuse Prevention and Treatment Act protects you against liability. If your report is bona fide (that is, if you file it in good faith), the law protects you from any suit filed by an alleged abuser.

2/8/07	1700	Circular burns 2 cm in diameter noted
		on lower ® and Ⓛ scapulae in various
		stages of healing while auscultating
		breath sounds. Pt. states these injuries
		occurred while playing with cigarettes
		he found at his babysitter's home. When
		parents were questioned separately as
		to the cause of injuries on child's back,
		mother stated the child told her he
		fell off a swing and received a rope
		burn. Father stated he had no idea of
		the child's injuries. Parents stated the
		child is being watched after school
		until they get home by the teenager
		next door, Sally Johnson. Parents
		stated that their son doesn't like being
		watched by her anymore, but they don't
		know why. Parents state they're looking
		into alternative care suggestions. Dr.
		Gordon notified of injuries and
		examined pt. at 1645. Social service
		department and nursing supervisor,
		Nancy Taylor, RN, notified at 1650.
		—————————— Joanne M. Allen, RN

Surgical nursing

Accurate documentation is essential for all surgical procedures. Data collection for surgical procedures begins during the preadmission period and continues throughout the preoperative, operative, and postanesthesia periods.

Preadmission assessment testing

The surgical process typically begins in the surgeon's office, where the surgeon discusses the procedure with the patient and his family. Legally, the surgeon who will perform the procedure is responsible for explaining the procedure and its risks as well as for obtaining the patient's informed consent. The consent form should state the specific procedure under consideration. After the surgeon informs the patient about the procedure, he may ask you to obtain the patient's signature on the consent form. In this case, you would sign the form as a witness, which means only that you have witnessed the patient's signature.

Before surgery, the patient undergoes laboratory and diagnostic tests to provide baseline data and detect problems that could increase the risk of postoperative complications. For elective surgery patients, tests are typically done in an outpatient setting during the week before surgery. Preoperative laboratory tests may include blood typing and crossmatching, blood urea nitrogen and creatinine levels, coagulation studies, complete blood count, electrolyte levels, human chorionic gonadotropin level, liver function studies, and urinalysis. The diagnostic tests performed depend on such factors as the patient's age, preexisting medical conditions or risk factors, and the type of surgery scheduled. Diagnostic studies may include a chest X-ray, electrocardiogram, or pulmonary function tests.

Preoperative nursing

A thorough preoperative nursing assessment helps to identify risk factors and establish a baseline for intraoperative and postoperative comparisons. During the assessment, focus on problem areas that the patient's history suggests and on body systems that surgery will directly affect. A preoperative physical examination is also performed and includes these items:

▶ general survey

▶ height and weight

▶ vital signs

▶ oxygen saturation

▶ head-to-toe assessment of major body systems.

The Joint Commission requires that all patients have a documented physical examination in their charts. The practitioner will document this in the clinic, office, or upon admission to the health care facility. The preoperative assessment includes both subjective and objective information. The nurse will conduct an interview to gather needed data. In addition to the information mentioned above, other pertinent data to be collected from the patient and documented include:

▶ allergies—List food, medications, and latex allergies that cause reactions. A wristband identifying all allergies is placed on the patient.

▶ health history—Include previous and current medical diagnoses, and past surgeries.

▶ medications—List prescription drugs, over-the-counter drugs, and herbs the patient is taking, including aspirin, warfarin (Coumadin), vitamin E, and clopidogrel (Plavix). It's helpful if the patient brings his medication bottles or a list with him for obtaining accurate drug names, strengths, and dosages. The anesthesiologist or surgeon may request that the patient stop taking specified medications and herbs 2 to 3 weeks before surgery.

▶ method of transportation—Document how the patient will be transported into the preoperative and intraoperative areas.

▶ NPO status—State whether or not the patient should have "nothing by mouth."

▶ valuables—This documentation should include rings, hearing aids, contact lenses, glasses, and dentures. Document which items stay with the patient and which ones are given to family members.

Other essential information that should be in the chart includes:

▶ preoperative orders—Document completeness.

▶ preoperative medications—Prophylactic I.V. antibiotics may be given as ordered preoperatively. The practitioner or anesthesiologist may have the patient take certain medications (such as blood pressure medication) before surgery despite NPO status.

▶ preoperative checklist—Check that each item has been completed for that procedure, which typically includes consent forms signed, preoperative orders and teaching completed, and laboratory and diagnostic test results attached to the patient's chart.

It's important that the preoperative nurse verify that all of these documents are complete and accurate. Lack of proper documentation or data may cause cancellation of the surgical procedure.

Patient teaching at the preadmission *and* preoperative stages is crucial. Effective teaching helps the patient cope with the physical and psychological stress of surgery, and helps him know what to expect during the peri- and postoperative periods. Adapt your teaching to the patient's age, understanding level, and cultural background. Consider the needs of the family or caregiver as well. Include these topics in your teaching:

► anesthesia concerns
► coughing and deep breathing exercises
► diagnostic tests
► dietary and fasting guidelines
► medications
► pain control
► postanesthesia care unit (PACU) experience
► postoperative exercises
► postoperative tubes and drains
► spirometer use
► surgical preparation
► surgical procedure
► use of assistive devices, such as crutches or a walker.

The patient typically waits in the preoperative holding area while the operating room is being prepared for surgery. When the patient arrives in the holding area, confirm his identity using two patient identifiers. The surgeon may see the patient and obtain consent if he hasn't already done so. You may start the patient's I.V. and, if ordered, perform hair removal. (The night before surgery, the patient usually showers or bathes with an antimicrobial soap.)

Before hair removal, you must verify the correct surgical site. Ideally, you should remove the patient's hair as close to the time of surgery as possible, preferably fewer than 2 hours before surgery. To remove hair, use a depilatory (after a patch test to check for skin reactions) or clip it with disposable clippers. Don't use a razor, which may cause skin trauma and increase infection risk.

Perioperative nursing care

Upon the patient's arrival in the operating room, you must confirm his identity again. The surgical site must be marked in an unambiguous manner by the individual performing the procedure. Immediately before starting the procedure, the surgical team must stop and take a "time out" to verify the correct patient, correct procedure, correct surgical site and, if applicable, any surgical implants required. You must document the time out on the perioperative flow sheet or per your facility's policy. The circulating nurse is responsible for perioperative documentation.

Also document the intraoperative nursing assessment and nursing diagnoses on the perioperative flow sheet. (See *Perioperative flow sheet.*)

A perioperative flow sheet should contain a place to document patient safety information. For example, a safety strap is placed across the patient's thighs, extremities are secured with safety straps, and padding is provided where needed. Another safety essential is placement of the electrosurgical grounding pad. Document the application of these safety items according to your facility's policy.

Medication safety is also crucial in the operating room. Each facility's policy and procedure manual should include a procedure to ensure safe operating room medication practices. All medications, containers, and solutions transferred from their original packaging must be labeled on and off the sterile field. The label should include the drug name, amount, strength, and expiration time or date. If the person preparing the label will not be administering the medication, two qualified individuals must verbally and visually verify the labels. When the procedure is completed, the labeled containers are discarded.

In some facilities, the instrument count sheet is another item included in the perioperative flow sheet. The count sheet may also be a separate form. (See *Instrument count sheet,* page 362.) Items to include on the count sheet may vary among facilities. See your facility's policy

Smarter charting

Perioperative flow sheet

Patient's full name: _Angela W. Ings_   Date: _10/1/06_

Procedure: _Laparoscopic cholecystectomy_

Suite #:	Procedure start:	Time patient in room:	Anesthesia start:	Anesthesia provider: _D. M. Walt, CRNA_
_2_	_1006_	_0928_	_0952_	Surgeon: _B. Georgi_ Assistant 1: _R. Berri_ Circulating nurse: _L. Honol_ Scrub assistant: _J. Engel_

ASA Score:	Procedure end:	Time patient out of room:	Anesthesia finish:	Pathology specimens:
_II_	_1040_	_1059_	_1058_	Routine: _one_ Frozen section: _0_ Cultures: _0_

INTRAOPERATIVE NURSING DATA

Risk for infection

☑ Skin intact pre-op ☐ Other: _____
☐ Surgical clippers: _____
 Area: _____
☑ Skin prep By: _L. Honol, RN_
  ☐ Povidone iodine ☑ Chlorhexidine
  ☐ Other _____
Wound classification:
  ☐ Clean ☑ Clean-contaminated
  ☐ Contaminated ☐ Dirty

☐ Urinary catheter:
 Size/type: _0_
 OR output _____ Inserted by: _____
☐ Drains/tubes (size/type/site): _0_
 OR drainage amount: _____
☐ Packing (size/type/site): _0_
☐ Cast (type/site): _0_
☑ Dressing (type/site): _4 X 4 and large bandaid –_
      umbilicus

Risk for hypothermia

☑ Apply warming blanket #: _6025_
 Temp setting: _high_   Applied by: _D. M. Walt_

☐ Warm I.V. fluid   ☐ Warm irrigation
☐ Other: _____

OPERATING ROOM PATIENT IDENTIFICATION:

Operative procedure and site: _Laparoscopic cholecystectomy_

Surgeon Circ Nurse
☑ ☑ Patient ID bracelet personally observed
☑ ☑ Patient questioned verbally regarding ID, Procedure, and Site
☑ ☑ Patient's chart reviewed to verify ID, Procedure, and Site
☑ ☑ Surgical site confirmed
☑ ☑ Time-out performed

Surgeon's Signature _B. Georgi, MD_   Time _0950_
Circulating Nurse's Signature _L. Honol, RN_   Time _0950_

Implants/Prosthesis ☐ Yes ☑ No
Exp. Date: _____
Manufacturer: _____
Type: _____
Size: _____
Lot/Serial #: _____

Risk for impaired skin integrity

Position for surgery: ☑ Supine ☐ Prone ☐ Lithotomy ☐ L lateral ☐ R lateral ☐ Other: _____
Positioning devices: ☐ Chest roll ☐ Shoulder roll ☐ Axillary roll ☐ Pillow ☐ Stirrups ☐ Leg holder ☐ Foot board
Pad bony prominences: ☑ Elbows ☑ Heels ☐ Arms tucked Other: _____

Risk for injury

☑ Apply safety strap to: _Ant. mid thigh_   ☑ Apply grounding pad Site: _Ant. left thigh_
☑ Electrosurgical unit #: _22_   ☐ Bipolar #: _____   _Setting:_ Coag: _35_   Cut: _35_
☐ Laser Type: _0_   Unit #: _____   Settings: _____   Time: _____
☐ Safety measures implemented Operator: _____
☐ Tourniquet checked & applied #: _0_   Site: _____
Applied by: _____   ☐ Inflated: _____   ☐ Deflated: _____   Pressure: _____
Sequential stockings: ☑ Yes ☐ No ☐ Other: _____   Unit #: _4_

RN's Signature _L. Honol, RN_   Time _1059_

Smarter charting

Instrument count sheet

Patient's full name: _Angela W. Ings_   Procedure: _Laparoscopic cholecystectomy_ Date: _10/1/06_

INSTRUMENTS	SET COUNT	FIRST COUNT	ADD	FINAL COUNT
Allis	6	6	—	6
Criles	12	12	—	12
Forceps	6	6	—	6
Hemostats	12	12	—	12
Kellys	12	12	—	12
Knife handles	3	3	—	3
Needle holders	3	3	1	4
Prep sticks	2	2	—	2
Scissors	4	4	—	4
Towel clips	6	6	—	6

Count verification:

First count correct ☑ Yes ☐ No   If incorrect, X-ray taken ☐ Yes ☐ No

Final count correct ☑ Yes ☐ No   Circulating RN's signature: _L. Hanel, RN_

and procedure manual for which items must be counted, the number of times the count must be performed, and other required documentation.

Postanesthesia nursing care

The immediate perianesthesia period starts when the patient arrives in the postanesthesia care unit (PACU), accompanied by the anesthesiologist or nurse anesthetist. During this critical phase, the patient's vital physiologic functions must be supported until the anesthesia wears off. When the patient arrives in the PACU, confirm his identity, document the arrival time, and obtain a report from the anesthesia provider.

In the PACU, conduct a rapid assessment immediately after the patient arrives. Continue to perform ongoing assessments and interventions based on your findings. Remember to document your assessment findings on the PACU flow sheet, according to your facility's policy. This flow sheet usually includes several assess-

Postanesthesia recovery scoring system

CRITERION	EXPLANATION	SCORE
Activity	Moves four extremities voluntarily or on command	②
	Moves two extremities voluntarily or on command	1
	No movement (moves no extremities)	0
Respiration	Able to cough and deep breathe freely	②
	Dyspnea or hypoventilation	1
	Apnea	0
Circulation	Blood pressure within 20% of preanesthesia level	②
	Blood pressure within 21% to 49% of preanesthesia level	1
	Blood pressure within 50% of preanesthesia level	0
Consciousness	Fully awake	②
	Responds to verbal stimuli (including name)	1
	No response	0
Oxygen saturation	Maintains oxygen saturation (Spo_2) > 92% on room air	2
	Needs supplemental oxygen to maintain Spo_2 > 92%	①
	Spo_2 < 92% with supplemental oxygen	0

TOTAL SCORE: 9

ment parameter tools, such as tools for assessing the patient's postanesthesia recovery, peripheral pulses, muscle strength, neurologic status, and pain. (See *Postanesthesia recovery scoring system*.)

Always monitor and promote your patient's comfort postoperatively. Because pain is a subjective experience, the most valid pain assessment comes from the patient. Use an age-appropriate pain assessment scale, give prescribed analgesics (such as an opioid, nonopioid analgesic, or an adjuvant analgesic such as an anticonvulsant), and teach him techniques to reduce incisional pain. Pain management may also involve epidural analgesia or patient-controlled analgesia (PCA). For the postoperative patient who can't find a comfortable position, use physi-

cal measures, such as positioning, back rubs, and environmental modifications, to promote comfort and enhance analgesic drug effectiveness. Your documentation should include pain assessment findings, interventions taken to manage pain, pain reassessment times, and effectiveness of pain management interventions.

In addition to monitoring for pain, PACU nurses must also assess their patients for additional postanesthesia complications. These include such potential respiratory complications as hypoventilation and laryngospasm. Examples of cardiovascular complications include hypotension, hypertension, and cardiac arrhythmias. A patient experiencing metabolic complications may develop hypothermia or malignant hyperthermia. Additional complications include central nervous system depression, nausea, and vomiting.

Typically, the patient must meet these criteria before he can be discharged from the PACU:

▶ adequate control of nausea and vomiting
▶ adequate pain control
▶ downward progression of the level of blockade from spinal anesthesia, with return of movement and sensation
▶ postanesthesia recovery score of 8 or above
▶ stable fluid balance status
▶ stable vital signs and oxygen saturation
▶ surgical site that's free from complications, with a dry, intact dressing or minimal drainage and patent drainage tubes.

Make sure your documentation reflects that the patient meets these discharge criteria.

The PACU practitioner is responsible for giving report to the unit before transfer of the patient. Time and contents of report, or hand-off, given to the receiving unit should be documented as well as the name of the receiving practitioner. If the patient is going home, the method of transfer, discharge teaching, follow-up office visits, and to whom the patient is being released must be documented.

Psychiatric nursing

In 1973, the American Nurses Association Coalition of Psychiatric Nursing Organizations issued standards to improve the quality of care provided by psychiatric and mental health nurses. These standards, last revised in 2000, apply to generalists and specialists working in any setting in which psychiatric and mental health nursing is practiced.

Psychiatric nursing documentation should encompass all of the standards of care as designated by the Coalition of Psychiatric Nursing Organizations. Standard I (assessment) is data collection related to the psychiatric and mental health of the patient. In this step, you gather subjective and objective information to develop a care plan, which determines the best possible care for the patient. You compile this data from information obtained during the interview, by observing the patient, consulting with other members of the health care team, reviewing past medical and psychiatric records, and analyzing the results of the physical and mental examination.

Standard II addresses diagnosis. During this step, the psychiatric mental health nurse analyzes the assessment data to determine the nursing diagnoses and potential problem statements. These diagnoses and problem statements must be prioritized according to the needs of the patient and conform to accepted classifications systems, such as the North American Nursing Diagnosis Association International's (NANDA-I) Nursing Diagnosis Classification and the *Diagnostic and Statistical Manual of Mental Disorders,* Fourth Edition, Text Revision.

Standard III describes outcome identification. Expected outcomes must be measurable and designate a specified time frame. They're patient-oriented, therapeutically sound, realistic, attainable, and cost-effective. Additionally, they're derived from the diagnosis and must be realistic for the patient.

Standard IV entails the planning or development of a care plan. A care plan is best tailored to the patient when it involves collaboration among the patient, family, significant others, and all members of the interdisciplinary health care team. It's used to guide therapeutic interventions, document progress, and achieve the expected outcomes. The care plan should include an educational program related to the patient's health problems, treatment regimen, and self-care activities. The format of the plan must allow for modification, interdisciplinary access, and retrieval of data.

Standard V involves implementation of the interventions identified in the care plan. A wide range of interventions is used to maintain or restore mental and physical health. They must be safe, timely, appropriate, ethical, and performed according to the psychiatric–mental health nurse's level of education, practice, and certification. Interventions must be evaluated and modified based on continued assessment of the patient's response. Subcategories of Standard V include counseling, milieu therapy, promotion of self-care activities, psychobiological interventions, health teaching, case management, health promotion and maintenance, and advanced practice interventions.

Standard VI evaluates the patient's progress in attaining expected outcomes. Needed revisions to the care plan, based on the ongoing assessment, are documented.

Confidentiality in the psychiatric setting

Because our society continues to attach a stigma to anyone labeled with a diagnosis of mental illness, it's essential that the confidentiality of written and verbal communication be maintained. Any breach of confidentiality can affect the rest of the patient's life in terms of relationships, employment and promotions, and insurance as well as in many other aspects. You can never be too careful with medical records.

Confidentiality can be breached only under the "duty to warn" and "duty to protect," which are closely related. These are legal obligations based on a Supreme Court case in 1976. The court determined that if a professional believes a patient may be dangerous to himself or to others, then that professional has a legal responsibility to take the necessary steps to protect the potential victim. This includes threats to an identified person and threats from contagious diseases (in some states). In this case, it's important for you to document all details, including the nursing interventions.

Special documentation considerations

Psychiatric nurses face a number of issues requiring special documentation. These include seclusion and restraints, substance abuse and withdrawal, and extrapyramidal adverse effects of therapeutic medications.

SECLUSION AND RESTRAINTS

When a patient becomes dangerously out of control, you may have to employ seclusion or restraints. You'll usually accomplish restraint through the application of such devices as cloth or leather wrist and ankle restraints. To employ seclusion, you'll usually isolate a patient in a locked room. The use of these devices is a very complex issue involving ethical, legal, and therapeutic issues and must be very carefully documented. Most states have laws that prohibit the use of unnecessary physical restraint or seclusion. (See *Using seclusion and restraints: What to document,* page 366.)

Seclusion

During seclusion, a patient is separated from others in a safe, secure, and contained environment with close nursing supervision to protect himself, other patients, and staff members from imminent harm. Seclusion is used when non-physical interventions are ineffective. Follow your facility's policy when placing a patient in

Legal eagle

Using seclusion and restraints: What to document

The use of seclusion and restraints poses a very sensitive legal issue. Precise documentation is a legal necessity. You must document the following:

▶ behaviors leading up to the use of seclusion or restraints

▶ actions taken to control the behavior before the use of seclusion or restraints

▶ the time the client's behavior became uncontrollable, and the time the client was placed in seclusion or restraints

▶ assessment of the client's behavior and vital signs as well as any nursing care provided (document this every 15 minutes)

▶ medications that were given, their effectiveness, and the time they were administered.

Objective documentation should show evidence of proper procedures or facts on which decisions were based. In court, it can be assumed that only those things documented were done.

2/21/07	2000	Approached by pt. at 1930, crying
		and saying loudly, "I can't stand it,
		they will get me." Repeated this
		statement several times. Unable to
		say who "they" were. Pt. asked to sit
		in a seclusion room saying, "It's
		quiet and safe there. That's what
		I do at the psych. hospital." Called
		Dr. Wright at 1935 and told him of
		pt. request. Verbal order given for
		seclusion as requested by pt. Dr.
		Wright will be in to evaluate pt. at
		2100. Pt. placed in empty pt. room
		on unit in close proximity to
		nurse's station. Told her that
		because seclusion was voluntary she
		was free to leave seclusion when
		she felt ready. Rita Summers, CNA,
		assigned to continuously observe
		pt. P 82, BP 132/82, RR 18, oral
		T 98.7° F. Family notified of pt.'s
		request for seclusion, that pt. is
		free to leave seclusion on her
		own, will be continuously observed
		by CNA and assessed frequently by
		RN and that doctor will be by to
		see her at 2100. Family stated
		they were comfortable with this
		decision. ———— Donna Blau, RN

seclusion. Also, familiarize yourself with the new standards on the use of seclusion for behavioral health care reasons in nonbehavioral health care settings set forth by The Joint Commission. These standards originally became effective January 1, 2001.

Seclusion is based on three principles: containment, isolation, and decreased sensory input. In containment, the patient is restricted to an area in which he can be protected from harm. Moreover, others are protected from impulsive acts by the patient. Isolations permits the pa-tient to withdraw from situations that are too intense for him to handle at that point. Decreased sensory input reduces external stimulation and sensory overload, allowing the patient to regroup and reorganize coping skills.

Restraints

Restraints are defined as any method of physically restricting a person's freedom of movement, physical activity, or normal access to his body. Restraints can cause numerous problems, including limited mobility, skin breakdown, impaired circulation, incontinence, psychological distress, and strangulation.

Effective January 1, 2001, The Joint Commission issued revised standards that were intended to reduce the use of restraints. According to revised standards in 2005, restraints are to be limited to emergencies in which the patient is at risk for harming himself or others. However, because they're used only in emergencies, your facility may authorize qualified nurses to initiate restraint use. The revised standards also emphasize staff education.

Time limitations also have been set on the use of restraints. Within 1 hour after placing the patient in restraints, the qualified staff member must notify and obtain a verbatim written order from the licensed independent practitioner. Within 4 hours of placing an adult patient in restraints (or within 2 hours for children younger than age 17), a licensed independent practitioner must conduct an initial evaluation in person and give an order for restraints. (If the patient is no longer in restraints when the initial verbal order expires, the independent licensed practitioner must evaluate the patient within 24 hours of the initiation of restraints.) This order must be renewed every 4 hours for patients age 18 and older, every 2 hours for children ages 9 to 17, and every 1 hour for children younger than age 9. If a patient requires the use of restraints for at least 2 separate episodes in a 12-hour time period, or if a patient remains in restraints for more than 12 hours, The Joint Commission requires notification of the clinical leaders.

The Joint Commission's revised standards require continuous monitoring by an assigned staff member who is competent and appropriately trained to ensure patient safety. The patient's family members also must be notified of the use of restraints if the patient consented to have them informed of his care. Moreover, the patient must be informed of the conditions necessary for his release from restraints.

2/21/07	1400	Pt. extremely agitated, cursing, and swinging fists and kicking feet at nurse and staff. Attempted to calm patient through nonthreatening verbal communication. No I.V. access available. Ativan 2 mg I.M. given per Dr. Miller's order. After evaluation, Dr. Miller ordered 4-point restraints applied to prevent harm to patient and staff. Pt. informed that restraints would be removed when he could remain calm and refrain from hitting or kicking. Pt. doesn't want his family to be notified of restraint application. See restraint monitoring sheet for frequent assessments and intervention notations. ——— Carol Sacks, RN

SUBSTANCE ABUSE AND WITHDRAWAL

As a psychiatric nurse, you're commonly faced with the care of patients addicted to substances. These patients may have multiple legal problems, recurrent social and interpersonal problems, and repeated absences or poor performances at work or school.

It's common for patients with alcohol and drug addictions to use defense mechanisms when discussing their disease. They may deny the amount and frequency of drug and alcohol use or its relationship to significant areas of their lives. This makes your nursing assessment very difficult to accomplish. Look to information from alternate sources, such as family, friends, coworkers, and past medical records, to provide reliable data. (See *Using the CAGE questionnaire,* page 368.)

Special federal rules address confidentiality related to patients treated or referred for substance abuse. These rules apply to any facility receiving federal funding. Information may be released only with the patient's written consent.

Substance withdrawal occurs when a person who's addicted to alcohol or drugs suddenly stops taking the substance he's addicted to. Withdrawal symptoms may include tremors, insomnia, and seizures. Substance withdrawal can also result in death.

2/2/07	1000	Pt. admitted to Chemical Dependency Unit for withdrawal from ethanol. Has a 30-year history of alcohol dependence and states, "I can't keep this up anymore. I need to get off the booze." Reports drinking a fifth of vodka per day for the last 2 months and that her last drink was today shortly before admission. Her blood alcohol level is 0.15%. She reports having gone through the withdrawal process 4 times before but has never completed rehabilitation. Reports the following symptoms during previous withdrawals: anxiety, nausea, vomiting, irritability and tremulousness. Currently demonstrates no manifestations of ethanol withdrawal. Dr. Jones notified of pt.'s admission and blood alcohol level results. Lorazepam 2 mg P.O. given at 0930. Pt. instructed regarding s/s of ethanol withdrawal and associated nursing care. She expressed full understanding of the information. Will reinforce teaching when blood tests reveal no alcohol in blood. ————————— Brian Winters, RN

If your patient is at risk for substance withdrawal or shows signs of withdrawal, contact the practitioner immediately and anticipate a program of detoxification, followed by long-term therapy to combat drug dependence.

Using the CAGE questionnaire

The CAGE (**C**utting down alcohol consumption, **A**nnoyance by criticism of drinking, **G**uilty feelings associated with alcohol use, **E**ye-openers or early morning drinks) questionnaire used to identify alcohol abuse has been tested in many clinical settings and is quick and easy to use. It consists of four questions:

▶ Have you ever felt you should cut down on your drinking?

▶ Have people annoyed you by criticizing your drinking?

▶ Have you ever felt bad or guilty about your drinking?

▶ Have you ever had a drink first thing in the morning to steady nerves or get rid of a hangover (eye-opener)?

At least two affirmative responses indicates alcohol addiction.

EXTRAPYRAMIDAL ADVERSE EFFECTS

Nurses frequently administer antipsychotic drugs to patients in psychiatric settings. Therefore, it's your responsibility to know the adverse effects of the medications that the patient is receiving and to recognize and report any adverse reactions that may occur.

Many of the antipsychotic medications are capable of causing profound motor effects known as extrapyramidal adverse effects. Haloperidol (Haldol), clozapine (Clozaril), fluphenazine (Prolixin), risperidone (Risperdal), and olanzapine (Zyprexa) are just a few of the drugs that may cause these adverse effects.

Tardive dyskinesia (TD) is one of the most common of the extrapyramidal adverse effects. It's an abnormal movement disorder characterized by involuntary movements of the tongue, face, mouth or jaw, trunk, or extremities. Examples include protrusion of the tongue, puffing of the cheeks, puckering of the mouth, or chewing movements. TD may be temporary, permanent, or even fatal. Symptoms usually become apparent when the medication is reduced or discontinued.

Early detection of tardive dyskinesia is critical. Several assessment tools are useful in identifying TD. These include the Abnormal Involuntary Movement Scale (AIMS) and the Simpson-Angus Neurologic Rating Scale.

The AIMS tool is designed to assess abnormal involuntary movements in the face, upper and lower extremities, and trunk. Observe the patient for movements such as grimacing, puckering, smacking, chewing, involuntary tongue thrusting, and for abnormal movements of the extremities. It's important to ascertain if the patient has any current problems with his teeth or dentures and to make sure that there's nothing in his mouth (such as gum). The AIMS tool scores the patient based on the movements observed. The highest severity observed is a 4 and the minimum is a 1, with 0 being no abnormal movements observed.

Selected references

Adams, B.L. "Assessment of Child Abuse Risk Factors by Advanced Practice Nurses," *Pediatric Nursing* 31(6):498-502, November-December 2005.

Angelini, D.J., and Mahlmeister, L.R. "Liability in Triage: Management of EMTALA Regulations and Common Obstetric Risks," *Journal of Midwifery & Women's Health* 50(6):472-8, November-December 2005.

Brown, G. "Wound Documentation: Managing Risk," *Advances in Skin & Wound Care* 19(3):155-65, April 2006.

Bruce, K., and Suserud, B.O. "The Handover Process and Triage of Ambulance-Borne Patients: The Experiences of Emergency Nurses," *Nursing in Critical Care* 10(4):201-9, July-August 2005.

Charting Made Incredibly Easy, 3rd. ed. Philadelphia: Lippincott Williams and Wilkins, 2006.

ChartSmart: An A-to-Z Guide to Better Nursing Documentation, 2nd ed. Philadelphia: Lippincott Williams and Wilkins, 2007.

Comprehensive Accreditation Manual for Hospitals: The Official Handbook. Oakbrook Terrace: Joint Commission Resources, Inc., 2007.

Doyle, M. "Promoting Standardized Nursing Language Using an Electronic Medical Record System," *AORN Journal* 83(6):1336-42, June 2006.

Ghulam, A.T., et al. "Patients' Satisfaction with the Preoperative Informed Consent Procedure: A Multicenter Questionnaire Survey in Switzerland," *Mayo Clinic Proceedings* 81(3):307-12, March 2006.

Joint Commission on Accreditation of Healthcare Organizations: www.jointcommission.org/PatientSafety/NationalPatientSafetyGoals

Junttila, K., et al. "Perioperative Nurses' Attitudes toward the Use of Nursing Diagnoses in Documentation," *Journal of Advanced Nursing* 52(3):271-80, November 2005.

Murray, R.B. "The Subpoena and a Day in Court: Guidelines for Nurses," *Journal of Psychosocial Nursing and Mental Health Services* 43(3):38-44, March 2005.

Parrish, E. "Pulling Together to Document Evidence," *Reflections on Nursing Leadership* 31(2):28-9, 42, 2005.

Porter, S.C., et al. "Getting the Data Right: Information Accuracy in Pediatric Emergency Medicine," *Quality & Safety in Health Care* 15(4):296-301, August 2006.

Rayner, L. "Language, Therapeutic Relationships and Individualized Care: Addressing These Issues in Mental Health Care Pathways," *Journal of Psychiatric and Mental Health Nursing* 12(4):481-7, August 2005.

Repasky, T.M. "A Frequently Used and Revised ED Chest Pain Pathway," *Journal of Emergency Nursing* 31(4):368-70, August 2005.

Silfen, E., Documentation and coding of ED patient encounters: an evaluation of the accuracy of an electronic medical record [white star]. *American Journal of Emergency Medicine* 24(6):664-678, October 2006.

Simpson, K.R., et al. "Nurse-Physician Communication during Labor and Birth: Implications for Patient Safety," *Journal of Obstetric, Gynecologic, and Neonatal Nursing* 35(4):547-56, July-August 2006.

Surgical Care Made Incredibly Visual. Philadelphia: Lippincott Williams & Wilkins, 2007.

Wickham, S. "Is the Apgar a Flexible Friend?" *The Practising Midwife* 8(7):35, July-August 2005.

Wolf, N.L. "Embracing the Role of the Advanced Practice Nurse in the Perinatal Setting," *AWHONN Lifelines* 10(3):226-33, June-July 2006.

LEGALLY PERILOUS CHARTING PRACTICES

12

If you're ever named in a malpractice suit that proceeds to court, your documentation may be your best defense. It provides a running record of your patient care. How and what you documented—and even what you didn't document—will heavily influence the outcome of the trial.

Credible evidence

Typically, the outcome of every malpractice trial boils down to one question: Whom will the jury believe? The answer usually depends on the credibility of the evidence. In a malpractice suit, a plaintiff presents evidence designed to show that he was harmed or injured because care provided by the defendant (in this case, the nurse) failed to meet accepted standards of care. The nurse, of course, strives to present evidence demonstrating that she provided an acceptable standard of care. However, if she can't offer believable evidence, the jury may have no choice but to accept the plaintiff's evidence. Even worse, if the nurse's evidence—including the medical record—is discredited, the plaintiff's attorney may convince a jury of her negligence.

In a malpractice suit, jurors may view the medical record as the best evidence of what really happened. It may be the hinge that swings the jury's verdict.

Negligent or not?

If you've actually been negligent and have truthfully documented the care given, the medical record will naturally be the plaintiff's best evidence, as it should be. In such instances, the case will probably be settled out of court.

If you haven't been negligent, the medical record should be your best defense, providing the best evidence of quality care. If the charted record makes you *seem* negligent, however, the jurors may conclude that you *were* negligent because they base their decision on the evidence. The lesson: A "bad" medical record can be used to make a good nurse look bad. A "good" medical record should defend those who wrote it.

By knowing how to chart, what to chart, when to chart, and even who should chart, you'll create a solid record. Knowing how to handle legally sensitive situations, such as difficult and nonconforming patients, and how to avoid misinterpreting written records will offer additional safeguards.

How to chart

You may assume that every nurse knows how to chart, but this isn't necessarily true. Charting is a craft that's refined with experience. A skilled nurse knows that she needs to document that the standard of care was delivered, keeping in mind that it isn't only *what* she charts but *how* she charts that's important.

Chart objectively
The medical record should contain descriptive, objective information: what you see, hear, feel, smell, measure, and count—not what you suppose, infer, conclude, or assume. The chart may also contain subjective information, but only when it's supported by documented facts.

STICK TO THE FACTS
To make sure that you keep the medical record factual, follow these simple rules:

Record only what you see and hear
For example, don't record that a patient pulled out his I.V. line if you didn't witness his doing so. Do, however, describe your findings—for example, "Found pt., arm board, and bed linens covered with blood. I.V. line and venipuncture device were untaped and hanging free."

Similarly, don't record that a patient fell out of bed if you didn't see him fall. If you saw him lying on the floor, record that. If the patient says he fell out of bed, record that. If you heard a muffled thud, went to the patient's room, and found him lying on the floor, record that. (See *Avoiding assumptions.*) An example of how to document a patient's fall appears below.

2/28/07	0600	Heard pt. scream. Found pt.
		lying beside bed. Pt. has lacer-
		ation 2 cm long on forehead.
		Side rails up. Pt. stated he
		climbed over side rails to go
		to the bathroom. BP 184/92,
		P 96, R 24. Dr. Phillips notified
		and ordered X-ray. Pt. c/o
		pain in Ⓡ hip. Pt. taken for
		X-ray of Ⓡ hip.
		— Sonia Benoit, RN

Describe—don't label—events and behavior
Expressions such as "appears spaced out," "flying high," "exhibiting bizarre behavior," or "using obscenities" have different meanings to different people. If a plaintiff's attorney asked you to define those terms, could you do it? Even if you could, would you be likely to gain or lose credibility in the process?

Facts, accurately reported, reflect professionalism. Subjective conclusions force you into the uncomfortable position of having to defend your own words. You'll almost always lose credibility and distract the jury from the fact that you provided the standard of care to the patient.

Be specific
Your goal in documenting is to describe facts clearly and concisely. To do so, use only ap-

proved abbreviations, and express your observations in quantifiable terms.

For example, the conclusion "output adequate" is vague. Give an exact measurement such as "1,200 ml." Similarly, "Pt. appears to be in pain" is vague. Ask yourself why he "appears to be in pain" and document the specific findings—for example, "Pt. requested pain medication after complaining of severe but slow-onset lower back pain radiating to his right leg, 6 on a scale of 0 to 10. No numbness or tingling, no edema. Color of extremity pink, temperature warm."

Similarly, avoid catchall phrases such as "Pt. comfortable." Instead, describe his comfort. Is he resting, reading, or sleeping? This type of information is more helpful and informative.

Here's an example of specific, clear documentation:

2/18/07	1400	Dressing removed from ®
		mastectomy site. Incision is
		pink. No drainage. Measures
		12.5 cm long and 2 cm wide.
		Slight bruising noted near cen-
		ter of incision. Dressing dry.
		Drain site below mastectomy
		incision measures 2 cm x 2 cm.
		Bloody, dime-sized drainage
		noted on drain dressing. No
		edema noted. Betadine dress-
		ings applied. Pt. complaining of
		mild incisional pain, 3 on a
		scale of 0 to 10. 2 Tylox P.O.
		given at 1330 hours. Pt. re-
		ports relief at 1355. ———
		——— Joan Delaney, RN

USE NEUTRAL LANGUAGE

Avoid including inappropriate comments or language in your notes. Such comments are unprofessional and can trigger difficulties in legal cases.

For example, one elderly patient's family became upset after the patient developed pressure

Legal eagle

Avoiding assumptions

Always aim to record the facts about a situation — not your assumptions or conclusions. In the following example, a nurse failed to document the facts and instead charted her assumptions about a patient's fall. As a result, she had to endure this damaging cross-examination by the plaintiff's attorney.

ATTORNEY: Would you read your fifth entry for January 6, please?
NURSE: Patient fell out of bed. . . .
ATTORNEY: Thank you. Did you actually see the patient fall out of bed?
NURSE: Actually, no.
ATTORNEY: Did the patient tell you he fell out of bed?
NURSE: No.
ATTORNEY: Did anyone actually see the patient fall out of bed?
NURSE: Not that I know of.
ATTORNEY: So these notes reflect nothing more than conjecture on your part. Is that correct?
NURSE: I guess so.
ATTORNEY: Is it fair to say then, that you charted something as fact even though you didn't know it was?
NURSE: I suppose so.
ATTORNEY: Thank you.

ulcers. They complained that the patient wasn't receiving adequate care. The patient later died of natural causes.

However, because the patient's family was dissatisfied with the care the patient received, they sued. In the patient's chart, under prognosis, the physician had written "PBBB." After learning that this stood for "pine box by bedside," the insurance company was only too happy to settle for a significant sum.

Legal eagle

Consequences of missing records

The case of *Battocchi v. Washington Hospital Center*, 581 A.2d 759 (D.C. App. 1990) underscores the significance of keeping the medical record intact. In this case, the plaintiffs brought a medical malpractice suit against the hospital and a physician for injuries sustained by their son during forceps delivery.

The nurse in attendance documented the events and her observations of the delivery immediately after the delivery. Later, the hospital's risk management personnel obtained the chart for analysis but apparently lost the nurse's notes from the record.

The court ruled in favor of the hospital and physician, holding that the jury couldn't presume negligence and causation against them simply because the hospital lost the attending nurse's notes.

However, on appeal, the District of Columbia Court of Appeals sent the case back to the trial court so that the lower court could rule whether the hospital's loss of the records stemmed from negligence or impropriety.

AVOID BIAS

Don't use words that suggest a negative attitude toward the patient. For example, don't use unflattering or unprofessional adjectives, such as *obstinate, drunk, obnoxious, bizarre,* or *abusive,* to describe the patient's behavior.

Remember, the chart is a legal document. Imagine how your harsh words would sound in court. They most certainly would invite the plaintiff's attorney to attack your professionalism with an argument such as this: "Look at how this nurse felt about my client—she called him 'rude, difficult, and uncooperative.' It's right here

in her own handwriting. No wonder she didn't take good care of this patient—she didn't like him." Also, remember that the patient has a legal right to see his chart. If he spots a derogatory reference, he'll be hurt, angry, and more likely to sue.

If a patient is difficult or uncooperative, document the behavior objectively. That way, the jurors will draw their own conclusions.

2/19/07	1400	I attempted to give pt. medication, but he said, "I've had enough pills. Now leave me alone." Explained the importance of the medication and attempted to determine why he would not take it. Pt. refused to talk. Dr. Ellis notified that medication was refused. ——— Anne Curry, RN

Keep the medical record intact

Take special care to keep the patient's chart complete and intact. Discarding pages from the medical record, even for innocent reasons, is bound to raise doubt in the jury's mind about the chart's reliability.

Suppose, for example, you spill coffee on a page, blurring several entries. You remove the original page from the chart, copy it, and place the copy in the chart. Then you discard the original. Imagine having to admit to a jury that you destroyed original evidence.

You could try to explain that you did so for an innocent reason, but the jury could be difficult to convince. Jurors are skeptical; they must be. Giving them a reason to doubt you makes the plaintiff's job a lot easier and yours much more difficult.

When something is considered part of the official record, never discard or destroy it. If you replace an original sheet with a copy, cross-reference it with lines such as these: "Recopied from page 4" or "Recopied on page 6." Be sure to attach the original. If a page is damaged, note "Reconstructed charting," and attach the damaged page. (See *Consequences of missing records.*)

What to chart

When you're busy, getting your work done may seem more important than documenting every detail. However, from a jury's viewpoint, an incomplete chart suggests incomplete nursing care. This is one of the most serious and common charting errors. It's no accident that a popular saying among malpractice attorneys is "If it wasn't charted, it wasn't done."

That isn't literally true, of course, but it's an easy conclusion for a jury to draw. You may have performed a nursing procedure that you simply forgot to chart. However, if the chart doesn't back you up, you'll have a hard time convincing a jury to accept your version of events.

Ask yourself, *What's my responsibility to the patient?* This should be your answer: to deliver the accepted standard of care and to document it in order to communicate with other health care providers and establish a permanent record of care. If this is done, you can defend yourself. Areas of documentation that are frequently reviewed in malpractice cases include timely vital signs, reporting changes in the patient's condition, medications given, patient responses, and discharge teaching.

Failure to document diminishes your ability to testify confidently and persuasively about the details—any one of which could be critical to the verdict. Of course, you should never document some situations, such as conflicts among the staff. (See *Keeping the record clean,* pages 376 and 377.)

Record critical and extraordinary information

When you encounter a critical or an extraordinary situation, take pains to document the details thoroughly. Failure to chart such situations can have serious repercussions. (See *What you don't document can hurt you,* pages 378 and 379.)

Consider the case of Tommy York, who was left partially paralyzed and severely brain damaged after an accident. He was admitted to the hospital for intensive rehabilitation.

Soon after he arrived, his parents told his nurse that a support from the right side of his wheelchair was missing and that they had noticed scratches on their son's right arm. The nurse failed to record the parents' or her own observations.

Later, the patient's hip became red, swollen, and increasingly painful. Although Tommy's mother pointed this out to the nurse, she again failed to record any observations.

Finally, the patient was diagnosed with a broken hip. The parents sued and the court ruled the hospital negligent in record keeping. The plaintiff was awarded $250,000, the maximum allowable in the state where the lawsuit was filed. (See *Recording critical information: A case in point,* page 380.)

The example below shows how to document extraordinary information correctly.

2/2/07	0920	Digoxin 0.125 mg P.O. not given because of nausea and vomiting. Dr. Kelly notified that digoxin not given. Dr. Kelly gave order for digoxin 0.125 mg I.V. Administered at 0915 hours.— Ruth Bullock, RN

Keeping the record clean

What you say and how you say it are of utmost importance in documentation. Keeping the patient's chart free of negative, inappropriate information — potential legal bombshells — can be quite a challenge when you're writing detailed narrative notes. Here are some guidelines to help you sidestep charting pitfalls and record an accurate account of your patient's care and status.

AVOID REPORTING STAFFING PROBLEMS

Even though staff shortages may affect patient care or contribute to an incident, you shouldn't refer to staffing problems in a patient's chart. Instead, discuss them in a forum that can help resolve the problem. Call the situation to the attention of the appropriate personnel, such as your nurse-manager, in a confidential memo or an incident report. Also, review your hospital's policy and procedure manuals to determine how you're expected to handle this situation.

KEEP STAFF CONFLICTS AND RIVALRIES OUT OF THE RECORD

Entries about disputes with nursing colleagues (including characterization and criticism of care provided), questions about a practitioner's treatment decisions, or reports of a colleague's rude or abusive behavior reflect personality clashes and don't belong in the medical record. They aren't legitimate concerns about patient care.

As with staffing problems, address concerns about a colleague's judgment or competence in the appropriate setting. After making sure that you have the facts, talk with your nurse-manager. Consult with the practitioner directly if an order concerns you. Share your opinions, observations, or reservations about colleagues with your nurse-manager only; avoid mentioning them in a patient's chart.

If you discover personal accusations or charges of incompetence in a chart, discuss this with your supervisor.

HANDLING INCIDENT REPORTS

An incident report is a confidential, administrative communication that's filed separately from the patient's chart. Some facilities require the notation, "Incident form completed," while others require you not to document in the chart that an incident report was filed. Be familiar with your facility's policy so you'll know how to accurately chart this.

You should always document the facts of an incident in the patient's chart. For example, "Found pt. lying on the floor at 1250 hours. No visible bleeding or trauma. Pt. returned to bed with side rails up and bed in low position. Vital signs: BP 120/80, P 76, T 98.2°. Notified Dr. Gary Dietrich at 1253 hours, and he saw pt. at 1300 hours" is a sufficient and accurate statement of the facts.

STEER CLEAR OF WORDS ASSOCIATED WITH ERRORS

Terms such as *mistake, accidentally, somehow, unintentionally, miscalculated,* and *confusing* can be

Chart full assessment data

Failing to document an adequate physical assessment is a key factor in many malpractice suits. When initially assessing your patient, focus on his chief complaint, but also document all his concerns and your findings.

After completing the initial assessment, establish your nursing care plan. A well-written interpreted as admissions of wrongdoing. Instead, let the facts speak for themselves — for example, "Pt. was given Demerol 100 mg I.M. at 1300 hours for abdominal pain VAS 7/10. Dr. was notified at 1305 and gave no new orders. Pt.'s vital signs are BP 120/82, P 80, R 20, T 98.4°."

If the ordered drug dose was 50 mg, this entry will let other health care providers know that the patient was overmedicated.

AVOID NAMING NAMES

Naming another patient in someone else's chart violates confidentiality. Use the word *roommate,* initials, or a room and bed number to describe the other patient.

NEVER CHART THAT YOU INFORMED A COLLEAGUE OF A SITUATION IF YOU ONLY MENTIONED IT

Telling your nurse-manager in the elevator or rest room about a patient's deteriorating condition doesn't qualify as informing her, but it *does* violate patient confidentiality. The nurse-manager is likely to forget the details and may not even realize that you expect her to intervene. You need to clearly state why you're notifying her so she can focus on the facts and take appropriate action. Otherwise, you can't say you've informed her. Chart the patient's deterioration in the record, and chart the time you notified your supervisor.

care plan provides a clear approach to the patient's problems and can assist in your defense— *if* it was carried out.

Phrase each patient problem statement clearly, and don't be afraid to modify the statement as you gather new assessment data. Also, state the care plan for solving each problem and then identify the actions you intend to implement. (See *Using good interview techniques to improve documentation,* page 381.)

Document discharge instructions

Hospitals today commonly discharge patients earlier than in years past. As a result, the patient and his family must change dressings; assess wounds; deal with medical equipment, tube feedings, and I.V. lines; and perform other functions that a nurse traditionally performed.

To perform these functions properly, the patient and his home caregiver must receive adequate instruction. The responsibility for these instructions is usually yours. If a patient receives improper instructions and an injury results, you could be held liable.

Many facilities distribute printed instruction sheets describing treatments and home care procedures that provide adequate instruction. The chart should indicate which materials were given and to whom.

Courts typically consider these teaching materials as evidence that instruction took place. However, to support testimony that instructions were given, the materials should be tailored to each patient's specific needs and include any verbal or written instructions that were provided. If caregivers practice procedures with the patient and family in the hospital, this should be documented too, along with the results.

Legal eagle

What you don't document can hurt you

Only careful documentation can substantiate your version of events. Consider the situations below.

THE CASE OF THE SUPPOSED PHONE CALL

A patient was admitted to the hospital for surgery for epicondylitis (tennis elbow). After the surgery, a heavy cast was applied to his arm. The patient complained to the nurse of severe pain, for which the nurse repeatedly gave pain medication.

The next morning, when the surgeon visited, he split the patient's cast. By that time, the ulnar nerve was completely paralyzed and the patient was left with a permanently useless, clawed hand.

The patient subsequently sued the nurse for failing to notify the surgeon about his pain. At the deposition, the dialogue between the nurse and the plaintiff's attorney sounded like this:

ATTORNEY: Did you call the doctor?
NURSE: I must have called him.
ATTORNEY: Do you remember calling him?
NURSE: Not exactly, but I must have.
ATTORNEY: Do you have a record of making that call?
NURSE: No, I don't.
ATTORNEY: If you had made such a call, shouldn't there be a record of it?
NURSE: Yes, I guess so.
ATTORNEY: "Guess" is right; you can't really say that you made that call. You can only "guess" that you "must have."

THE CASE OF THE DOCUMENTATION DEFICIT

In the case of *Sweeney v. Purvis*, 665 So. 2d 926 (Ala., 1995), a 42-year-old woman was transferred to a rehabilitation facility 10 days after being admitted to the hospital with a brain infarction. On her first day there, she attended therapy sessions without a problem.

The next day, after therapy, she had cramping in her left leg that wasn't relieved by analgesics. She also complained of pain in her left heel. The nursing staff called the physician, who ordered a heating pad applied to the affected leg.

The patient reported little pain that evening, but the next day her left leg appeared swollen so she stayed in bed. When she tried to get out of bed, she again had pain. The LPN caring for her noted a positive Homans' sign, which may indicate the presence of a blood clot. The RN on duty also got a positive response and reported it to her manager. Believing that the manager would notify the physician, the RN didn't document the positive Homans' sign or tell the next shift about it.

The next morning, a nurse practitioner and an RN examined the patient. Because her left calf appeared enlarged, the nurses were concerned about her undergoing therapy — if a clot were present, movement could cause it to move to her lung. When told about her condition, the physician told the nurses to get her up for therapy.

When to chart

Finding the time to chart can be a problem during a busy shift. But timely entries are crucial in malpractice suits.

Ideally, you'll document your nursing care and other relevant activity when you perform it or not long after—but never before performing it.

Documenting ahead of time makes your notes inaccurate and also omits information about the patient's response to intervention. Even though you may subsequently do what you charted, this practice can lead the plaintiff's attorney to pose a question such as: "Is it your regular or even occasional practice to chart something in anticipation of doing it?" If you answer "yes," the jury

That afternoon at lunch, the patient shook, turned blue, and developed pinpoint pupils. Then her breathing and pulse stopped. Paramedics transported her to the hospital, where she died.

The administrator of the patient's estate sued the physician and his professional corporation for wrongful death. In court, the RN who noted the positive Homans' sign testified that she told her manager about it and the manager told her she would contact the physician. However, the RN didn't chart her actions or tell the next shift of her findings.

The nurse-manager testified that she didn't recall the RN telling her about the patient's condition and she didn't remember contacting the physician. The physician testified that he didn't recall the nurse-manager notifying him of the positive Homans' sign. Additionally, no documentation in the nurses' notes, the physician's orders, or the interdisciplinary progress notes supported the RN's claim that the physician was notified.

The jury decided in favor of the plaintiff and awarded $500,000 in damages.

The lesson? Appropriate nursing assessments aren't enough if you don't document your findings. This patient's death might have been averted if the nurse had written "positive Homans' sign" in the chart.

Who should chart?

You, and only you, should chart your nursing care and observations. At times, because of understaffing or other circumstances, you may be tempted to ask another nurse to complete your portion of the medical record. However, doing so is illegal and prohibited by your state's nurse practice act.

Do your own charting

Having someone else chart for you can result in disciplinary actions that range from a reprimand to the suspension of your nursing license. It may also cause harm to your patient if your coworker makes an error or misinterprets information.

If the patient sues you for negligence, you could be held accountable, along with your employer, because delegated documentation is illegal and may constitute fraud.

Delegating documentation duties has another consequence. It destroys the credibility and value of the medical record, leading reasonable nurses and practitioners to doubt the accuracy of the chart, and it diminishes the record's value as legal evidence. A judge will give little, if any, weight to a medical record that contains second-hand observations or hearsay evidence. To avoid this unsafe practice, do your own charting and refuse to do anyone else's.

won't perceive the chart as a reliable indicator of what you actually did. From that point on, your credibility and that of the medical record will be compromised. (See *Understanding the importance of timely documentation,* pages 382 and 383.)

Countersign cautiously

Countersigning, or signing off on someone else's entry, requires good judgment. Although countersigning doesn't imply that you performed the procedure, it does imply that you reviewed the entry and approved the care given.

Recording critical information: A case in point

This case illustrates the significance of documenting critical information accurately as proof that you provided the accepted standard of care.

FAILURE TO DOCUMENT

Patti Bailey was admitted to the hospital to deliver her third child. During her pregnancy, she had gained 63 lb, her blood pressure had risen from 100/70 in her first trimester to 140/80 at term, and an ultrasound done at 22 weeks showed possible placenta previa.

In the 4 hours after her admission, she received 10 units of oxytocin in 500 ml of dextrose 5% in lactated Ringer's solution. Documentation during this period was scant — her blood pressure was never recorded, and there were only single notations of the fetal heart rate and how labor was progressing. The nurses failed to record the baby's reaction to the drug as well as the nature of the mother's contractions.

Suddenly, after complaining of nausea and epigastric pain, Mrs. Bailey suffered a generalized tonic-clonic seizure. Because her condition was so unstable, she couldn't undergo a cesarean section, and her baby girl was delivered by low forceps. Mrs. Bailey developed disseminated in-

travascular coagulation and required 20 units of whole blood, platelets, and packed red blood cells within 8 hours of delivery.

Incredibly, Mrs. Bailey's nurse had documented nothing in the labor or delivery records or the progress notes.

DEFICIENT POLICY AND PROCEDURE MANUALS

When the unit's policy and procedure manuals were reviewed, no protocol for administering oxytocin and assessing the patient was included. At the very least, the manuals should have recommended using an oxytocin flow sheet to record vital signs, labor progress, fetal status, and changes in the drug administration rate.

THE RESULT

Although Mrs. Bailey recovered, her daughter has seizures and is developmentally disabled. Now age 15, the daughter can't walk or talk and has a gastrostomy tube for nutrition. The case was settled out of court for $450,000; the nurse and hospital were held responsible for one-third of the judgment and the physician paid the rest.

To act correctly and to protect yourself, review your employer's policy on countersigning and proceed accordingly. Does your facility interpret countersigning to mean that the licensed practical nurse (LPN), graduate nurse, or nurse's aide performed the nursing actions in the countersigning registered nurse's presence? If so, don't countersign unless you were there when the actions occurred.

On the other hand, if your facility acknowledges that you don't necessarily have time to witness your coworkers' actions, your countersignature implies that the LPN or nurse's aide had

the authority and competence to perform the care described. In countersigning, you verify that all required patient care procedures were carried out.

If policy requires you to countersign a subordinate's entries, be careful. Review each entry, and make sure that it clearly identifies who did the procedure. If you sign off without reviewing an entry, or if you overlook a problem the entry raises, you could share liability for any patient injury that results.

What should you do if another nurse asks you to document her care or sign her notes? In a

Using good interview techniques to improve documentation

Assessing a patient's condition adequately is part of your professional and legal responsibility. That means following up and documenting each of the patient's complaints. Documenting your data can be easier when you know how to ask questions that elicit the most information from your patient. What follows is an example of an open-ended interview with a patient being assessed for abdominal pain.

NURSE: How would you describe the pain in your abdomen?
PATIENT: It's dull but constant. Actually, it doesn't bother me as much as my blurry eyesight.
NURSE: Tell me about your blurry eyesight.
PATIENT: When I work long hours at my computer, all the words and lines seem to blend together. Sometimes it also happens when I watch television. I probably should see my eye doctor, but I haven't had the time.

NURSE: We'll be sure to follow up on your blurred vision. Now, how about that abdominal pain. How does it affect your daily routine and your sleep?

A lot of things went right in this interview.
▶ First, the nurse didn't dismiss the patient's vision problem. If she had and it turned out to be serious, she might have been judged negligent.
▶ Second, she asked open-ended questions so that the patient could explain his answers rather than simply saying "yes" or "no."
▶ Third, she didn't put words in the patient's mouth. For example, she avoided saying, "The abdominal pain bothers you when you try to sleep, doesn't it?" That would have been a leading question. And the patient, assuming the nurse knows the right answer because she's a nurse, might have answered "yes"—even if the correct answer was "no."

---

word, don't. Unless your facility's policy authorizes or requires you to witness someone else's notes, your signature will make you responsible for anything written in the notes above it.

Charting legally sensitive situations

Among the most legally charged situations are those involving dissatisfied patients, suicidal patients, violent patients, and patients who carry out "nonconforming" behavior, such as refusing treatment, leaving the health care facility against medical advice, or mishandling equipment.

Handle difficult patients with care

No doubt you've cared for dissatisfied patients and heard remarks such as these: "I've been ringing and ringing for a nurse. I could have died before you got here!" or "This food is terrible—take it away!" or "I've never seen such filth in my life. What kind of a hospital is this, anyway?" These are the sounds of unhappy patients. If you tend to dismiss them, you may be increasing your risk of a lawsuit.

TRY TO PUT OUT THE FIRE
The first step in defusing a potentially troublesome situation is to recognize that it exists. Most nurses know the signs of a difficult patient: constant grumpiness, endless complaints, no re-

Legal eagle

Understanding the importance of timely documentation

Although you would never document care before providing it, you may wait until the end of your shift or until your dinner break to complete your nurse's notes. That's what one nurse did. Some time later she was summoned to court as a witness in a malpractice suit. She took the witness stand, answered the attorney's questions, and regularly referred to and read from the chart while doing so. She relied heavily on it for her defense and, in the process, implicitly asked the jury to do the same.

The plaintiff's attorney began his cross-examination by asking the nurse to read from her entries. After a few minutes, here's what happened:

ATTORNEY: Excuse me, may I interrupt? As I listened to you read these entries, a question occurred to me. Maybe it occurred to the jury, too. Would you tell us whether you make the entries you are reading at the time of the events they describe?

NURSE: Well, no, I would have made them sometime later.

ATTORNEY: You're sure?

NURSE: Yes.

ATTORNEY: Thank you. Now, I'd like you to look at the chart and tell the jury whether you noted the time that you actually gave the patient his medication.

NURSE: No, I didn't.

ATTORNEY: Now, I'd like you to look at the chart again and tell the jury whether you indicated the time that you made the entry.

NURSE: No.

ATTORNEY: Given the absence of those two pieces of information, how could you so promptly and confidently respond to my original question? How can you remember so clearly now that you made the entry sometime after the event it describes? Is it because your regular practice is to wait until the end of your shift to chart each and every detail of every event that transpired over your entire shift,

and that you rely solely on your memory when making all these entries?

NURSE: Well, yes, that's true.

ATTORNEY: Would you tell the jury how long a shift you worked that day?

NURSE: A 10-hour shift.

ATTORNEY: And how many patients did you see over that 10-hour period?

NURSE: About 15.

ATTORNEY: Now, each of these 15 patients was different, correct? Each had his own individualized care plan that corresponded to his particular health problems, isn't that right?

NURSE: That's right.

ATTORNEY: And how many different times did you see each of these different patients over the 10-hour period?

NURSE: I probably saw each one, on average, about once an hour.

ATTORNEY: In other words, you probably had 150 patient contacts on that shift alone, is that correct?

NURSE: I suppose so.

ATTORNEY: Now, during the course of your shift, do unexpected events sometimes develop? Unanticipated developments that must be attended to?

NURSE: Sometimes, yes.

ATTORNEY: And when these situations occur, do they distract you from things you had planned to do?

NURSE: Sometimes.

ATTORNEY: After working such a long shift, do you sometimes feel tired?

NURSE: Yes.

ATTORNEY: And at the end of a shift, are you sometimes in a hurry? With things to do, places to go, people to see?

NURSE: Yes.

ATTORNEY: Now, would you tell the jury the purpose of the chart you keep for each patient?

NURSE: Well, we want to communicate information about the patient to others on the health care team, and we want to develop a historic account of the patient's problems, what has been done for him, and his progress.

ATTORNEY: So, other people rely on the information in this chart when they make their own decisions about the patient's care?

NURSE: Yes, that's true.

ATTORNEY: So you would agree that the chart must be reliable?

NURSE: Yes.

ATTORNEY: And you would agree that it must be factual and accurate in all respects?

NURSE: Yes.

ATTORNEY: And you would agree that it needs to be comprehensive and complete, wouldn't you?

NURSE: Yes, I would.

ATTORNEY: So you're trying to develop a record that is factual, accurate, and complete at a time when you're sometimes tired, sometimes in a hurry, after working 10 consecutive hours and seeing 15 different patients 10 different times, and after having dealt with unexpected and distracting events. Is that the essence of your testimony?

NURSE: Well. . . yes.

ATTORNEY: Thank you. You may continue to read your entries to the jury.

By attacking the timeliness of charted entries, the attorney undermined their reliability, accuracy, and completeness. The jurors will now probably be skeptical of the chart and the nurse as well.

HOW TO PREVENT UNTIMELY ENTRIES

So, how do you prevent this situation? By timely charting. Some nurses may carry a notepad to keep working notes of events while they're fresh in their minds. This isn't recommended because during a lawsuit a plaintiff's attorney could subpoena your notes, hoping to find discrepancies between them and the chart. If he succeeds, he'll use those discrepancies to discredit the chart. This will also corroborate that timely charting doesn't exist.

sponse to friendly remarks, and not a trace of a smile when you try a little humor. You don't have to accept the situation; instead, try to improve it. Here are three simple strategies:

▶ Continue reaching out to the patient, even if he doesn't respond.

▶ Ask your colleagues to support and reinforce your efforts.

▶ Record the details of all patient contacts. (See *Documenting precisely,* page 384.)

RECORD SIGNIFICANT PATIENT COMMUNICATIONS

If a patient suggests that he's going to sue you and other caregivers, document this on the progress notes and report it to your nurse-manager or your employer's legal department or attorney. An example of an entry in the progress notes appears below.

2/8/07	1000	Pt. stated that he plans to file suit against this facility for causing his bed sores. ———— ————————Dave Bevins, RN

Assess intent to commit suicide

Take all self-destructive behaviors and comments about suicide seriously. People with suicidal intent not only have thoughts about committing suicide, they also have a concrete plan. They may give evidence of their intent either by self-destructive behaviors or comments about suicide. Follow your facility's policy on caring for a patient with a suicidal intent. If you suspect a patient is at risk for self-destructive behavior or a suicide attempt, immediately notify the practitioner and assess the patient for suicide clues.

Legal eagle

Documenting precisely

Patients or their families may believe a bad outcome is due to poor care. As you know, this isn't always the case. Here's an example of how precise documentation saved the day for one nurse.

A son wanted to sue a hospital and nurse for an incident involving his elderly father, who had been hospitalized for a cholecystectomy. Several days after surgery, his father became disoriented and disorderly, fell out of bed, and broke both hips. He never walked again.

In talking with his attorney, the son claimed, "That nurse either didn't know or didn't care that Dad was confused and agitated. She did nothing to protect him from harm. I want to sue."

The son's description of the father's care sounded like nursing negligence — until the attorney reviewed the patient's record and the nurse's notes. The nurse provided a detailed account of the events preceding the fall. Clearly, she knew about the patient's problem and did everything she could to protect him. Specifically, she:

► confined him to bed with a Posey restraint in compliance with the physician's order
► assigned an aide to stay with him when he became agitated
► made sure that the side rails were always up
► notified coworkers and asked them to watch the patient (his bed was visible from the nurses' station)
► charted all times that the patient and restraint were checked.

The record established that the nurse acted properly and showed concern for the patient. The patient's son was convinced that this unfortunate accident was just that — an accident.

Even if the case had gone to court, that nurse would have been well prepared to meet any challenge to her memory. The details were all there, in black and white.

2/21/07	1100	Pt. reports that she lost her job yesterday. 3 months ago she had a miscarriage. She states, "I don't think I'm supposed to be here." Speaks with a low-toned voice, appears sad, avoids eye contact, and has an unkempt appearance. Reports getting no more than 3 hours of sleep per night for several weeks and states, "That's why I lost my job — I couldn't stay awake at work." Pt. reports having thoughts about suicide but declares, "I would never kill myself." She denies having a suicide plan. Has no history of previous suicide attempts. Pt. lives alone with no family nearby. Doesn't belong to a church and denies having any close friends. Denies having a history of drug or alcohol abuse or psychiatric illness. Dr. Patterson called at 1045 and told of this conversation with pt. She states that she will see pt. for further evaluation at 1130. Will maintain constant observation of pt. until evaluated by Dr. Patterson. — Roger C. Trapley, RN

USE SUICIDE PRECAUTIONS

Patients who have been identified as at risk for self-harm or suicide are placed on some form of suicide precautions based on the gravity of the suicide intent. If your patient has suicidal ideations or makes a suicidal threat, gesture, or attempt, contact the practitioner immediately and institute suicide precautions, making sure to follow your facility's policy. Notify the nursing supervisor, other members of the health care team, and the risk manager and update the patient's care plan.

2/21/07	1600	Pt. stated, "Every year about this
		time, I think about offing myself."
		History of self-harm 1 year ago
		when he lacerated both wrists on
		the 3rd anniversary of his father's
		suicide. States that he has been
		thinking about cutting his wrists
		again. Dr. Gordon notified and pt.
		placed on suicide precautions. Leah
		Halloran, RN, nursing supervisor
		and Michael Stone, risk manager,
		also notified. Pt. placed in room
		closest to nurse's station, verified
		that the sealed window can't be
		opened. With pt. present, personal
		items inventoried and those
		potentially injurious were placed
		in the locked patient belongings
		cabinet. Instructed pt. that he
		must remain in sight of the
		assigned staff member at all
		times, including being accompanied
		to the bathroom and on walks on
		the unit. Betsy Richter is assigned
		to constantly observe pt. this shift.
		Pt. contracted for safety stating,
		"I won't do anything to hurt
		myself." See flow sheet for
		q15min assessments of mood,
		behavior, and location. ————
		———————— Sandy Peres, RN

Safely respond to violent patients

When a patient demonstrates violent behavior, quick action is needed to protect him, other patients, and the staff from harm. Follow your facility's policy for dealing with a violent patient. Call for help immediately and contact security. The practitioner, nursing supervisor, and risk manager should also be informed of the patient's violence. Stay with the patient, without crowding him.

If your own safety is threatened, have a coworker stay with you, if necessary. Remove dangerous objects from the area. Never block your exit or the patient's exit from a room. Use your communication skills to try to calm the patient. Don't challenge him or argue with him. Use a calm and nonthreatening tone of voice and stance. Listen to the patient and acknowledge his anger.

2/6/07	1715	Heard shouts and a crash from pt.'s
		room at 1645. Upon entering room,
		saw dinner tray and broken dishes on
		floor. Pt. was standing, red-faced,
		with fist in air yelling, "My dog gets
		better food than this." Called for
		help and maintained a distance of
		approx. 5' from pt. When other
		nurses arrived, I told them to wait
		in hall. Pt. was throwing books and
		other items from nightstand to floor.
		Firmly told pt. to stop throwing
		things and that I wanted to help
		him. I stated, "I can see you're angry.
		How can I help you?" Pt. responded,
		"Try getting me some decent food."
		Asked a nurse in the hall to call
		dietary office to see what other
		choices were on menu for tonight.
		Told pt. I would try to get him
		other food choices. Asked pt. to sit
		down with me to talk. Pt. sat on edge
		of his bed and I sat on chair approx.
		4' from pt. Pt. started to cry and
		said, "I'm so scared. I don't want to
		die." Listened to pt. verbalize his
		fears for several minutes. When
		asked, pt. stated he would like to
		speak with chaplain and would agree
		to talk with a counselor. He
		apologized for his behavior and
		stated he was embarrassed. Contacted
		Dr. Hartwell at 1705 and told him of
		pt.'s behavior. Doctor approved of
		psych. consult and gave verbal order.
		On-call psychiatrist paged at 1708.
		Hasn't yet returned call. Nursing
		supervisor, Jack Fox, RN, also
		notified of incident. ————————
		———————— Kristen Burger, RN

Depending on their policies, some facilities prepare to handle violent individuals by mobilizing personnel. You may be required to call a specific code through the paging operator such as "code orange room 462B." Specific staff members, such as security personnel, male staff members, and individuals trained to handle volatile situations, would respond to the call. The patient would then be approached and physically subdued and restrained enough to ensure safety without harming himself, staff, or other patients. When the patient is restrained, he'll need to be closely monitored and assessed, and the cause of the episode will need to be determined. He may also require continued chemical or physical restraints if his behavior persists and no physical causation is determined.

Chart patient's nonconforming behavior

Occasionally, a patient does something—or fails to do something—that may contribute to an injury or explain why he hasn't responded to nursing and medical care. Document these behaviors and the outcomes.

Although patients have the right to refuse medical and nursing care, be sure to document on the progress notes any behavior that contradicts medical instructions and the fact that you informed the patient of the possible consequences of his actions.

FAILURE TO PROVIDE INFORMATION

You may occasionally encounter a patient who refuses to provide accurate or complete information about his health history, current medications, or treatments. He may be uncooperative for various reasons: He thinks too many caregivers have asked him the same questions too many times, he doesn't understand the significance of the information, he's fearful or disoriented, or he's suspicious of why you want him to divulge personal information. Alternatively, he may have severe pain, a psychiatric problem, or a language barrier.

In such situations, try to obtain the information from other sources or forms. Clearly document any trouble you've had in communicating with the patient.

Here's an example of what to chart when a patient refuses to answer questions:

2/5/07	0830	When asked for a list of his current medications, the pt. said, "Why do you want to know? What business is it of yours? I don't know why I have to answer that question."
		— Nora Martin, RN

UNUSUAL POSSESSIONS

Document any unauthorized personal belongings discovered in the patient's possession (including alcoholic beverages, tobacco, heating pads, medications, vitamins, and other items that should be checked by the biomedical department before use). Describe the object and how you disposed of it. Here's an example:

2/9/07	1150	Found 3 cans of unopened beer in pt.'s bedside table when checking his soap supply. Explained to pt. that beer was not allowed in the hospital. Took beer to nurse's station to be sent home with family. Dr. Kennedy notified at 1140 hours. He stated he would discuss this with pt. on rounds later today. Pt. denied having drunk any alcohol during hospitalization. No alcohol odor on breath. No empty cans in the trash or room.
		— Elaine Kasmer, RN

Firearms at bedside

If you observe or have reason to believe that your patient has a firearm in his possession, follow your facility's policy and contact security and your nursing supervisor immediately. Keep other patients, staff, and visitors away from the area and let the security guard deal with the firearm.

1/18/07	1000	When reaching in bedside table at 0930 to retrieve basin to assist pt. with a.m. care, noted black gun, approx. 6" long. Closed bedside table door, pushing table back out of reach of bed, left room and closed door. Called security at 0931 and reported gun in bedside table of Rm. 312 to Officer Halliday, who responded that a security guard would be sent up immediately, to keep out of pt.'s room, and to keep staff, visitors, and other patients away from area. Called Mary Delaney, RN, nursing supervisor, at 0933, who reported she's on her way to the floor immediately. Security officer Moore spoke with pt., who produced license to carry gun and turned unloaded gun over to the officer to be locked in hospital safe until discharge. Ms. Delaney reinforced hospital policy on firearms to pt. who stated he understood. ———— Tom O'Brien, RN

MISUSE OF EQUIPMENT

At times, a patient may manipulate equipment or misuse supplies (such as pressing keys on a pump or monitor, detaching tubing, or playing with switches) without understanding the consequences. If your patient misuses equipment, explain that such misuse can harm him. Tell him to call for the nurse if he feels that equipment isn't working properly, is causing him discomfort, or if he has other concerns.

When misuse occurs, document in the progress notes what you saw the patient do (or what he told you he did) and what you did about the problem. Here's an example:

2/6/07	0930	I.V. rate set at 60 ml/hr, 1,000 ml D₅W 1,000 ml in bag. ———— K. Comerford, RN
2/6/07	1020	Checked I.V. at 1000 840 ml left in bag. Pt. stated, "I flicked the switch because I didn't see anything happening. Then I pressed the green button and the arrow." BP 110/82, P 80, T 98.4°. No signs of fluid overload. Breath sounds clear bilaterally. Instructed pt. not to touch the pump or I.V. Repositioned pump to limit pt. access. Dr. Huang notified at 1015 hours. ———— K. Comerford, RN

AMA DISCHARGES AND ELOPEMENTS

If a patient decides to leave the hospital against medical advice (AMA), notify your nurse-manager, the patient's practitioner, and possibly a member of the patient's family, who may be able to persuade the patient to stay.

Expect the patient's practitioner to inform the patient of the risks posed by refusing further treatment. Then, if the patient still intends to leave, complete the paperwork required by your facility, and chart the time and the patient's condition in the chart. Chart the patient's desire for leaving AMA and any reason he gave. Also, document how he left, such as by cab, with a friend or family member, or by wheelchair. (For more information on documenting AMA discharges, see chapter 10, Documentation of Everyday Events.)

If the patient elopes from the health care facility without having said anything about leaving, look for him on your unit immediately and notify security, your nurse-manager, and the patient's practitioner and his family. If the patient is at risk for harming himself or others, notify the police. Document the time you discovered the patient missing, your attempts to find him, and the times and people notified. The legal consequences of a patient's leaving the facility without medical permission can be particularly severe if he's confused or mentally incompetent, especially if he's injured or dies of exposure as a result of his absence.

Interpreting medical record entries

Keeping your own documentation neat and legible should be a primary goal. However, what about other caregivers who aren't careful about their handwriting? Misinterpreting medical record entries can lead to mistakes in care. If you can't read handwritten notes or orders, ask for clarification.

To avoid making an error, always make sure that you clearly understand a written order before carrying it out. If you have questions, clarify the order with the practitioner who wrote it. Don't ask other nurses or practitioners on the unit—they would be guessing, too.

An assistant director of nursing at a well-known general hospital learned this lesson when she decided to help out on an understaffed pediatric unit. A physician ordered 3 ml of a cardiac glycoside for an infant. Not realizing that he meant the pediatric elixir, she administered 3 ml of an injectable, adult-strength cardiac glycoside. This was equivalent to about five times what the physician intended. When the infant died, her parents successfully sued the nurse and the hospital. (See chapter 10, Documentation of Everyday Events, for more on clarifying orders.)

Selected references

Charting Made Incredibly Easy, 3rd. ed. Philadelphia: Lippincott Williams & Wilkins, 2006.

ChartSmart: An A-to-Z Guide to Better Nursing Documentation, 2nd ed. Philadelphia: Lippincott Williams & Wilkins, 2007.

Helms, L., et al. "Disability Law and Nursing Education: An Update," *Journal of Professional Nursing* 22(3):190-6, May-June 2006.

Murray, R.B. "The Subpoena and a Day in Court: Guidelines for Nurses," *Journal of Psychosocial Nursing and Mental Health Services* 43(3):38-44, March 2005.

Parrish, E. "Pulling Together to Document Evidence," *Reflections on Nursing Leadership* 31(2): 28-29, 42, 2005.

Porter, S.C., et al. "Getting the Data Right: Information Accuracy in Pediatric Emergency Medicine," *Quality & Safety in Health Care* 15(4):296-301, August 2006.

Summers, A. "Stating the Facts," *Emergency Nurse* 13(10):14-17, March 2006.

Zimring, S.D. "Health Care Decision-Making Capacity: A Legal Perspective for Long-Term Care Providers," *Journal of the American Medical Directors Association* 7(5):322-326, June 2006.

ELECTRONIC DOCUMENTATION

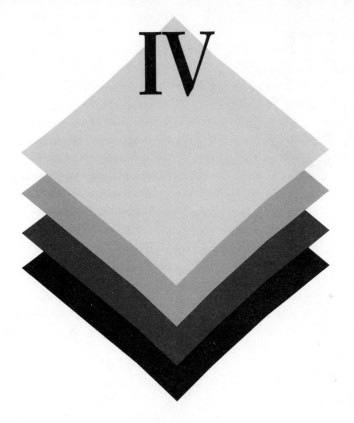
IV

ELECTRONIC MEDICAL RECORDS 13

The electronic medical record (EMR) is the patient-centered product of a complex, interconnected set of clinical software applications that processes, inputs, and sends data. The EMR ormats and categorizes this information, making it readily available to provide guidance to clinicians and act as a record of the patient's care. The EMR also provides a longitudinal record of the patient's health care history in a particular facility and beyond. It includes ambulatory and inpatient records that can be accessed in a variety of ways to fill information needs. Whether you're a seasoned advanced practice nurse or a nursing student tackling your first clinical assignment, it's up to you to learn how to incorporate the EMR into your daily practice, even as its importance becomes tinged with new relevance and character, thanks to other emerging technologies and changes within the health care industry.

What's different? A lot. No doubt you've realized that you have access to more clinical data than ever before, and although that's a benefit, it also comes with more responsibility. In order to utilize this wealth of data properly, you've had to become familiar with new tools that help you access and interpret data quickly and, most important, accurately. These new tools are coming from the information technology that's being built and implemented for caregivers.

The nationwide nursing shortage presents challenges to the health care industry. Nurses are expected to care for more patients, and they're dissatisfied with the amount of nonclinical responsibilities they're responsible for, such as satisfying regulatory and accreditation agency bookkeeping. One of the brighter sides to this glum picture is the development and acceptance of new technologies that enable nurses to better cope with their changing responsibilities. Internet-based self-scheduling, real-time clinical and operational report writing, electronic order entry, the ability to transfer and discharge a patient themselves, and a nurse-clinician documentation system are just a few examples of technology that can help better serve nurses' needs.

As the shortage worsens, hospitals are finding themselves using every means possible to support their nurses, including the use of new, exciting technologies. By increasing efficiency and alleviating some of the burden on nurses, technology can free nurses to concentrate on direct patient care. As part of a comprehensive strategy to support nurses within the hospital, it can also help make the care environment more rewarding and thus help improve recruitment and retention.

The move toward electronic documentation

The nursing shortage is certainly not the sole engine driving the development and implementation of electronic nursing documentation systems, but it's a significant factor. Without the shortage and the strain it creates on their nursing staffs, hospitals and other health care facilities probably wouldn't be so quick to proceed with the purchase or internal development of such systems.

Of course, other factors are also behind this move toward implementation. When many institutions were spending large amounts of capital funds on laboratory management, pharmacies, admissions, and billing systems, clinical documentation seemed fairly easy. Fifteen years ago, it was hard to find a hospital that was relying on an EMR as its primary repository of patient clinical information. Back then, nursing admin-

Documentation: A time of transition

By the end of the 20th century, sky-high medical costs had broken the back of the health care system, and managed care had arrived, putting the business of health care primarily in the hands of insurance companies and regulatory agencies. As a result, there are now increased demands from payers and regulators for stricter adherence to governmental and third-party-payer rules and regulations. With this in mind, the government enacted the Health Insurance Portability and Accountability Act to help standardize the processes and language of the business transactions between health care providers and third-party payers. By standardizing formats and coding, all parties—third-party payers, health care facilities, and patients—receive benefits in saved time and money. Computerized documentation plays a big role in this important transition.

istrators, managers, and staffers were reluctant to take on the risks of such a massive change in a documentation system that had been in place for nearly half a century. They were more than happy with the status quo.

What's changed? Let's just say that in today's modern health care environment, facilities have been driven toward EMRs. (See *Documentation: A time of transition.*) Standardization of health care billing transactions demands far more accurate documentation to satisfy third-party payers, and the needs of the business functions of the hospital are also in play. The most compelling reason for the development of a proficient EMR system, however, is better patient care.

A work in progress

Definitions and parameters for workable EMRs remain a work in progress. Informatics—the merging of medical and nursing science with computer science in order to better manage data—continues to see its role expand in all health care environments, and several medical-nursing informatics organizations are working to create standards. National organizations, such as the Healthcare Information and Management Systems Society, the American Nursing Informatics Association, the North American Nursing Diagnosis Association International, and the American Medical Informatics Association, are convening standing EMR committees to accomplish this task.

Advantages of an EMR

Even in this relatively early stage of the EMR, there are far more reasons than not for all clinical documentation to be incorporated into a EMR. The advantages include improvement in the standardization of charting, the quality of the medical record, information accessibility, medical management, data retrieval, legibility, and error correction. (See *Benefits of EMRs.*)

Standardization

Standardization of clinical data and reporting has been pushed to the forefront by the Health Insurance Portability and Accountability Act–mandated changes and accurate and timely reports required for accrediting, regulatory, and third-party payers. This increased demand for reports requires computerization of the report writer, which in turn requires clinical data input.

Benefits of EMRs

This list highlights the key benefits of using an electronic medical record (EMR):

- ▶ ability for all providers to see each other's documentation
- ▶ access by different providers at different locations
- ▶ access by different providers at the same time
- ▶ access to clinical information
- ▶ access EMRs at appropriate workstations
- ▶ automated reports for quality indicators
- ▶ clinical decision making easier and more accurate
- ▶ ease in auditing charting
- ▶ ease of access—"where to look"
- ▶ increased quality of documentation
- ▶ legibility
- ▶ multidisciplinary access
- ▶ on-line clinical support information
- ▶ patient-driven care planning
- ▶ point-of-care charting (no more waiting until the end of your shift)
- ▶ "real-time" diagnostic results and reports
- ▶ reduced redundant charting
- ▶ remote access.

Quality

With a properly designed and implemented clinical information system, EMR documentation improves the overall caliber of clinical information and returns the focus of nurses to providing patient care.

Accessibility

A well-developed electronic documentation system makes accessing patient data quick and painless by filing clinical information in the same location from patient to patient and department to department. This across-the-board universality saves time in the short and long runs and contributes to more accurate assessment of recorded data.

Different members of the health care team can also have access to different types of patient information. For example, a dietitian who logs into the patient's record with her username and password may see dietary orders but not physical therapy orders. When used correctly, this access feature can help maintain a patient's privacy.

Medication management

Electronic documentation allows for direct order transmittal that cuts down medication errors by eliminating order transcription errors. It also alerts the practitioner to the patient's allergies. Additionally, the system's medication order screens typically provide the practitioner with choices of dosages and administration routes, which can help prevent dosing errors.

Data retrieval

After the practitioner's orders are entered, you can log into the electronic documentation system to update the patient record as needed. To display the patient's electronic chart on the screen, enter the patient's name or account number, or choose the patient's name from a patient census list. After retrieving the patient's information, you can choose the function you want to perform. For example, you can enter new data into the care plan or progress notes, sign out medications that you have administered, or compare data on the patient's vital signs, laboratory test results, or intake and output.

Typically, electronic documentation systems allow health care providers to retrieve information more quickly than traditional documenta-

tion systems do. Most systems allow you to print a patient Kardex each shift that contains information to guide your care. (See "Characteristics of a computer-generated Kardex," in chapter 6.)

Legibility

In 1999, the Institute of Medicine published a report that recommended the move toward a universal system of electronic order entry because medication errors were commonly caused by the inability to properly decipher handwritten orders. The report's recommendation makes perfect sense. With electronic documentation, legibility is a nonissue and improved patient safety is the likely result.

Error correction

Most electronic documentation systems have a special feature that allows you to correct a charting error. Be sure to follow your facility's protocol for correcting such errors. Electronic entries are part of the patient's permanent record and, as such, can't be deleted. You simply access a screen that prompts you to make the correction. Then you enter the date and time the error was made, locate the error in the record, and correct it. Just as with traditional charting, the correction is shown along with the original error.

Disadvantages of an EMR

EMRs are still fairly new. Every day, we learn how to improve their use a little bit more. If we're to make use of them fully, we must become proficient in their strengths and adapt to their weaknesses.

Maintaining patient confidentiality

The American Nurses Association and the American Records Association offer these guidelines for maintaining confidentiality of electronic medical records.

NEVER SHARE

Never give your personal password or computer code to anyone—including another nurse in the unit, a nurse serving temporarily in the unit, or a doctor. Your health care facility can issue a short-term password that allows infrequent users to access certain records.

LOG OFF

After you log on to a computer terminal, don't leave the terminal unattended. Although some computer systems have a timing device that automatically logs off the user after an idle period, you should get in the habit of logging off the system before leaving the terminal.

DON'T DISPLAY

Don't leave information about a patient displayed on a monitor where others can see it. Also, don't leave print versions or excerpts of the medical record unattended.

Computer crashes

Computer systems can "crash," or break down, making information temporarily unavailable. However, with today's more reliable technology and more sophisticated software, these occurrences are becoming less and less frequent. Downtimes will happen and, in fact, they're occasionally necessary to back up the system (a planned downtime procedure can alleviate a lot of the fear of such occurrences as well as ensure continuity of the patient's record). However, as

technology improves, computer crashes are becoming less of an issue.

Unfamiliarity

As new nurses graduate college and enter the workforce, the use of computers becomes more of an expectation and less of an alien concept. However, there are still segments of the nursing population that aren't comfortable with computer usage. This is an important issue. Used improperly, electronic documentation systems can scramble patient information and threaten a patient's right to privacy if appropriate security measures are neglected. They can also yield inaccurate or incomplete information if they use standardized, limited vocabulary or phrases.

HIPAA and patient confidentiality

Preventive measures must be taken to prevent breaches in patient confidentiality when using electronic documentation and technology. (See *Maintaining patient confidentiality*.) One of the drawbacks of electronic documentation is the potential for unauthorized personnel to access confidential medical records. The Health Insurance Portability and Accountability Act (HIPAA) of 1996 was enacted by the U.S. government to ensure the privacy of individual health information, both paper and electronic.

The electronic security provisions of HIPAA are meant to maintain the protection of patient information by prohibiting clinicians from using facility computers for online recreation, shopping, or other pursuits not related to patient care. Not allowing these activities helps to safeguard facility computers from viruses that could allow unauthorized access to confidential patient information. HIPAA gives patients more control over their health information, sets limits on the use of health records, and establishes safeguards that health care providers must achieve. It also provides for penalties when a patient's privacy is violated and dictates when health care information can be disclosed for the purpose of public safety.

An important part of HIPAA is the Administrative Simplification Act (ASA), which requires standard formats be used when health information is transmitted electronically. Electronic data exchange can help to improve the efficiency and effectiveness of the health care delivery system. The U.S. federal government is playing an important role in the adoption of health data standards and in the security of a patient's EMR.

Maintaining patient confidentiality is equally important when it comes to the use of other electronic devices. Disclosing patient information to unauthorized personnel may have significant legal implications. Be sure to keep this in mind when using printers, copiers, phones, fax machines, and pagers.

Raising the standards and value of documentation

The 2006 standards for accreditation of hospitals developed by The Joint Commission include the identification of goals, functions, and standards for providing patient care. The purpose of The Joint Commission's National Patient Safety Goals is to promote specific improvements in patient safety. These goals highlight problematic areas in health care and describe evidence and expert-based solutions to these problems. Because The Joint Commission recognized that sound system design is intrinsic to the delivery of safe, high-quality health care, the goals focus on system-wide solutions wherever possible.

One way electronic documentation can assist nurses in meeting The Joint Commission's National Patient Safety Goals is by improving the safety of medication administration. As mentioned earlier in this chapter, the adoption of an electronic order entry system has the potential to reduce medication errors that occur from mistakes in the transcription and interpretation of handwritten medication orders. Bar code technology is another new feature some facilities have incorporated into their computer systems that has greatly reduced medication errors. (See chapter 14, Electronic Nursing Documentation.)

Nursing organizations and regulatory and accrediting entities are leaning toward a greater dependency on electronic documentation. The Joint Commission regularly focuses its attention on aspects of care and documentation that it views as lacking. Nursing continues to grapple with the Nursing Minimum Data Set (NMDS) as a codified data set that will lend itself to better evaluation of patient interventions and outcomes as well as for research. In addition, task-oriented documentation is no longer sufficient. (See chapter 14 for more information.) Clinical documentation must be patient and patient-outcome supportive.

The clinical documentation system is an ideal platform for the implementation of new standards. A great example of this was The Joint Commission initiative to improve the documentation of patient and family teaching. Before the initiative, documentation of patient teaching tended to be spotty. However, new electronic systems in the hands of nurses now present on-line forms that prompt caregivers to address the many facets of patient teaching and provide a sharp picture of the experience and results of the teaching in the CPR.

Another aspect of The Joint Commission's initiative is its mandate to standardize patient-teaching documentation across multidisciplinary services and departments, resulting in a multi-disciplinary teaching record that everyone can access and use. Electronic documentation should help facilitate this change.

Access to reports and trends demonstrating the changing nursing interventions and charting is key for managers and auditors. Therefore, having the ability to easily change and upgrade the tools for nursing documentation is of great importance. Information technology will allow for the implementation of NMDS to build a universal nursing decision support system, making the electronic clinical system and resultant EMR a mandatory documentation medium.

Nursing research and education

Nurses are actively involved in the research and development of electronic nursing documentation systems. Nurses are charged with gathering the most up-to-date research on patient care and nursing processes and integrating this evidence into interdisciplinary computer documentation systems. It's nursing research that guides this function and is at the core of a well-designed system.

The National League of Nursing (NLN) has formed a task group to examine informatics competencies in nursing education. The NLN has recognized the increased use of technology in health care and is making recommendations to nurse educators to develop student and faculty informatics competencies. Information tech-nology has wide-ranging uses in nursing education. From computer tutorials to learning management systems to simulation manikins, computers and the Internet have transformed the classroom environment. These additions to the curricula are preparing nursing students for the technology-laden health care environment.

Future of IT in nursing documentation

In 2004, President Bush helped to solidify the future of information technology (IT) in nursing documentation when he directed the U.S. Department of Health and Human Services (HHS) to create the new position of National Health Information Technology (HIT) coordinator. The HHS appointed David J. Brailer, MD, PhD, as the nation's first HIT coordinator. The major goal of this position is to develop standards and an infrastructure to support the government and the public in implementing IT into the health care system. The HIT coordinator will ensure the privacy and security of health care information. He will also create incentives within the government to encourage the use of IT. It's believed that these efforts will improve the quality of patient care and reduce health care costs.

The president set as a 10-year goal for his 2004 initiative that a majority of Americans will have an electronic health record (EHR). This record will reside on the National Health Information Network and contain information about care the patient received in different health care settings. The HIT coordinator will develop strategies to ensure that this goal is met within this timeframe.

To help with the goals of the HIT coordinator, the HHS has licensed a standardized medical vocabulary, developed by the College of American Pathologists, called the Systematized Nomenclature of Medicine (SNOMED). This language has created a common clinical language that is an integral part of the health care information infrastructure. In addition, HHS is also working with the international standards-setting organization known as Health Level 7 (HL-7) to standardize functions needed for an electronic medical record. These initiatives, as well as many others, are helping to ensure the uniform, ongoing IT development in health care that results in information exchange between the government and the public.

In conjunction with the development of the EHR, nurses will also increase their role in ensuring accurate electronic documentation at the point of care, which will become a part of the patient's EHR for his lifetime.

Additional future advances currently under development for the future of nursing documentation include an expanded use of bar coding technology as well as computers that recognize speech. What's more, high-speed computer networks have made the Internet readily available at the patient's bedside for use by the patient and the nurse. The trend is toward real-time point-of-care documentation with computer terminals at the bedside. These computer terminals may be in the form of computers-on-wheels, laptops, notebook computers, personal data assistants (PDAs), and stationary computer terminals. In addition, biometrics—the ability to recognize humans by a physical or behavioral trait—will also be more widely used in health care.

Selected references

Allan, K., and Ribbons, B. "Nurses Combine IT and Nursing Skills to Improve Discharge Communication," *Australian Nursing Journal* 14(1):30, July 2006.

Anderson, H.J. "With Shortage of Nurses, I.T. Becomes More Essential," *Health Data Management* 14(7):4, July 2006.

Charting Made Incredibly Easy, 3rd. ed. Philadelphia: Lippincott Williams & Wilkins, 2006.

ChartSmart: An A-to-Z Guide to Better Nursing Documentation, 2nd ed. Philadelphia: Lippincott Williams & Wilkins, 2007.

Conn, J. "Embedded Trouble. Link in Software Inherited through Acquisition Left Patient Data Vulnerable," *Modern Healthcare* 36(32):28, 30, August 2006.

Cross, M. "Web Lends a Hand with Nurse Training," *Health Data Management* 14(6):84-85, June 2006.

Doyle, M. "Promoting Standardized Nursing Language Using an Electronic Medical Record System," *AORN Journal* 83(6):1336-42, June 2006.

Kaufman, D., et al. "Applying an Evaluation Framework for Health Information System Design, Development, and Implementation," *Nursing Research* 55(2 Suppl):S37-42, March-April 2006.

Lunney, M., et al. "Advocating for Standardized Nursing Languages in Electronic Health Records" *The Journal of Nursing Administration* 35(1):1-3, January 2005.

Nicol, N., and Huminski, L. "How We Cut Drug Errors. At One Hospital, IT and Changed Culture Saves Lives," *Modern Healthcare* 36(34):38, August 2006.

Smith, K., et al. "Evaluating the Impact of Computerized Clinical Documentation," *CIN: Computers, Informatics, Nursing* 23(3):132-38, May-June 2005.

ELECTRONIC NURSING DOCUMENTATION 14

Electronic health record information systems can increase efficiency and accuracy in all phases of the nursing process and can help nurses meet the standards set by the American Nurses Association (ANA) and The Joint Commission. Current computerized systems not only collect, transmit, and organize the information but also suggest nursing diagnoses and provide standardized patient status and nursing interventions, which you can use for care plans and progress notes. Computerized systems may even interact with you, prompting you with questions and suggestions about the information that you enter.

Depending on your facility's software, you might use computers for all five steps of the nursing process: assessment, nursing diagnosis, planning, implementation, and evaluation. (See *Electronic charting and the nursing process.*)

Care plans

A complex function of computerized nursing documentation is the integration of nursing care plans. Care plans can be solely nursing generated or can be generated based on the patient's medical diagnosis. Once a care plan is chosen within a computer system, the assessment and intervention parameters are defined based on the nursing diagnosis. Evidence-based practice guides the input of standardized nursing care plans, which results in customized screens based upon the patient's individual needs. (See *Electronic charting system,* page 400.)

Electronic charting and the nursing process

A computer information system can either stand alone or be a subsystem of a larger hospital system. Nursing information systems (NISs) can increase efficiency and accuracy in all phases of the nursing process—assessment, nursing diagnosis, planning, implementation, and evaluation—and can help nurses meet the standards established by the American Nurses Association and The Joint Commission. In addition, NISs can help nurses spend more time meeting patient needs. Consider these uses of computers in the nursing process.

ASSESSMENT

You can use the computer terminal to record admission information. As you collect data, enter additional information as prompted by the computer's software program. Enter data about the patient's health status, history, chief complaint, and other assessment factors.

Some software programs prompt you to ask specific questions and then offer pathways for gathering further information. Other programs flag assessment values that are outside the acceptable range to call attention to them.

NURSING DIAGNOSIS

Most current programs list standard diagnoses with associated signs and symptoms as references. However, you must still use clinical judgment to determine a nursing diagnosis for each patient. With this information, you can rapidly obtain diagnostic information. For example, the computer can generate a list of possible diagnoses for a patient with selected signs and symptoms, or it may enable you to retrieve and review the patient's records according to the nursing diagnosis.

PLANNING

To help you begin to write a care plan, some computer programs display recommended expected outcomes and interventions for the selected diagnosis. Computers can also track outcomes for large patient populations. You can use computers to compare large amounts of patient data, help identify outcomes the patient is likely to achieve based on his problems and needs, and estimate the time frame for reaching outcome goals.

IMPLEMENTATION

You can also use the computer to record actual interventions and patient-processing information, such as transfer and discharge instructions, and to communicate this information to other departments. Computer-generated progress notes automatically sort and print out patient data—such as medication administration, treatments, and vital signs—making documentation more efficient and accurate.

EVALUATION

During evaluation, you can use the computer to record and store observations, patient responses to nursing interventions, and your own evaluation statements. You may also use information from other members of the health care team to determine future actions and discharge planning. If a desired patient outcome hasn't been achieved, record new interventions taken to ensure desired outcomes. Then reevaluate the second set of interventions.

Electronic charting system

SYSTEM	USEFUL SETTINGS	PARTS OF RECORD	ASSESSMENT	CARE PLAN	OUTCOMES AND EVALUATIONS	PROGRESS NOTES FORMAT
Electronic	• Acute care • Long-term care • Home care • Ambulatory care	• Progress notes • Flow sheets • Nursing care plan • Database • Teaching plan	• Initial: baseline assessment • Ongoing: progress notes	• Database • Care plan	• Outcome-based care plan	• Evaluative statements • Expected outcomes • Learning outcomes

Laboratory and diagnostic test results

One of the earliest clinical uses of computers in the health care arena was for retrieving laboratory results. In an electronic system it's possible for authorized personnel to enter and retrieve test results from various ancillary departments. As one of The Joint Commission's National Patient Safety Goals, it's essential that you follow your facility's policy regarding the reporting of critical test results and values.

Systems and functions

Depending on which type of computer hardware and software your health care facility has, you may access information by using a keyboard, light pen, touch-sensitive screen, mouse, or voice activation. In addition to having a mainframe computer, most health care facilities place personal computers or terminals at workstations throughout the facility so that departmental staff will have quick access to vital information. Some facilities put terminals at patients' bedsides, making data even more accessible.

Most electronic documentation systems provide a menu of words or phrases you can choose from to individualize documentation on standardized formats. Some systems permit you to use a series of phrases to quickly create a complete narrative note. You can then elaborate on a problem or clarify flow sheet documentation in the comment section of an electronic form by entering standardized phrases or typing in comments.

Some current electronic systems are the Nursing Information System (NIS), the Nursing Minimum Data Set (NMDS), the Nursing Outcomes Classification (NOC) system, and voice-activated systems.

Nursing Information System

Currently available NIS software programs allow nurses to record nursing actions in the patient's electronic medical record. These systems reflect most or all of the components of the nursing process so they can meet the standards of the ANA and The Joint Commission. Each NIS provides different features and can be customized to conform to a facility's documentation forms and formats. For example, some systems offer automated drug information, guidelines regarding facility policies and procedures, and intranet access. Other systems may provide the capability for online literature searches, which keeps the latest health care information at the nurse's fingertips.

Some NISs manage information passively—that is, they collect, transmit, organize, format, print, and display information that you can use to make a decision, but they don't suggest decisions for you. However, some systems can suggest nursing diagnoses based on predefined assessment data that you enter. The more sophisticated systems provide you with standardized patient status and nursing intervention phrases that you can use to construct your progress notes. These systems let you change the standardized phrases, if necessary, and allow room for you to add your own notes.

NEW DEVELOPMENTS

The most recent NISs are interactive, meaning that they prompt you with questions and suggestions that are in accordance with the information you enter. These systems require only a brief narrative, and the questioning and diagnostic suggestions that the systems provide ensure quick but thorough documentation. The programs also allow you to add or change information so that you can tailor your documentation to fit each individual patient. Ultimately, this sequential decision-making format should lead to more effective nursing care and documentation.

Nursing Minimum Data Set

The NMDS is a means of standardizing nursing information. It contains three categories of data: nursing care, patient demographics, and service elements. (See *Elements of the Nursing Minimum Data Set.*)

Elements of the Nursing Minimum Data Set

The Nursing Minimum Data Set contains three elements—nursing care, patient demographics, and service. These elements are the core data needed to support decision making in clinical nursing and to implement the electronic medical record.

NURSING CARE
► Nursing diagnoses
► Nursing interventions
► Nursing outcomes
► Nursing intensity

PATIENT DEMOGRAPHICS
► Personal identification
► Date of birth
► Sex
► Race and ethnicity
► Residence

SERVICE
► Unique facility or service agency number
► Unique health record number of patient
► Unique number of principal registered nurse providers
► Episode admission or encounter date
► Discharge or termination date
► Disposition of patient
► Expected payer of medical bills

NURSING BENEFITS

The NMDS allows you to collect nursing diagnoses and intervention data and identify the nursing needs of various patient populations. It also lets you track patient outcomes and describe nursing care in various settings, including the patient's home. This system helps establish accurate estimates for nursing service costs and provides data about nursing care that may influence health care policy and decision making.

With the NMDS, you can compare nursing trends locally, regionally, and nationally, allowing you to compare nursing data from various clinical settings, patient populations, and geographic areas. However, the NMDS does more than provide valuable information for research and policy making. It also helps you provide better patient care. For instance, examining the outcomes of patient populations will help you set realistic outcomes for an individual patient as well as formulate accurate nursing diagnoses and plan interventions.

The standardized format of the NMDS also encourages more consistent nursing documentation. All data are coded, making documentation and information retrieval faster and easier. Currently, the North American Nursing Diagnosis Association International assigns numerical codes to all nursing diagnoses so they can be used with the NMDS.

Nursing Outcomes Classification

The NOC system provides the first comprehensive, standardized method of measuring nursing-sensitive patient outcomes. The NOC has major implications for nursing administrative practice and the patient care delivery system. It allows you to compare your patients' outcomes to the outcomes of larger groups according to such parameters as age, diagnosis, or health care setting.

NOC implementation is essential to support ongoing nursing research. This system makes possible the inclusion of patient data-related outcomes that have been absent from computerized medical information databases in the past.

Voice-activated systems

Some hospitals have instituted voice-activated nursing documentation systems, which are most useful in hospital departments that have a high volume of structured reports, such as the operating room.

The software program uses a specialized knowledge base—nursing words, phrases, and report forms, combined with automated speech recognition (ASR) technology. This system allows the user to record prompt and complete nurse's notes by voice. The ASR system requires little or no keyboard use; you simply speak into a telephone handset and the text appears on the computer screen.

The software program includes information on the nursing process, nursing theory, nursing standards of practice, report forms, and a logical format. The system uses trigger phrases that cue the system to display passages of report text. You can use the text displayed to design an individualized care plan or to fill in standard facility forms.

Although voice-activated systems are designed to work most efficiently with these trigger phrases, they also allow word-for-word dictation and editing. The system increases the speed of reporting and frees the nurse from paperwork so that she can spend more time at the bedside.

Additional system features

Depending on the system type, an electronic documentation system may provide the ability to print out patient schedules. The system may also be equipped with bar code technology.

PATIENT SCHEDULES

Most systems have the ability to print out schedule lists for patients. For example, you can print out a schedule of patients who require fingerstick glucose level tests. If the situation requires you to delegate the task, the list may be given to ancillary staff members. The list lets them know exactly when they're supposed to obtain the fingerstick glucose level for each patient.

BAR CODE TECHNOLOGY

Bar code technology is a new feature some facilities have incorporated into their computer systems, and it has greatly reduced medication errors. With this technology, you scan a drug's bar code, scan the patient's identification bracelet, and then scan your own identification badge before administering the drug to the patient. As soon as the medication and patient's identification bracelet are scanned, the information immediately appears on a mobile computer screen, documenting the administration.

Bar code technology helps keep track of discontinued medications. The system connects to the order-entry system, so if a practitioner discontinues a medication, it won't show up on the patient's listed medications when you scan the patient's wristband.

Scanning of medications also ensures that the nurse hasn't inadvertently chosen the wrong medication out of the medication drawer or received the wrong medication from the pharmacy. Other advantages of bar code technology include saved time and streamlined documentation. If a patient refuses a medication, the nurse can document it immediately into the mobile computer. At the end of the shift, the nurse-manager can print a report to identify patients who didn't receive their medications.

Nursing informatics

In 2001 the ANA defined nursing informatics (NI) as a specialty that integrates nursing science, computer science, and information science to manage and communicate data, information, and knowledge in nursing practice.

With the growing interest in the development of a national electronic health record, nurses have played an integral role in the development of data standards used in these records. An NI expert has an acute understanding of the nursing process and is also knowledgeable regarding how technology can advance the practice of nursing. As the government and the public collaborate to promote the expanded use of technology in the health care environment, nurses must be extensively involved in current policy and future development of these systems.

The role of the NI expert is extremely broad. Software vendors who design electronic documentation systems employ nurses in this specialty. They work in the health care environment helping to choose the proper system for a particular facility. An NI expert also can work within a health care organization to administer and customize a purchased system. These nurses can use the system to extract data for research to help advance the nursing profession. NI experts work in education to utilize technology in the classroom and to ensure that nurses entering the profession are competent in the increasing technological demands involved in patient care. NI specialists also develop computer-based educational materials for the purpose of training and continuing education.

Selected references

Angermo, L.M., and Ruland, C.M. "Increasing the Usability of Nursing Intervention Classification in EHRs," *Studies in Health Technology and Informaties* 122:985-86, 2006.

Briggs, B. "Nursing I.T.: From Stations to Bedside," *Health Data Management* 14(7):28, 30, 32-35, July 2006.

Charting Made Incredibly Easy, 3rd. ed. Philadelphia: Lippincott Williams & Wilkins, 2006.

ChartSmart: An A-to-Z Guide to Better Nursing Documentation, 2nd ed. Philadelphia: Lippincott Williams & Wilkins, 2007.

Cross, M. "Web Lends a Hand with Nurse Training," *Health Data Management* 14(6):84-85, June 2006.

Guenther, J.T. "Mapping the Literature of Nursing Informatics," *Journal of the Medical Library Association* 94(2 Suppl):E92-98, April 2006.

Kaufman, D., et al. "Applying an Evaluation Framework for Health Information System Design, Development, and Implementation," *Nursing Research* 55(2 Suppl):S37-42, March-April 2006.

Moody, L. E., et al. "Electronic Health Records Documentation in Nursing: Nurses' Perceptions, Attitudes, and Preferences," *CIN: Computers, Informatics, Nursing* 22(6):337-344, November-December 2004.

Roemer, L. K., et al. "Redundancy in a Computer-Generated Order List: Meeting the Needs of Nurses at Various Levels of Practice Expertise," *CIN: Computers, Informatics, Nursing* 23(2): 73-82, March-April 2005.

Saba, V. K., and McCormick, K. A. *Essentials of Nursing Informatics,* 4th ed. New York: McGraw-Hill, 2006.

Strople, B., and Ottani, P. "Can Technology Improve Intershift Report? What the Research Reveals," *Journal of Professional Nursing* 22(3):197-204, May-June 2006.

Wright, M.J., et al. "Maintaining Excellence in Physician Nurse Communication with CPOE: A Nursing Informatics Team Approach," *Journal of Healthcare Information Management* 20(2):65-70, Spring 2006.

APPENDICES
INDEX

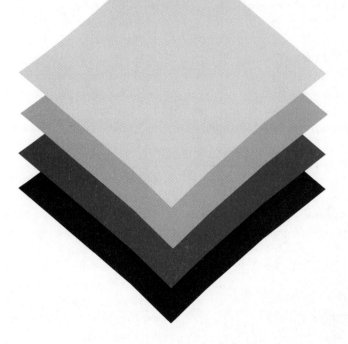

NANDA-I NURSING DIAGNOSES BY DOMAIN

The following is a list of the 2007-2008 current nursing diagnosis classifications according to domain. The 2007 revised and new diagnoses are in *italics*.

1. DOMAIN: HEALTH PROMOTION
- ▶ Effective therapeutic regimen management
- ▶ Health-seeking behaviors (specify)
- ▶ Impaired home maintenance
- ▶ Ineffective community therapeutic regimen management
- ▶ Ineffective family therapeutic regimen management
- ▶ Ineffective health maintenance
- ▶ Ineffective therapeutic regimen management
- ▶ *Readiness for enhanced immunization status*
- ▶ Readiness for enhanced nutrition
- ▶ Readiness for enhanced therapeutic regimen management

2. DOMAIN: NUTRITION
- ▶ Deficient fluid volume
- ▶ Excess fluid volume
- ▶ Imbalanced nutrition: Less than body requirements
- ▶ Imbalanced nutrition: More than body requirements
- ▶ Impaired swallowing
- ▶ Ineffective infant feeding pattern
- ▶ Readiness for enhanced fluid balance
- ▶ Risk for deficient fluid volume
- ▶ Risk for imbalanced fluid volume
- ▶ Risk for imbalanced nutrition: More than body requirements
- ▶ *Risk for impaired liver function*
- ▶ *Risk for unstable glucose level*

3. DOMAIN: ELIMINATION/EXCHANGE
- ▶ Bowel incontinence
- ▶ Constipation
- ▶ Diarrhea
- ▶ Functional urinary incontinence
- ▶ Impaired gas exchange
- ▶ Impaired urinary elimination
- ▶ *Overflow urinary incontinence*
- ▶ Perceived constipation
- ▶ Readiness for enhanced urinary elimination
- ▶ Reflex urinary incontinence
- ▶ Risk for constipation
- ▶ Risk for urge urinary incontinence
- ▶ Stress urinary incontinence
- ▶ Total urinary incontinence
- ▶ Urge urinary incontinence
- ▶ Urinary retention

4. DOMAIN: ACTIVITY/REST
- ▶ Activity intolerance
- ▶ Bathing or hygiene self-care deficit
- ▶ Decreased cardiac output
- ▶ Deficient diversional activity
- ▶ Delayed surgical recovery
- ▶ Dressing or grooming self-care deficit
- ▶ Dysfunctional ventilatory weaning response
- ▶ Energy field disturbance

- Fatigue
- Feeding self-care deficit
- Impaired bed mobility
- Impaired physical mobility
- Impaired spontaneous ventilation
- Impaired transfer ability
- Impaired walking
- Impaired wheelchair mobility
- Ineffective breathing pattern
- Ineffective tissue perfusion (specify: renal, cerebral, cardiopulmonary, gastrointestinal, peripheral)
- *Insomnia* (formerly Disturbed sleep pattern)
- *Readiness for enhanced self-care*
- Readiness for enhanced sleep
- Risk for activity intolerance
- Risk for disuse syndrome
- Sedentary lifestyle
- Sleep deprivation
- Toileting self-care deficit

5. DOMAIN: PERCEPTION/COGNITION
- Acute confusion
- Chronic confusion
- Deficient knowledge (specify)
- Disturbed sensory perception (specify: visual, auditory, kinesthetic, gustatory, tactile, olfactory)
- Disturbed thought processes
- Impaired environmental interpretation syndrome
- Impaired memory
- Impaired verbal communication
- Readiness for enhanced communication
- *Readiness for enhanced decision making*
- Readiness for enhanced knowledge (specify)
- *Risk for acute confusion*
- Unilateral neglect
- Wandering

6. DOMAIN: SELF-PERCEPTION
- Chronic low self-esteem
- Disturbed body image
- Disturbed personal identity
- Hopelessness
- Powerlessness
- *Readiness for enhanced hope*
- *Readiness for enhanced power*
- Readiness for enhanced self-concept
- *Risk for compromised human dignity*
- Risk for loneliness
- Risk for powerlessness
- Risk for situational low self-esteem
- Situational low self-esteem

7. DOMAIN: ROLE RELATIONSHIPS
- Caregiver role strain
- Dysfunctional family processes: Alcoholism
- Effective breast-feeding
- Impaired parenting
- Impaired social interaction
- Ineffective breast-feeding
- Ineffective role performance
- Interrupted breast-feeding
- Interrupted family processes
- Parental role conflict
- Readiness for enhanced family processes
- Readiness for enhanced parenting
- Risk for caregiver role strain
- Risk for impaired parent/infant/child attachment
- Risk for impaired parenting

8. DOMAIN: SEXUALITY
- Ineffective sexuality pattern
- Sexual dysfunction

9. DOMAIN: COPING/STRESS TOLERANCE
- Anxiety
- Autonomic dysreflexia
- Chronic sorrow

▶ *Complicated grieving* (formerly Dysfunctional grieving)
▶ Compromised family coping
▶ Death anxiety
▶ Decreased intracranial adaptive capacity
▶ Defensive coping
▶ Disabled family coping
▶ Disorganized infant behavior
▶ Fear
▶ *Grieving* (formerly Anticipatory grieving)
▶ Ineffective community coping
▶ Ineffective coping
▶ Ineffective denial
▶ Post-trauma syndrome
▶ Rape-trauma syndrome
▶ Rape-trauma syndrome: Compound reaction
▶ Rape-trauma syndrome: Silent reaction
▶ Readiness for enhanced community coping
▶ Readiness for enhanced coping (individual)
▶ Readiness for enhanced family coping
▶ Readiness for enhanced organized infant behavior
▶ Relocation stress syndrome
▶ Risk for autonomic dysreflexia
▶ Risk for disorganized infant behavior
▶ *Risk for complicated grieving* (formerly Risk for dysfunctional grieving)
▶ Risk for post-trauma syndrome
▶ Risk for relocation stress syndrome
▶ *Risk prone health behavior* (formerly Impaired adjustment)
▶ *Stress overload*

10. DOMAIN: LIFE PRINCIPLES
▶ Decisional conflict (specify)
▶ Impaired religiosity
▶ *Moral distress*
▶ Noncompliance (specify)
▶ *Readiness for enhanced decision making*
▶ *Readiness for enhanced hope*

▶ Readiness for enhanced religiosity
▶ Readiness for enhanced spiritual well-being
▶ Risk for impaired religiosity
▶ Risk for spiritual distress
▶ Spiritual distress

11. DOMAIN: SAFETY/PROTECTION
▶ *Contamination*
▶ Hyperthermia
▶ Hypothermia
▶ Impaired dentition
▶ Impaired oral mucous membrane
▶ Impaired skin integrity
▶ Impaired tissue integrity
▶ Ineffective airway clearance
▶ Ineffective protection
▶ Ineffective thermoregulation
▶ Latex allergy response
▶ *Readiness for enhanced immunization status*
▶ Risk for aspiration
▶ *Risk for contamination*
▶ Risk for falls
▶ Risk for imbalanced body temperature
▶ Risk for impaired skin integrity
▶ Risk for infection
▶ Risk for injury
▶ Risk for latex allergy response
▶ Risk for other-directed violence
▶ Risk for perioperative positioning injury
▶ Risk for peripheral neurovascular dysfunction
▶ Risk for poisoning
▶ Risk for self-directed violence
▶ Risk for self-mutilation
▶ Risk for sudden infant death syndrome
▶ Risk for suffocation
▶ Risk for suicide
▶ Risk for trauma
▶ Self-mutilation

12. DOMAIN: COMFORT

▶ Acute pain
▶ Chronic pain
▶ Nausea
▶ *Readiness for enhanced comfort*
▶ Social isolation

13. DOMAIN: GROWTH/DEVELOPMENT

▶ Adult failure to thrive
▶ Delayed growth and development
▶ Risk for delayed development
▶ Risk for disproportionate growth

THE JOINT COMMISSION NURSING CARE AND DOCUMENTATION STANDARDS

The 2006 standards for accreditation of hospitals that were developed by The Joint Commission include identification of goals, functions, and standards for the provision of patient care. The guidelines emphasize the integration of services from many providers so that goals, functions, and standards reflect the combined responsibilities of those providing patient care. The standards are written to address patient needs rather than identify discrete responsibilities of separate providers.

In addition, the standards stress the value of continuous, rather than episodic, accreditation so that ongoing data collection, assessment, intervention, and evaluation can be performed.

The selected standards presented here cover the assessment of patients, care of patients, leadership, management of human resources, and nursing.

Assessment of patients

The standards associated with the assessment of patients clearly show the focus on performance-improvement processes, while addressing the hospital's responsibility to collect data about each patient's physical and psychosocial status and health history, to analyze that data, and to make patient care decisions based on the following information:

- Each patient's physical, psychological, functional, and social status is assessed.
- Nutritional status is assessed when warranted by the patient's needs or condition.
- Pain is assessed in all patients.
- Functional status is assessed when warranted by the patient's needs or condition.
- Diagnostic testing necessary for determining the patient's health care needs is performed.
- The need for discharge planning assessment is determined.
- Each admitted patient's initial assessment is conducted within a time frame specified by hospital policy.
- Possible victims of abuse, neglect, or exploitation are identified using criteria developed by the hospital.
- Each patient is reassessed at points designated in hospital policy.
- Staff members integrate the information from various assessments of the patient to identify and assign priorities to his care needs.
- The hospital has defined patient assessment activities in writing.
- A registered nurse assesses the patient's need for nursing care in all settings where nursing care is provided.

▶ The assessment process is individualized to meet each patient's needs.

▶ The assessment process addresses the special needs of patients who are receiving treatment for emotional or behavioral disorders.

▶ The assessment process addresses the special needs of patients who are receiving treatment for alcoholism or other substance use disorders.

▶ The assessment process addresses the special needs of patients who are possible victims of alleged abuse.

Care of patients

The selected standards presented here apply to any organization that provides care to patients, and the standards are to be applied collaboratively to ensure that care is integrated and continuous. The responsibilities of individual providers are determined by their professional credentials, licensure, and scope of practice; the type of care being provided; the experience level of the individual provider; and hospital policies and job descriptions.

▶ Care, treatment, and rehabilitation are planned to ensure that they're appropriate to the patient's needs and severity of disease, condition, impairment, or disability.

▶ Care is planned and provided in an interdisciplinary, collaborative manner by qualified individuals.

▶ Patient care procedures (such as bathing) are performed in a manner that respects privacy.

▶ The patient's progress is periodically evaluated against care goals and the care plan and, when indicated, the plan or goals are revised.

▶ Patients are informed in a timely manner of the need to plan for discharge or transfer to another facility or level of care.

▶ Continuing care at the time of discharge is based on the patient's assessed needs.

▶ Medication use processes are organized and systematic throughout the hospital.

▶ Each patient's nutritional care is planned.

▶ Restraint or seclusion use is limited to situations with adequate, appropriate, clinical justification.

▶ Patients are educated about pain and pain management.

Leadership

The selected leadership standards presented here clearly show the focus on patient care and the integration of services. The Joint Commission specifies that leadership should be inclusive, not exclusive; should encourage staff participation in shaping the hospital's vision and values; should develop leaders at every level who help to fulfill the hospital's mission, vision, and values; should accurately assess the needs of patients and other users of the hospital's services; and should develop an organizational culture that focuses on continuously improving performance to meet these needs:

▶ Each hospital department, service, or program has effective leadership.

▶ The leaders provide for both short-term and long-term hospital planning.

▶ Essential services are provided in a timely manner.

▶ The hospital leaders set expectations, develop plans, and manage processes to measure, assess, and improve the quality of the hospital's governance, management, clinical, and support activities.

▶ The leaders support the coordination and provision of patient education activities.

▶ The leaders allocate adequate resources for measuring, assessing, and improving the hospital's performance.

▶ The leaders ensure the implementation of an integrated patient safety program.

Management of human resources

Efficient management of human resources requires making provisions for the right number of competent staff members to meet patient needs. Adequate staffing is the responsibility of all hospital leaders, not just that of the human resources department. Hospital leaders are responsible for considering many factors when identifying how patient care will be delivered, including the hospital's mission, the patient population (including degree and complexity of care), the treatment and services used in patient care, and the expectations of the patients:

▶ The organization defines the qualifications and performance expectations for all staff positions.

▶ The hospital provides an adequate number of staff members whose qualifications are consistent with job responsibilities.

▶ The leaders ensure that the competence of all staff members is assessed, maintained, demonstrated, and improved continually.

▶ The hospital verifies the credentials, education, and competence of staff members according to assigned responsibilities at the time of hire and upon expiration of the credentials.

▶ An orientation process provides initial job training and information and promotes effective and safe job performance.

▶ Ongoing in-service and other education and training maintain and improve staff competence.

▶ The hospital assesses each staff member's ability to meet the performance expectations stated in his job description.

Nursing

Standards related to the nurse-executive position focus on responsibilities. Qualifications for the position are outlined in the intent statements and include education at the master's level or equivalent (such as another appropriate postgraduate degree). The nurse-executive, registered nurses, and other designated nursing staff members write nursing policies and procedures, nursing standards of patient care, standards of nursing practice, and standards to measure, assess, and improve patient outcomes:

▶ Nursing services are directed by a nurse-executive who is a registered nurse qualified by advanced education and management experience.

▶ The nurse-executive has the authority and responsibility for establishing standards of nursing practice, nursing policies and procedures, and nursing staffing plans.

▶ Nursing policies and procedures, nursing standards of patient care, and standards of nursing practice are approved by the nurse-executive or a designee.

▶ The nurse-executive and other nursing leaders participate with leaders from the governing body, management, and medical staff in the hospital's decision-making structures and processes.

▶ The nurse-executive implements an effective, ongoing program to evaluate and improve patient care and treatment.

Outcomes and Interventions for Common Nursing Diagnoses

After you've explored your patient's chief complaint, performed an assessment, and analyzed the findings, you can formulate your nursing diagnoses (or problem list) and develop a care plan. This plan will specify patient outcomes and the interventions to achieve them. Completing the process requires documenting your findings and activities.

Risk for **Activity intolerance**

related to immobility

Definition

Extreme fatigue or other physical symptoms during or following simple activity

Key outcomes

Record appropriate patient outcomes on the care plan. Possible outcomes include:

- ▶ Patient maintains muscle strength and ROM, as indicated by use of functional mobility scale.
- ▶ Patient carries out isometric exercise regimen.
- ▶ Patient communicates understanding of rationale for maintaining activity level.
- ▶ Patient avoids risk factors that may lead to activity intolerance.
- ▶ Patient performs self-care activities to tolerance level.
- ▶ Vital signs remain within prescribed range during periods of activity (specify).

Nursing interventions

Document interventions related to:

- ▶ patient's expressed motivation to maintain maximum activity level within restrictions imposed by illness
- ▶ patient's physiologic response to increased activity (times and dates of vital signs: blood pressure, respirations, heart rate and rhythm)
- ▶ patient repositioning and turning (including times and assistive devices used)
- ▶ patient's functional level (use a functional mobility scale)
- ▶ prescribed ROM and other exercises (including times and assistive devices used such as trapezes)
- ▶ patient teaching (including reason for treatment regimen and signs and symptoms of overexertion, such as dizziness, chest pain, and dyspnea) and patient's response
- ▶ patient's ability to perform activities of daily living (ADLs)
- ▶ evaluation of expected outcomes.

Ineffective **Airway clearance**

related to decreased energy or fatigue

Definition

Anatomic or physiologic obstruction of the airway that interferes with the maintenance of a clear airway

Key outcomes

Record appropriate patient outcomes on the care plan. Possible outcomes include:
▶ Airway remains patent.
▶ Adventitious breath sounds are absent.
▶ Chest X-ray shows no abnormality.
▶ Oxygen level is in normal range.
▶ Patient breathes deeply and coughs to remove secretions.
▶ Patient expectorates sputum.
▶ Patient demonstrates controlled coughing techniques.
▶ Ventilation is adequate.
▶ Patient demonstrates skill in conserving energy while attempting to clear airway.
▶ Patient states understanding of changes needed to diminish oxygen demands.

Nursing interventions

Document interventions related to:
▶ patient's perception of ability to cough
▶ observed respiratory status and other physical findings
▶ patient positioning and repositioning (including times)
▶ airway and pulmonary clearance maneuvers (such as coughing and deep breathing, suctioning to stimulate cough and clear airways, aerosol treatments, postural drainage, percussion and vibration) and patient's response
▶ sputum characteristics (including amount, odor, consistency)
▶ prescribed medication administration (including expectorants, bronchodilators, and other drugs)
▶ amount of fluid intake to help liquefy secretions
▶ oxygen administration (including times, dates, equipment, and supplies)
▶ test results, including ABG levels and hemoglobin values, and reportable deviations from baseline levels
▶ endotracheal intubation
▶ patient teaching
▶ evaluation of expected outcomes.

Anxiety

related to situational crisis

Definition

Feeling of threat or danger to self arising from an unidentifiable source

Key outcomes

Record appropriate expected outcomes on the care plan. Possible outcomes include:
▶ Patient identifies factors that elicit anxious behaviors.
▶ Patient discusses activities that tend to decrease anxious behaviors.
▶ Patient practices progressive relaxation techniques _____ times a day.
▶ Patient copes with current medical situation (specify) without demonstrating severe signs of anxiety (specify for individual).

Nursing interventions

Document interventions related to:

► patient's expressions of anxiety and feelings of relief
► observed signs of patient's anxiety
► time spent with patient, duration of anxious episodes, and emotional support given to patient and family
► comfort measures
► patient teaching (including clear, concise explanations of anything about to occur and relaxation techniques, such as guided imagery, progressive muscle relaxation, and meditation)
► referrals to community or professional mental health services
► patient's involvement in making decisions related to care
► evaluation of expected outcomes.

Disturbed **Body image**

Related to biophysical changes

Definition

Negative perception of self that makes healthful functioning more difficult

Key outcomes

Record appropriate expected outcomes on the care plan. Possible outcomes include:

► Patient acknowledges change in body image.
► Patient communicates feelings about change in body image.
► Patient participates in decision making about his care (specify).
► Patient talks with someone who has experienced the same problem.

► Patient demonstrates ability to practice two new coping behaviors.
► Patient expresses positive feelings about self.

Nursing interventions

Document interventions related to:

► patient's observed coping patterns and responses to change in structure or function of body part (such as touching or not touching)
► patient's participation in self-care
► patient's perception of self, prostheses, adaptive equipment, and limitations
► patient's focus on or denial of specific body parts
► patient's involvement in decision making related to care
► patient's response to nursing interventions
► patient teaching (including information on how bodily functions are improving or stabilizing and specific coping strategies)
► referrals to a mental health professional, a support group, or another person who has had a similar problem
► positive reinforcement of patient's efforts to adapt and use coping strategies
► evaluation of expected outcomes.

Ineffective **Breathing pattern**

related to decreased energy or fatigue

Definition

Change in rate, depth, or pattern of breathing that alters normal gas exchange

Key outcomes

Record appropriate expected outcomes on the care plan. Possible outcomes include:

▶ Patient's respiratory rate stays within 5 breaths per minute of baseline.

▶ ABG levels return to baseline.

▶ Patient reports feeling comfortable when breathing.

▶ Patient reports feeling rested each day.

▶ Patient demonstrates diaphragmatic pursed-lip breathing.

▶ Patient achieves maximum lung expansion with adequate ventilation.

▶ Patient demonstrates skill in conserving energy while carrying out ADLs.

Nursing interventions

Document interventions related to:

▶ patient's expressions of comfort in breathing, emotional state, understanding of medical diagnosis, and readiness to learn

▶ physical condition related to pulmonary assessment (including respiratory rate and depth, breath sounds, and reportable changes)

▶ test results such as ABG levels

▶ prescribed medication and oxygen administration (including dates, times, dosages, routes, adverse effects, equipment, and supplies)

▶ comfort measures (including supporting upper extremities with pillows, providing an overbed table with a pillow to lean on, or elevating the head of the bed)

▶ airway suctioning to remove secretions

▶ patient teaching (including pursed-lip breathing, abdominal breathing, relaxation techniques, medications [dosage, frequency, reportable adverse effects], activity and rest, and diet)

▶ scheduling of activities to allow periods of rest

▶ evaluation of expected outcomes.

▶ # Decreased **Cardiac output**

related to reduced stroke volume as a result of mechanical or structural problems

Definition

Cardiovascular or respiratory symptoms resulting from insufficient blood being pumped by the heart

Key outcomes

Record appropriate expected outcomes on the care plan. Possible outcomes include:

▶ Patient maintains hemodynamic stability: pulse not less than _____ and not greater than _____ beats/minute; blood pressure not less than _____ and not greater than _____ mm Hg.

▶ Patient exhibits no arrhythmias.

▶ Skin remains warm and dry.

▶ Patient exhibits no pedal edema.

▶ Patient achieves activity within limits of prescribed heart rate.

▶ Patient expresses sense of physical comfort after activity.

▶ Heart's workload diminishes.

▶ Patient maintains adequate cardiac output.

▶ Patient performs stress-reduction techniques every 4 hours while awake.

▶ Patient states understanding of signs and symptoms, prescribed activity level, diet, and medications.

Nursing interventions

Document interventions related to:

▶ patient's needs and perception of problem
▶ observed physical findings (including LOC, heart rate and rhythm, blood pressure, and auscultated heart and breath sounds)
▶ reports of abnormal findings (including times, dates, and names)
▶ intake and output measurements, daily weight
▶ observation of pedal or sacral edema
▶ interventions for life-threatening arrhythmias, as ordered
▶ skin care measures to enhance skin perfusion and venous flow
▶ increasing patient's activity level within limits of prescribed heart rate
▶ observed pulse rate before and after activity
▶ patient's response to activity
▶ dietary restrictions as ordered
▶ patient teaching (including desired skills related to diet, prescribed activity, and stress-reduction techniques; procedures and tests; chest pain and other reportable symptoms; medications [name, dosage, frequency, therapeutic and adverse effects]; and simple methods for lifting and bending)
▶ administration of and response to oxygen therapy
▶ evaluation of expected outcomes.

Impaired verbal Communication

related to decreased circulation to brain

Definition

Deficient ability to speak, understand, or use words appropriately.

Key outcomes

Record appropriate expected outcomes on the care plan. Possible outcomes include:

▶ Staff consistently meets patient's needs.
▶ Patient maintains orientation.
▶ Patient maintains effective level of communication.
▶ Patient answers direct questions correctly.

Nursing interventions

Document interventions related to:

▶ patient's current level of communication, orientation, and satisfaction with communication efforts
▶ changes in speech pattern or level of orientation
▶ observed speech deficits, expressiveness and receptiveness, and ability to communicate
▶ diagnostic test results
▶ supplies or equipment used to promote orientation (TV, radio, calendars, reality orientation boards)
▶ promoting effective communication and patient's response
▶ evaluation of expected outcomes.

Constipation

related to personal habits

Definition

Interruption of normal bowel movements resulting in infrequent or absent stools

Key outcomes

Record appropriate expected outcomes on the care plan. Possible outcomes include:

▶ Elimination pattern returns to normal.
▶ Patient moves bowels every _____ day(s) without laxative, suppository, or enema.
▶ Patient states understanding of causative factors of constipation.
▶ Patient gets regular exercise.
▶ Patient describes changes in personal habits to maintain normal elimination pattern.
▶ Patient states plans to seek help resolving emotional or psychological problems.

Nursing interventions

Document interventions related to:
▶ frequency of bowel movements and characteristics of stools
▶ administration of laxatives or enemas and their effectiveness
▶ patient's weight (weekly)
▶ referrals to or consultations with nutritional staff
▶ patient's expressions of concern about change in diet, activity level, use of laxatives or enemas, and bowel pattern
▶ establishment of daily schedule
▶ adherence to dietary recommendations
▶ observed diet, activity tolerance, and characteristics of stools
▶ patient teaching (high-fiber diet, increased fluid intake, exercise, importance of responding to urge to defecate, and long-term effects of laxatives or enemas)
▶ evaluation of expected outcomes.

Ineffective **Coping**

related to situational crisis

Definition

Inability to use adaptive behaviors in response to difficult life situations, such as loss of health, a loved one, or job

Key outcomes

Record appropriate expected outcomes on the care plan. Possible outcomes include:
▶ Patient communicates feelings about the present situation.
▶ Patient becomes involved in planning own care.
▶ Patient expresses feeling of having greater control over present situation.
▶ Patient uses available support systems, such as family and friends, to aid in coping.
▶ Patient identifies at least two coping behaviors.
▶ Patient demonstrates ability to use two healthful coping behaviors.

Nursing interventions

Document interventions related to:
▶ patient's perception of current situation and what it means
▶ patient's efforts at self-care
▶ patient's coping behaviors and his evaluation of their effectiveness
▶ patient's verbal expression of feelings indicating comfort or discomfort
▶ observed patient behaviors
▶ nursing interventions to help patient cope and his responses

▶ patient teaching (about treatments and procedures)
▶ referrals to counselors and support groups
▶ patient's verbalization of factors that exacerbate the inability to cope
▶ evaluation of expected outcomes.

Ineffective **Denial**

related to fear or anxiety

Definition

The conscious or unconscious attempt to disavow the knowledge or meaning of an event to reduce fear or anxiety to the detriment of health

Key outcomes

Record appropriate expected outcomes on the care plan. Possible outcomes include:
▶ Patient describes knowledge and perception of present health problem.
▶ Patient describes lifestyle and reports any recent changes.
▶ Patient expresses knowledge of stages of grief.
▶ Patient demonstrates behavior associated with grief process.
▶ Patient discusses present health problem with physician, nurses, and family members.
▶ Patient indicates by conversation or behavior an increased awareness of reality.

Nursing interventions

Document interventions related to:
▶ patient's perception of health problem, including its severity and potential impact on lifestyle

▶ patient's verbalization of feelings related to present problem
▶ mental status (baseline and ongoing)
▶ communications with physician (to assess what patient has been told about illness)
▶ patient's knowledge of grief process
▶ patient's behavioral responses
▶ interventions implemented to assist patient
▶ patient's response to nursing interventions
▶ patient teaching and patient's response
▶ evaluation of expected outcomes.

Diarrhea

related to malabsorption, inflammation, or irritation of bowel

Definition

Passage of loose, unformed stools

Key outcomes

Record appropriate expected outcomes on the care plan. Possible outcomes include:
▶ Patient controls diarrhea with medication.
▶ Elimination pattern returns to normal.
▶ Patient regains and maintains fluid and electrolyte balance.
▶ Skin remains intact.
▶ Patient discusses causative factors, preventive measures, and changed body image.
▶ Patient practices stress-reduction techniques daily.
▶ Patient seeks persons with similar condition or joins a support group.
▶ Patient demonstrates ability to use ostomy devices if diarrhea results from colorectal surgery.

Nursing interventions

Document interventions related to:

▶ patient's expressions of concern about diarrhea, causative factors, and adaptation to changes in body image if diarrhea results from colorectal surgery

▶ administration and observed effects of antidiarrheal medications

▶ intake and output measurements and daily weight

▶ observed stool characteristics and frequency of defecation

▶ skin condition (especially decreased skin turgor or excoriation)

▶ bowel sounds (auscultation findings)

▶ patient teaching (including causes, prevention, cleaning of perineal area and comfort, dietary restrictions, stress reduction, preoperative instruction about ileostomy or colostomy and abdominal surgery, and postoperative instructions about ostomy equipment)

▶ referrals to support groups (such as ostomy clubs) if appropriate

▶ evaluation of expected outcomes.

Deficient **Fluid volume**

related to active loss

Definition

Excessive loss of body fluid and electrolytes

Key outcomes

Record appropriate expected outcomes on the care plan. Possible outcomes include:

▶ Vital signs remain stable.

▶ Skin color and temperature are normal.

▶ Electrolyte levels stay within normal range.

▶ Patient produces adequate urine volume.

▶ Patient has normal skin turgor and moist mucous membranes.

▶ Urine specific gravity remains between 1.005 and 1.010.

▶ Fluid and blood volume return to normal.

▶ Patient expresses understanding of factors that caused deficient fluid volume.

Nursing interventions

Document interventions related to:

▶ vital signs

▶ patient's complaints of thirst, weakness, dizziness, and palpitations

▶ interventions to control fluid loss and patient's response

▶ observed skin and mucous membrane condition and other physical findings (including signs of fluid and electrolyte imbalances, such as tachycardia, dyspnea, or hypotension)

▶ intake and output and significant changes (including amount and characteristics of urine, stools, vomitus, wound drainage, NG drainage, chest tube drainage, or other output)

▶ urine specific gravity (including times and dates)

▶ administration of any fluids, blood or blood products, or plasma expanders and patient's response

▶ patient's daily weight and abdominal girth

▶ patient teaching (about fluid loss and ways to monitor fluid volume at home such as by measuring intake and output and body weight daily)

▶ evaluation of expected outcomes.

Impaired **Gas exchange**

related to altered oxygen supply

Definition

Interference in cellular respiration resulting from inadequate exchange or transport of oxygen and carbon dioxide

Key outcomes

Record appropriate expected outcomes on the care plan. Possible outcomes include:
- ▶ Patient maintains respiratory rate within 5 breaths per minute of baseline.
- ▶ Patient expresses feeling of comfort.
- ▶ Patient coughs effectively.
- ▶ Patient expectorates sputum.
- ▶ Patient maintains sufficient fluid intake to prevent dehydration: _____ ml/24 hours.
- ▶ Patient performs ADLs to level of tolerance.
- ▶ Patient has normal breath sounds.
- ▶ Patient's ABG levels return to baseline: _____ pH; _____ PaO_2; _____ $PaCO_2$.
- ▶ Patient performs relaxation techniques every 4 hours.
- ▶ Patient correctly uses breathing devices to improve gas exchange and increase oxygenation.

Nursing interventions

Document interventions related to:
- ▶ patient's complaints of dyspnea, headache, or restlessness or expression of well-being
- ▶ observed physical findings (including vital signs, auscultation results, pulmonary status, and cardiac rhythm)
- ▶ medication and oxygen administration (including times, dates, dosages, route, adverse effects, and equipment and supplies) and patient's response
- ▶ patient positioning and repositioning and times; bronchial hygiene measures, such as coughing, percussion, postural drainage, suctioning
- ▶ intake and output measurements
- ▶ reportable signs of dehydration or fluid overload
- ▶ test results, including ABG levels
- ▶ endotracheal intubation and mechanical ventilation measures (including equipment and supplies used)
- ▶ patient teaching (including relaxation techniques and other measures to lower demand for oxygen)
- ▶ patient's ability to perform ADLs
- ▶ evaluation of expected outcomes.

Hopelessness

related to failing or deteriorating physiologic condition

Definition

Subjective state in which an individual sees few or no available alternatives or personal choices and can't mobilize energy on own behalf

Key outcomes

Record appropriate expected outcomes on the care plan. Possible outcomes include:
- ▶ Patient identifies feelings of hopelessness regarding current situation.
- ▶ Patient demonstrates more effective communication skills, including direct verbal responses to questions and increased eye contact.

▶ Patient resumes appropriate rest and activity pattern.

▶ Patient participates in self-care activities and in decisions regarding care planning.

▶ Patient participates in diversional activities (specify).

▶ Patient identifies social and community resources for continued assistance.

Nursing interventions

Document interventions related to:

▶ patient's mental status

▶ patient's verbal and nonverbal communication

▶ patient's medical regimen

▶ increasing patient's feelings of hope and self-worth and involvement in self-care and his response (including time spent communicating, talking, or sitting with patient)

▶ medication administration and comfort measures

▶ referrals to ancillary services, such as dietitian, social worker, clergy, mental health clinical nurse specialist, or support groups

▶ patient teaching (including diversional activities, self-care instruction, and discharge planning)

▶ patient's response to comfort measures

▶ evaluation of expected outcomes.

▶ Functional urinary
Incontinence

related to sensory or mobility deficits

Definition

Involuntary and unpredictable passage of urine in socially unacceptable situations, where patient usually doesn't recognize warning signs of bladder fullness

Key outcomes

Record appropriate expected outcomes on the care plan. Possible outcomes include:

▶ Patient discusses impact of incontinence on self and others.

▶ Patient voids in appropriate situation using suitable receptacle.

▶ Patient voids at specific times.

▶ Patient has no wet episodes.

▶ Patient maintains fluid balance; intake equals output.

▶ Complications are avoided or minimized.

▶ Patient and family members demonstrate skill in managing incontinence.

▶ Patient and family members identify resources to assist with care following discharge.

Nursing interventions

Document interventions related to:

▶ patient's expression of concern about incontinence and motivation to participate in self-care

▶ voiding pattern

▶ intake and output

▶ hydration status

▶ bladder elimination procedures (including bladder training, commode use times, toileting regimen, episodic wetness or dryness, use of external catheter, and use of protective pads and garments)

▶ skin condition and care (including use of protective pads and garments)

▶ patient teaching (including toileting environment, time, and place; alcohol and fluid in-

take; techniques for stimulating voiding reflexes; and techniques for reducing anxiety)
▶ patient's response to treatment regimen and
patient teaching
▶ referrals to appropriate counselors and support groups
▶ family involvement in assisting patient with
toileting
▶ evaluation of expected outcomes.

Risk for **Infection**

related to external factors

Definition

Presence of internal or external hazards that
threaten physical well-being

Key outcomes

Record appropriate expected outcomes on the
care plan. Possible outcomes include:
▶ Temperature stays within normal range.
▶ WBC count and differential stay within nor-
mal range.
▶ No pathogens appear in cultures.
▶ Patient maintains good personal and oral hy-
giene.
▶ Respiratory secretions are clear and odorless.
▶ Urine remains clear yellow and odorless and
exhibits no sediment.
▶ Patient shows no evidence of diarrhea.
▶ Wounds and incisions appear clean, pink, and
free from purulent drainage.
▶ I.V. sites show no signs of inflammation.
▶ Patient shows no evidence of skin break-
down.
▶ Patient consumes _____ ml of fluid and _____ g
of protein daily.

▶ Patient states infection risk factors.
▶ Patient identifies signs and symptoms of infection.
▶ Patient remains free from all signs and symptoms of infection.

Nursing interventions

Document interventions related to:
▶ temperature readings (including dates and
times and reporting of elevations)
▶ test procedures (including dates, times, and
sites of obtained test specimens)
▶ test results (including WBC count and cultures of urine, blood, respiratory secretions,
and wound drainage) and reporting of any abnormal results
▶ skin condition and wound care
▶ preventive measures (including personal hygiene, oral hygiene, airway suctioning, coughing, and deep-breathing measures)
▶ catheter management procedures (including
dates and times of all catheter insertions, re-
movals, and site care)
▶ equipment and supplies (including particu-
lars of humidification or nebulization of oxygen)
▶ sanitary measures (for example, providing tissues and disposal bag for expectorated sputum)
▶ fluid intake
▶ nutritional intake
▶ isolation and other precautions
▶ patient teaching (including toileting and hygiene, hand-washing technique, factors that
increase infection risk, and infection signs
and symptoms)
▶ patient's response to nursing interventions
▶ episodes of loose stools or diarrhea
▶ evaluation of expected outcomes.

Risk for **Injury**

related to sensory or motor deficits

Definition

Accentuated risk of physical harm caused by sensory or motor deficits

Key outcomes

Record appropriate expected outcomes on the care plan. Possible outcomes include:

▶ Patient identifies factors that increase potential for injury.

▶ Patient assists in identifying and applying safety measures to prevent injury.

▶ Patient and family members develop strategy to maintain safety.

▶ Patient performs ADLs within sensorimotor limitations.

Nursing interventions

Document interventions related to:

▶ observed factors that may cause or contribute to injury

▶ safety measures (side rails, positioning, use of call button and bed controls, orienting patient to environment, keeping bed in low position, and close night watch)

▶ statements by patient and family members about potential for injury due to sensory or motor deficits

▶ observed or reported unsafe practices

▶ interventions to decrease risk of injury to patient and his response

▶ patient teaching (including safe ways to improve visual discrimination, to decrease risk of burns from sensory loss, to use hearing aids and mobility assistive devices, and to en-

sure household, automobile, and pedestrian safety)

▶ evaluation of expected outcomes.

Insomnia

related to internal factors

Definition

Inability to meet individual need for sleep or rest arising from internal factors

Key outcomes

Record appropriate expected outcomes on the care plan. Possible outcomes include:

▶ Patient identifies factors that prevent or disrupt sleep.

▶ Patient performs relaxation exercises at bedtime.

▶ Patient sleeps _____ hours a night.

▶ Patient reports feeling well rested.

▶ Patient shows no physical signs of sleep deprivation.

▶ Patient exhibits no sleep-related behavioral symptoms, such as restlessness, irritability, lethargy, or disorientation.

Nursing interventions

Document interventions related to:

▶ patient's complaints about sleep disturbances

▶ patient's report of improvement in sleep patterns

▶ observed physical and behavioral sleep-related disturbances

▶ interventions used to alleviate sleep disturbances (such as pillows, bath, food or drink,

reading material, TV, soft music, quiet environment) and patient's response
▶ prescribed medication and patient's response
▶ patient teaching (including reason for treatment, relationship of regular exercise and sleep, and relaxation techniques, such as imagery, progressive muscle relaxation, and meditation)
▶ evaluation of expected outcomes.

Deficient **Knowledge (specify)**

related to lack of exposure

Definition

Inadequate understanding of information or inability to perform skills needed to practice health-related behaviors

Key outcomes

Record appropriate expected outcomes on the care plan. Possible outcomes include:
▶ Patient communicates a need to know.
▶ Patient states or demonstrates understanding of what has been taught.
▶ Patient demonstrates ability to perform new health-related behaviors as they are taught, and lists specific skills and realistic target dates for each.
▶ Patient sets realistic learning goals.
▶ Patient states intention to make needed changes in lifestyle, including seeking help from health care professionals when needed.

Nursing interventions

Document interventions related to:

▶ patient's statements of known or unknown information and skills, expressions of need to know, and motivation to learn
▶ patient teaching (including learning objectives, teaching methods used, information imparted, skills demonstrated) and patient's responses
▶ referrals to resources or organizations that can continue instructional activities after discharge
▶ evaluation of expected outcomes.

Impaired physical **Mobility**

related to pain or discomfort

Definition

Limitation of physical movement

Key outcomes

Record appropriate expected outcomes on the care plan. Possible outcomes include:
▶ Patient states relief from pain.
▶ Patient displays increased mobility.
▶ Patient shows no evidence of complications, such as contractures, venous stasis, thrombus formation, or skin breakdown.
▶ Patient attains highest degree of mobility possible within confines of disease.
▶ Patient or family member demonstrates mobility regimen.
▶ Patient states feelings about limitations.

Nursing interventions

Document interventions related to:
▶ patient's observed daily functional ability and changes (use functional mobility scale)

▶ patient's expressed feelings and concerns about immobility and its impact on his lifestyle, and his willingness to participate in care

▶ observed impairments and pain

▶ prescribed treatment regimen for underlying condition and patient's response to treatment and nursing interventions

▶ medication administration and other supportive measures (including padding extremities to prevent skin breakdown and ensuring correct height of crutches)

▶ prescribed ROM exercises

▶ patient repositioning (include times)

▶ progressive mobilization up to limits of patient's tolerance for pain (bed to chair to ambulation)

▶ patient and family teaching (including instructions for using crutches and walkers; practicing techniques to control pain, such as distraction and imaging; understanding need for mobility despite pain; performing ROM exercises, transfers, skin inspection, and mobility regimen) and patient's response

▶ referrals to counselor, support group, or social service agency

▶ evaluation of expected outcomes.

Noncompliance (specify)

related to patient's value system

Definition

Unwillingness to practice prescribed health-related behaviors

Key outcomes

Record appropriate expected outcomes on the care plan. Possible outcomes include:

▶ Patient identifies factors that influence noncompliance.

▶ Patient contracts with nurse to perform _____ (specify behavior and frequency).

▶ Patient uses support systems to modify noncompliant behavior.

▶ Patient demonstrates a level of compliance that doesn't interfere with physiologic safety.

Nursing interventions

Document interventions related to:

▶ patient's stated reasons for noncompliance

▶ observed specific noncompliant behaviors

▶ promoting compliance (including negotiations and terms agreed upon with patient as well as positive reinforcements provided) and patient's response

▶ daily progress in complying with treatment regimen

▶ referrals to counselors or support groups

▶ evaluation of expected outcomes.

Imbalanced **Nutrition: Less than body requirements**

related to inability to digest or absorb nutrients because of biological factors

Definition

Change in normal eating pattern that results in decreased body weight

Key outcomes

Record appropriate expected outcomes on the care plan. Possible outcomes include:

▶ Patient tolerates oral, tube, or I.V. feedings without adverse effects.

▶ Patient takes in _____ calories daily.

► Patient gains _____ lb weekly.
► Patient shows no further evidence of weight loss.
► Patient and family or significant other communicate understanding of special dietary needs.
► Patient and family or significant other demonstrate ability to plan diet after discharge.

Nursing interventions

Document interventions related to:
► daily weight
► daily fluid intake and output measurements (include volume and characteristics of any vomitus and stools—a clue to nutrient absorption)
► parenteral fluid administration
► daily food intake from prescribed diet
► electrolyte levels
► consultations with dietary department or nutritional support team
► any abnormal findings.
   If the patient receives tube feedings, document interventions related to:
► concentration and delivery of regular feeding formula or one containing food-coloring additives (especially in patient with altered LOC or diminished gag reflex)
► use of supportive equipment such as an infusion pump
► degree of elevation of head of bed during feeding
► feeding tube placement.
   If the patient receives total parenteral nutrition, document interventions related to:
► monitored blood glucose levels and urine specific gravity (at least once each shift)
► monitored bowel sounds (once each shift)
► oral hygiene

► patient teaching (including the reasons for the current treatment regimen, principles of nutrition suited to the patient's specific condition, meal planning, and preoperative instructions if applicable)
► evaluation of expected outcomes.

Acute **Pain**
related to physical, biological, or chemical agents

Definition
An unpleasant sensory and emotional experience arising from actual or potential tissue damage or described in terms of such damage; pain may be of sudden or slow onset, vary in intensity from mild to severe, and be constant or recurring; pain lasts less than 6 months; and period of pain has an anticipated or predictable end

Key outcomes
Record appropriate expected outcomes on the care plan. Possible outcomes include:
► Patient identifies pain characteristics.
► Patient articulates factors that intensify pain and modifies behavior accordingly.
► Patient states and carries out appropriate interventions for pain relief.
► Patient expresses a feeling of comfort and relief from pain.

Nursing interventions
Document interventions related to:
► patient's description of physical pain, pain relief, and feelings about pain

▶ observed physical, psychological, and socio-cultural responses to pain
▶ prescribed medication administration (including times, dates, dosages, routes, adverse effects) and comfort measures (such as massage, relaxation techniques, heat and cold applications, repositioning, distraction, and bathing)
▶ patient's response to nursing interventions
▶ patient teaching (about pain and pain-relief strategies) and patient's response
▶ evaluation of expected outcomes.

Risk for impaired **Skin integrity**

related to impaired mobility and the aging process

Definition

Presence of risk factors for interruption or destruction of skin surface

Key outcomes

Record appropriate expected outcomes on the care plan. Possible outcomes include:
▶ Patient maintains muscle strength and joint ROM.
▶ Patient sustains adequate food and fluid intake.
▶ Patient maintains adequate skin circulation.
▶ Patient communicates understanding of preventive skin care measures.
▶ Patient and family demonstrate preventive skin care measures.
▶ Patient and family correlate risk factors and preventive measures.
▶ Patient experiences no skin breakdown.

Nursing interventions

Document interventions related to:
▶ skin condition and any changes
▶ repositioning patient as scheduled and ordered (including dates and times)
▶ ambulation or active ROM exercises to improve circulation and mobility (including dates and times)
▶ use of skin care devices and supplies (such as foam mattress, sheepskin, alternating pressure mattress, lotions and powders) and effectiveness of interventions
▶ nutritional intake
▶ hydration status
▶ weekly risk factor potential and score (use the Braden scale)
▶ patient teaching (including the need to implement preventive measures to promote skin integrity, good personal hygiene habits, signs of skin breakdown, patient and responsible caregiver's demonstrated skill in carrying out preventive skin care measures) and patient's response
▶ evaluation of expected outcomes.

Impaired **Swallowing**

related to neuromuscular impairment

Definition

Inability to move food, fluid, or saliva from the mouth through the esophagus

Key outcomes

Record appropriate expected outcomes on the care plan. Possible outcomes include:
▶ Patient shows no evidence of aspiration pneumonia.

▶ Patient achieves adequate nutritional intake.

▶ Patient maintains weight.

▶ Patient maintains oral hygiene.

▶ Patient and responsible caregiver demonstrate correct eating or feeding techniques to maximize swallowing.

Nursing interventions

Document interventions related to:

▶ patient's expressed feelings about current condition

▶ observed and reported swallowing impairment, as evidenced by cyanosis, dyspnea, or choking

▶ nursing interventions and patient's response (include times of turning and repositioning and degree of elevation of head during mealtimes and for 30 minutes after)

▶ respiratory assessments and airway suctioning (including dates and times, instances of cyanosis, dyspnea, or choking)

▶ daily intake and output and weight measurements

▶ referrals to dietitian and other health services such as dysphagia rehabilitation team

▶ oral hygiene and comfort measures

▶ patient teaching (about positioning, dietary requirements, oral hygiene, and stimuli and feeding techniques to improve mastication, promote swallowing, and decrease aspiration)

▶ evaluation of expected outcomes.

Ineffective **Tissue perfusion, cardiopulmonary**

related to decreased cellular exchange

Definition

Decrease in cellular nutrition and respiration due to decreased capillary blood flow

Key outcomes

Record appropriate expected outcomes on the care plan. Possible outcomes include:

▶ Patient attains hemodynamic stability: pulse not less than ____ and not greater than ____ beats/minute; blood pressure not less than ____ and not greater than ____ mm Hg.

▶ Patient doesn't exhibit arrhythmias.

▶ Patient's skin remains warm and dry.

▶ Patient's heart rate remains within prescribed limits while he carries out ADLs.

▶ Patient maintains adequate cardiac output.

▶ Patient modifies lifestyle to minimize risk of decreased tissue perfusion.

Nursing interventions

Document interventions related to:

▶ patient's perception of health problems and health needs

▶ observed physical findings (including heart rate, blood pressure, central venous pressure, pulse rate, temperature, skin color, respiratory rate, and breath sounds)

▶ observed response to activity

▶ test procedures (including ECG to monitor heart rate and rhythm and results of creatine kinase, lactate dehydrogenase, and ABG analysis)

▶ prescribed medication administration and oxygen therapy (including dates, times, dosages, routes, adverse effects, equipment, and supplies)

▶ patient positioning and repositioning to enhance vital capacity and to avoid lung congestion and skin breakdown

▶ patient teaching (about need for low-fat, low-cholesterol diet; nitroglycerin or other medications, including possible adverse effects; activity level; stress management; risk factors for heart and lung disease; need to avoid straining with bowel movements; and benefits of quitting smoking)
▶ evaluation of expected outcomes.

Impaired **Urinary elimination**

related to sensory or neuromuscular impairment

Definition
Alteration or impairment of urinary function

Key outcomes
Record appropriate expected outcomes on the care plan. Possible outcomes include:
▶ Patient discusses impact of urologic disorder on self and others.
▶ Patient maintains fluid balance; intake equals output.
▶ Patient voices increased comfort.
▶ Complications are avoided or minimized.
▶ Patient and family members demonstrate skill in managing urinary elimination problem.
▶ Patient and family members identify resources to assist with care after discharge.

Nursing interventions
Document interventions related to:
▶ observed neuromuscular status
▶ observed voiding pattern
▶ patient's expression of concern about the urologic problem and its impact on body image and lifestyle

▶ patient's motivation to participate in self-care
▶ intake and output and fluid replacement therapy
▶ medication administration
▶ bladder training (including times and dates of commode use, Kegel exercises to strengthen sphincter)
▶ intermittent catheterization (record dates, times, volume eliminated spontaneously, volume eliminated via catheter, bladder balance)
▶ external catheterization of male patient (including time and date of condom catheter application and changes, supplies used, skin condition of penis, and hygiene)
▶ indwelling urinary catheterization (including time and date of catheter insertion and changes, condition and care of urinary meatus, type of drainage system used, and volume drained)
▶ suprapubic catheterization (including time and date of catheter insertion and changes, dressing changes, type of drainage system used, and supplies used)
▶ supportive care measures (including pain control and hydration, prompt response to call light, and bed in close proximity to bathroom), their effectiveness, and patient's response
▶ patient teaching (including signs and symptoms of full bladder, home catheterization techniques and management, signs and symptoms of autonomic dysreflexia, management of autonomic dysreflexia, and emergency measures)
▶ referrals of patient and family members to counselors and support groups
▶ evaluation of expected outcomes.

INDEX

i refers to an illustration; t refers to a table.

i refers to an illustration; t refers to a table.

Joint Commission (*continued*)
  restraint and seclusion standards of,
    366-367
  surgical site verification standards of,
    242, 243i
Jugular vein examination, 333
Jury trials, 29

K

Kardex, 10, 81, 156-160
  computer-generated, 156, 157-158i,
    393
  medication, 157, 255, 256-257i

L

Labor and delivery, 346-349
Laboratory tests, 281-283
  electronic documentation of, 400
Late entries, 308-309
Latex allergy, 95
Lavage, peritoneal, 273
Learning. *See* Patient teaching.
Legal issues, 371-388
  advance directives, 4, 33-37, 36i,
    318-319
  brain death, 296-297, 335
  causation, 19
  competence, 33
  confidentiality, 23-25, 38-40, 365,
    367, 394-395
  corrections and alterations in medical
    record, 11, 18, 26, 309
  damages, 19
  discharge against medical advice,
    325-327, 387-388
  documentation standards, 16-17
  do-not-resuscitate orders, 4, 36i,
    37-38, 318-319
  duty and breach of duty, 18
  errors and omissions in documenta-
    tion, 11, 17-18, 26, 28, 29, 307,
    393
  firearms, 387
  informed consent, 32-33, 38, 39-40,
    337, 341i, 358
  intent to sue, 383
  malpractice, 18-19, 25-29. *See also*
    Malpractice.
  missing patient, 327
  nurse practice acts, 11-12
  patient access to records, 13, 26, 40
  patient misbehavior, 386-388
  patient transfers, 345
  in pediatric nursing, 352-353
  power of attorney and, 37
  proximity, 19
  reasonable nurse standard, 18, 20
  restraints, 323-324, 324i, 325, 326i
  standards of care, 19-20
  suicide, 383-385

Legal issues, (*continued*)
  timeliness of practitioner notification,
    17, 378-379
  violent patients, 383-386
Liability. *See* Malpractice.
Licensed practical and vocational
    nurses, ethical code for, 30
Long-term care documentation, 12,
    185-205
  care plans in, 198
  discharge and transfer forms in, 199,
    203-204i
  guidelines for, 205
  initial nursing assessment in, 199
  levels of care and, 186
  minimum data set in, 188-198,
    189-197i
  nursing summaries in, 199
  Preadmission Screening and Annual
    Resident Review in, 188,
    198-199
  regulation of, 186-188
  Resident Assessment Instruments in,
    187
  resident assessment protocols in, 188,
    198
  risk assessment forms for, 199,
    201-204i
Lumbar puncture, 279-280

M

Malovec v. Santa Monica Hospital, 17
Malpractice, 18-19
  versus bad outcome, 19
  breach of duty and, 18-19
  causation and, 19
  comparative negligence in, 25
  contributory negligence in, 25
  damages for, 19
  standards of care and, 19-20
Malpractice insurance, 27
Malpractice lawsuits, 25-29
  avoidance of, 26
  complaint in, 26-27
  contingency fees in, 26
  courtroom hearings in, 28-29
  credible evidence in, 371-372
  depositions in, 27
  discovery in, 27-28
  expert witnesses in, 28
  incident report disclosure in, 23-25
  judge's role in, 29
  jury in, 29
  legal representation in, 27
  medical records in, 6, 26, 29
  nurse's response in, 28
  preliminary steps in, 26
  preparations for adjudication in, 26
  settlement of, 26, 29
Maslow's hierarchy of needs, 118, 119i

Maternal-neonatal nursing documenta-
    tion, 345-352
Mechanical ventilation, 275-276
Medicaid. *See* Medicare and Medicaid.
Medical history, 4
Medical records. *See also*
    Documentation.
  abbreviations in, 88-89, 90-91t
  in accreditation, 6-7
  admission notes in, 54
  bias in, 374
  charting by exception and, 9, 60-61t,
    72-78
  components of, 4
  requirements for, 6-7
  confidentiality of, 38-40
  corrections and alterations of, 11, 18,
    26, 309
  diagnosis-related group codes in, 7-8,
    51
  discharge notes in, 54
  electronic, 10, 86, 390-397
  errors and omissions in, 11, 17-18,
    26, 28, 29, 307, 309, 393
  as evidence, 371-372, 378-379. *See
    also* Malpractice lawsuits.
  formats for, 8-10
  incomplete, 28, 29, 374-375
  inconsistencies in, 54, 55
  late entries in, 308-309
  in lawsuits, 26, 29
  as legal documents, 6, 16-18. *See also*
    Legal issues.
  legible handwriting in, 87-88
  loss of, 374
  making entries in, 87-92
  narrative, 9
  neutral language in, 374
  objectivity in, 96, 372-374
  order of entries in, 87-89
  organization of, 8-10
  patient access to, 13, 26, 40
  peer review of, 7, 8, 22-23, 41, 48, 49
  in performance improvement, 7
  problem-oriented, 9-10, 60-61t,
    65-68, 66i
  purpose of, 5-8
  release of, 38, 39-40
  signing entries in, 92, 93i
  third-party access to, 40
  transfer notes in, 54
Medical Update and Patient
    Information Form (Form 486),
    209, 213i, 234
Medicare and Medicaid, 50-55,
    196-198. *See also* Reimburse-
    ment.
  ambulatory care and, 238-241
  case management and, 48-50, 136
  certification for, 52

---

i refers to an illustration; t refers to a table.